HEMATOLOGY TECHNIQUES AND CONCEPTS FOR VETERINARY TECHNICIANS

Hematology Techniques and Concepts for Veterinary Technicians

Editor:

Stephen Rego, Ph.D.

Delve Publishing
www.delvepublishing.com

Hematology Techniques and Concepts for Veterinary Technicians
Editor: **Stephen Rego, Ph.D.**

708 3rd Avenue, 6th Floor
New York, NY 10017
United States of America
www.delvepublishing.com

ISBN: 978-1-68095-867-6

Library of Congress Control Number: 2016951620

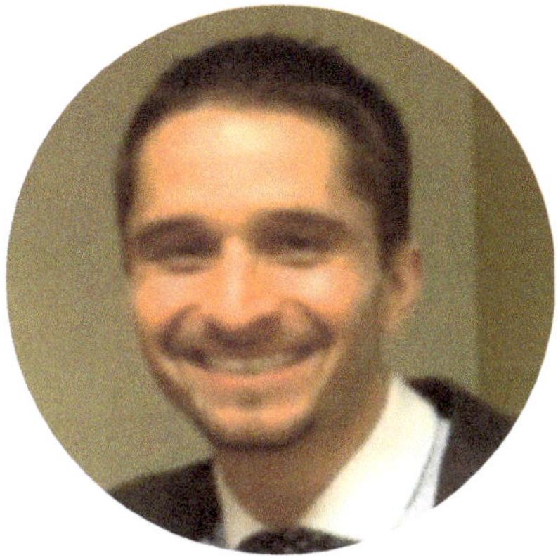

About the Editor

Stephen Rego, Ph.D.

Stephen obtained his PhD from the University of North Carolina at Charlotte in 2013 where his graduate research focused on cancer immunology and the tumor microenvironment. He received postdoctoral training in regenerative and translational medicine, specifically gastrointestinal tissue engineering, at the Wake Forest Institute of Regenerative Medicine. Currently, Stephen is an instructor for anatomy and physiology and biology at Forsyth Technical Community College.

Contents

List of Contributors

Giuseppe Musumeci
Department of Biomedical and Biotechnological Sciences, Human Anatomy and Histology Section, School of Medicine, University of Catania, Via S. Sofia 87, 95123 Catania, Italy

Yu Xiang
Morphometric Research Laboratory, North Sichuan Medical College, 234 Fujiang Road, Nanchong, Sichuan 637007, China

Zheng-Wei Yang
Morphometric Research Laboratory, North Sichuan Medical College, 234 Fujiang Road, Nanchong, Sichuan 637007, China

Al Jassim RAM
The University of Queensland, Gatton, St Lucia QLD-4072, Queensland, Australia

Shahsavari A
The University of Queensland, Gatton, St Lucia QLD-4072, Queensland, Australia

Owen H
The University of Queensland, Gatton, St Lucia QLD-4072, Queensland, Australia

Khamas W
Western University of Health Sciences, 309 E 2nd, St. Pomona, CA 91766, United States of America

Luciana Pacheco Golinelli
Instituto de Química, Universidade Federal do Rio de Janeiro, Av. Athos da Silveira Ramos 149 Cidade Universitária, Zip-code 21949-909, Rio de Janeiro-RJ, Brazil

Joab Trajano Silva
Instituto de Química, Universidade Federal do Rio de Janeiro, Av. Athos da Silveira Ramos 149 Cidade Universitária, Zip-code 21949-909, Rio de Janeiro-RJ, Brazil

Ana Carolina Carvalho
Instituto de Química, Universidade Federal do Rio de Janeiro, Av. Athos da Silveira Ramos 149 Cidade Universitária, Zip-code 21949-909, Rio de Janeiro-RJ, Brazil
Universidade Federal do Rio de Janeiro-Campus Macaé, Av. Aloízio da Silva Gomes, 50-Granja dos Cavaleiros, Macaé-RJ, Zip-code 27930-560, Rio de Janeiro-RJ, Brazil

Vânia Margaret Flosi Paschoalin
Instituto de Química, Universidade Federal do Rio de Janeiro, Av. Athos da Silveira Ramos 149 Cidade Universitária, Zip-code 21949-909, Rio de Janeiro-RJ, Brazil

Usman Khalid
Cardiff Transplant Unit, Department of Nephrology and Transplant Surgery, University Hospital of Wales, Heath Park, Cardiff, UK
Institute of Nephrology, Cardiff University, Cardiff, UK

Gilda Pino-Chavez
Institute of Nephrology, Cardiff University, Cardiff, UK

Prabhu Nesargikar
Cardiff Transplant Unit, Department of Nephrology and Transplant Surgery, University Hospital of Wales, Heath Park, Cardiff, UK
Institute of Nephrology, Cardiff University, Cardiff, UK

Robert H. Jenkins
Institute of Nephrology, Cardiff University, Cardiff, UK

Timothy Bowen
Institute of Nephrology, Cardiff University, Cardiff, UK

Donald J. Fraser
Institute of Nephrology, Cardiff University, Cardiff, UK

Rafael Chavez
Cardiff Transplant Unit, Department of Nephrology and Transplant Surgery, University Hospital of Wales, Heath Park, Cardiff, UK
Institute of Nephrology, Cardiff University, Cardiff, UK

Dalia A. Mohamed
Department of Histology and Cell Biology, Faculty of Medicine, Zagazig University, Egypt

Heba M. Elnegris
Department of Histology and Cell Biology, Faculty of Medicine, Zagazig University, Egypt

Rania A. Wahdan
Department of Histology and Cell Biology, Faculty of Medicine, Zagazig University, Egypt

Shashi Nandar Kumar
Environmental Toxicology Lab, National Institute of Pathology (ICMR), Safdarjung Hospital Campus, New Delhi-110029, India

Banajit Bastia
Environmental Toxicology Lab, National Institute of Pathology (ICMR), Safdarjung Hospital Campus, New Delhi-110029, India

Avinash Gopal Telang
Centre for Animal Disease Research and Diagnosis (CADRAD), Indian Veterinary Research Institute, Izatnagar, Bareilly-243122, (U.P.), India

Karam Pal Singh
Centre for Animal Disease Research and Diagnosis (CADRAD), Indian Veterinary Research Institute, Izatnagar, Bareilly-243122, (U.P.), India

Rambir Singh
Institute of Biomedical Sciences, Bundelkhand University, Kanpur Road, Jhansi 284001, Uttar Pradesh, India

Arun Kumar Jain
Environmental Toxicology Lab, National Institute of Pathology (ICMR), Safdarjung Hospital Campus, New Delhi-110029, India

Murtala M. Jibril
Department of Anatomy, Faculty of Medicine Ahmadu Bello University (A.B.U) Zaria, Nigeria

Ojo S. Adeniyi
Department of Veterinary Anatomy, Faculty of Veterinary Medicine, Ahmadu Bello University (A.B.U) Zaria, Nigeria

Bawa E. Kambai
Department of Theriogenology, Faculty of Veterinary Medicine, Ahmadu Bello University (A.B.U) Zaria, Nigeria

Zubairu S. Rayyan
Department of Anatomy, Faculty of Medicine Ahmadu Bello University (A.B.U) Zaria, Nigeria

Hagar A. Hashish
Department of Anatomy and Embryology, Faculty of Medecine, Mansoura University, Egypt

Abeer M. El-Mahalaway
Department of Histology and Cell Biology, Benha Faculty of Medicine, Benha University, Egypt

Amal A. Selim
Department of Biology, Faculty of Applied Sciences, Umm Al-Qura University, Makkah, Kingdom of Saudi Arabia

Faiza Abdul Razzak Mahboub
Department of Biology, Faculty of Applied Sciences, Umm Al-Qura University, Makkah, Kingdom of Saudi Arabia

Nikolaos Dervisis
Virginia Maryland College of Veterinary Medicine, 245 Duck Pond Dr., Blacksburg, VA 24061, USA

Shawna Klahn
Virginia Maryland College of Veterinary Medicine, 245 Duck Pond Dr., Blacksburg, VA 24061, USA

Gerhard J Molderings
Institute of Human Genetics, University Hospital of Bonn, Sigmund-FreudStr. 25, D-53127 Bonn, Germany

Stefan Brettner
Department of Oncology, Hematology and Palliative Care, Kreiskrankenhaus Waldbröl, Dr.-Goldenburgen-Str. 10, D-51545 Waldbröl, Germany

Jürgen Homann
Department of Internal Medicine, Evangelische Kliniken Bonn, Waldkrankenhaus, Waldstrasse 73, D-53177 Bonn, Germany

Lawrence B Afrin
Division of Hematology/Oncology, Medical University of South Carolina, Charleston, South Carolina, USA

Giuseppe musumeci
Department of Bio-medical Sciences, Anatomy and Histology Section, School of Medicine, University of Catania, Italy

Rania A. Zidan
Department of Histology and Cell Biology, Faculty of Medicine, Zagazig University, Egypt

Heba M. Elnegris
Department of Histology and Cell Biology, Faculty of Medicine, Zagazig University, Egypt

Zienab A. Gouda,
Department of Histology and Cell Biology, Faculty of Medicine, Zagazig University, Zagazig 44519, Egypt.

Samah M. Ahmed
Department of Histology and Cell Biology, Faculty of Medicine, Zagazig University, Zagazig 44519, Egypt.

Nabila M. Elghonaimy
Department of Histology and Cell Biology, Faculty of Medicine, Zagazig University, Zagazig 44519, Egypt.

Ahmed A.M. Abdel Hamid
Department of Histology and Cell Biology, Faculty of Medicine, Mansoura University, Egypt

Mona FM Soliman
Department of Histology and Cell Biology, Faculty of Medicine, Mansoura University, Egypt

Rachael Thomas
Department of Molecular Biomedical Sciences, College of Veterinary Medicine & Center for Comparative Medicine and Translational Research, North Carolina State University, Raleigh NC 27607, USA

Preface

Hematology is the study of blood, its chemistry, and components. The most common blood test is a complete blood count (CBC). This test determines the number and type of white and red blood cells circulating in the bloodstream. It is most often used to check for signs of inflammation or infection (revealed by changes in the number and appearance of different kinds of white blood cells). Determining the number, size, and hemoglobin content of red blood cells helps identify disorders such as anemia. Platelets are also examined during a CBC; changes in platelets can help identify blood clotting disorders. If a pet has a specific problem at the time of the examination, the veterinarian may perform additional tests that are not generally part of a routine physical examination. For example, examination of a dog with suspected vision problems might include tests that assess overall vision, examination with an ophthalmoscope and various stains, and determination of the pressure within the eye (intraocular pressure). Similarly, examination of a lame horse might include a hands-on examination of the affected leg, blood and biochemical tests, muscle biopsy, and various types of imaging techniques. Hematology techniques are important for the general and emergency care of animals and should be a commonly utilized tool for veterinary technicians. The field of hematology involves the study of normal and diseased conditions related to the blood. One of the primary techniques used to study the blood is histology, which involves studying the microscopic anatomy of the cells in the blood to determine their relative abundance, phenotype and function. Histology is a major focus of this book, although other techniques are discussed. Along with general overviews of histology and histopathology, numerous examples are provided regarding specific diseases and their diagnosis using hematology. Some of the diseases, conditions and treatments discussed in this book include Monensin Toxicosis infection, Kidney ischaemia reperfusion injury, hormone replacement therapies, endosulfan, tadalafil and ochratoxin-A therapies, hepatitis, burns and cancer which is discussed in detail. Along with veterinary technicians, animal owners and other veterinary professionals may gain insights into hematology through reviewing this material.

Editor

Stephen Rego, Ph.D.

INTRODUCTION

Hematology is that medical specialty which concerns itself with the blood, and the generation of blood in the bone marrow. Hematology studies the red and white blood cells, their relative proportions and general cell health, and the diseases that are caused by imbalances between them, notably leukemia and anemia. Red blood cells carry oxygen from the lungs to the various parts of the body, and white blood cells fight infections. Both are necessary, but they have to be in the body in the right proportions and systems will break down.

Anemia is a shortage of red blood cells, a condition which can be caused by a number of different factors. Women of childbearing age are more likely to be anemic than anyone else because they lose red blood cells monthly through menstruation. Anemia caused by a lack of iron in the diet is easily treated by iron supplements. Other types of anemia with less easily remedied causes can be harder to treat and life-threatening. Hematology diagnoses these conditions and prescribes appropriate treatments for them.

Leukemia is a condition in which the bone marrow produces too many white blood cells. These are typically abnormal white cells, and their sheer numbers crowd out the red blood cells, causing anemia and other dangerous symptoms. Hematology recognizes a number of different types of leukemia, with different causes and treatment protocols.

Acute leukemia needs immediate treatment, since it is immediately life-threatening, yet some forms of chronic leukemia can be watched without treatment until symptoms emerge. Chemotherapy can do much for leukemia sufferers and is currently one of the main tools in a doctor's leukemia toolbox. Bone marrow transplants, which are considerably more intrusive, are another.

Symptoms of diseases that fall under the hematology umbrella are widely varied and easily confused with other diseases. However, a quick blood test for cell counts can quickly tell a hematologist whether or not a patient has a disorder of the blood.

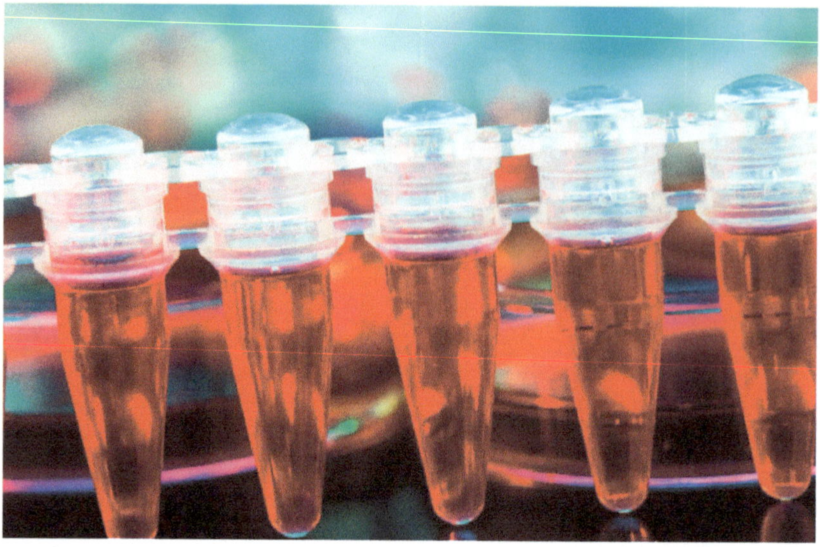

Hematology is the study of blood and the tissues that form, store, or circulate blood cells. Examination of the blood is a very common and useful procedure for several reasons. Blood bathes all the other cells of the body carrying nutrients, oxygen, and waste products, and is exposed to almost all metabolic processes of these cells, often reflecting any alteration from normal function. Blood is essential in water and electrolyte balance, temperature control, and the functioning of the immune system, which is the defense mechanism of the body. Obtaining, studying, and testing a blood sample is a relatively easy way of gathering information on many parts of the body. Even though the term "hematology" literally means "the study of blood," many of the techniques of collection, sample preparation, and cell identifications learned by the technician can be applied to other regions of the body, such as joint fluid, cerebrospinal fluid, thoracic and abdominal fluids, aspirants from abnormal growths or swellings, and cells collected from mucous membranes (e.g., the oral cavity, trachea, or vagina). Veterinary technicians should expect to encounter a wide range of laboratory facilities and instrumentation in various veterinary clinics. This can vary from a separate room fully equipped with the latest automated analyzers to a small area on one counter with a microscope, slides, and stains in smaller clinics. Even if the clinic sends out all of its hematology tests to a commercial lab, or to the local human hospital, the technician is still usually responsible for correctly collecting, preparing, and mailing or delivering the sample as well as reporting and recording the results. Hematology is one of several specialties in the field of clinical pathology, a field that encompasses any manual or automated laboratory procedure used on the animal to aid in diagnosing a clinical condition. Clinical chemistry, parasitology, and urinalysis are additional classical aspects of clinical pathology. Other diagnostic tools used by the veterinarian that qualify as clinical pathology under this definition are microbiology, diagnostic imaging (radiology and ultrasound), and the microscopic interpretation of biopsies (tissue samples).

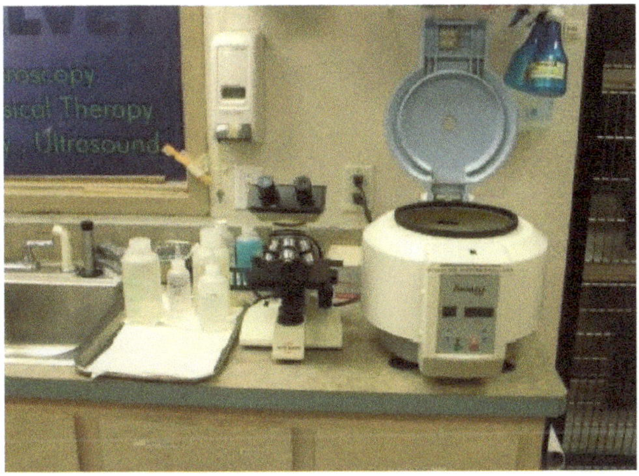

Uses and Benefits of Results

The most common use of the hematology laboratory is to screen the general health of an animal and to assess its overall ability to transport oxygen and defend against infectious agents. Hematology results provided by the technician are also used by the veterinarian as tools that, when combined with the history, physical examination, and other laboratory findings, help to form a diagnosis. Although occasionally a blood test will yield a definitive diagnosis (e.g., blood parasites), most laboratory results should be viewed as large or small pieces of a diagnostic puzzle that must be assembled. Hematology results may also indicate a course of treatment for the animal. An example of this is the use of hematology to differentiate between anemia caused by internal hemorrhage and that caused by bone marrow depression. Another example is finding specific infectious organisms within blood cells. Laboratory findings may also suggest other beneficial tests, such as a bone marrow biopsy. Serial sampling, which is the collection and testing of a series of blood nature of the cellular structure. Wright and Giemsa stains are examples of this type of staining technique and are the basis for the almost universal current use of commercial dip technique stains. These staining systems use

1. a fixative, such as methyl alcohol,
2. a red-colored, acidic dye (usually eosin), which is attracted to the basic components of cells, such as hemoglobin and the cytoplasmic granules in eosinophils, and
3. a dark blue to purple, alkaline, or basic dye (usually methylene blue), which will stain the more acid components, such as nucleic acids and the cytoplasmic granules in basophils.

It is worth noting here that this is the basis for the naming of the granulocytic leukocytes: eosinophils (also called acidophils, acid staining), basophils (basic staining), and neutrophils (neutral). These dyes may be present as three separate solutions or incorporated into one or two solutions by various manufacturers. Use of the stains involves dipping a slide into each solution for a length of time, or a certain number of times, specified by the manufacturers. The only maintenance needed for these stains is routine filtering to remove debris and replenishment or replacement from stock solutions. To prevent evaporation, the stains, and especially the fixative, must be tightly capped when not in use. One other staining technique that is commonly used to demonstrate erythrocyte alterations or inclusions is the reticulocyte stain. This is called a supravital stain and must be used on fresh blood that has not been placed in a fixative. New methylene blue (0.5 percent in distilled water) is most often used (a different dye from the methylene blue used in Romanowsky stains) and can be applied by two different, but extremely simple, methods. A drop of new methylene blue can be placed on a coverslip, which is then placed directly on an unfixed, unstained blood slide, or small, equal amounts of the stain and the blood sample are mixed prior to making the smear. The stain will outline the cells and incorporate into any DNA, RNA, or reticular fibers present.

Blood Film Preparation and Staining

Blood and bone marrow films that are well prepared and properly stained have a great value in haematology. They are used in: a) viewing cell morphology for diagnosing anemias and leukemias, b) WBC differential counts and c) estimating the number of platelets.

Technique of Spreading

Spreading is done on dust free glass microscope slides using a spreader, which is a microscope slide having one corner removed at each end.

Types of Blood Films

- Thick blood film which is used for parasitology e.g. malaria. It is prepared by handling the spreader by the edge, using the corner to spread the blood in a circular form with 3-6 movements.
- Thin blood film which is used in hematology and prepared as described below.

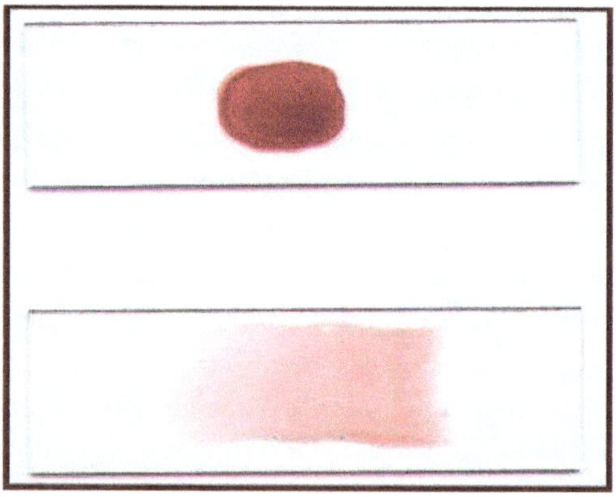

Blood Smear Preparation Method

1. EDTA anticoagulated blood is used. Blood is taken using capillary tubes.
2. Place a drop of blood near the end of the slide, about 1-2 cm from one end.
3. Place the spreading slide at an angle of 45° about 1 cm in front of the drop of blood.
4. Back the spreader into the drop of blood. The spreader catches the blood and it spreads by capillary action along its edge.
5. Maintaining the 45° angle, push the spreader smoothly across the slide. This pulls the blood across to makethe smear. It should take about one second to make the smear.
6. Allow the film to air dry.

Notes on method:

- The edge of the spreader must be very smooth, and narrower than that of the slide.
- The spreader must be cleaned and dried if it had been used for spreading more than five films.
- A smooth action is required, with the edge of the spreader held against the slide.
- Films may be prepared manually or automated slide spreaders.
- The blood film length shouldn't be too long nor should it be too short.
- All slides should be labeled for identification.

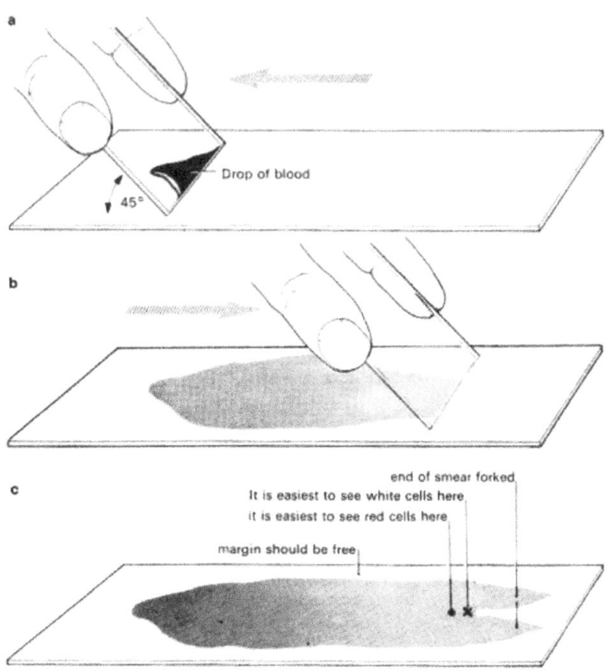

Types of Stains

Romanovwsky dyes are universally employed for routine staining of blood films. Romanowsky stains include leishman's stain, write stain, may grunwald stain, jenner's stain and giemsa stain. Romanowsky dyes consist of two components:

- Basic Part: azure blue or methylene blue which bind to the acidic part of the cell (nucleus) and stain it blue.
- Acidic Part: eosin Y which binds to the basic parts of the cell (proteins, cytoplasm and Hb) giving them a red color.

Azure B(basic)= nuclei (containing nucleic acid) = Blue

Azure B(basic) = Basophilic granules (containing heparin which is acidic) = Violet

Eosin Y(acidic) = Cytoplasm and Hb (basic) = Red

Eosin Y(acidic) = Eosinophilic granules (alkaline) = Red orange granules

Staining Steps

1. Fixation of blood cells to protect them from hemolysis due to washing. Well-fixed cells resist the action of water. Fixation is done by:
    - Methanol (1.5 min)
    - B-Undiluted stain (neat stain) as in leishman's & wright stain
2. Staining
3. Washing

Clinical Hematology

Hematology refers to the study of the numbers and morphology of the cellular elements of the blood the RBCs (erythrocytes), WBCs (leukocytes), and platelets (thrombocytes) and the use of these results in the diagnosis and monitoring of disease.

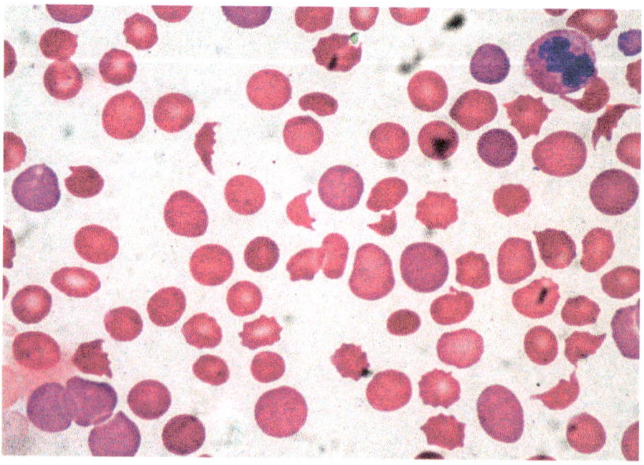

Red Blood Cells

Three RBC measurements are routinely done: packed cell volume (PCV), the proportion of whole blood volume occupied by RBCs; hemoglobin (Hgb) concentration of whole lysed blood; and RBC count, the number of RBCs per unit volume of whole blood. Although these are separate estimations, they are in effect three ways to measure the same thing, and it is incorrect to attempt to interpret them as separate variables. Inasmuch as they do vary in relation to each other, they allow calculation of two further meaningful parameters, mean corpuscular volume (MCV) and mean corpuscular hemoglobin concentration (MCHC).

$$\text{MCV (fL)} = \frac{\text{PCV(decimal fraction)} \times 1{,}000}{\text{RBC}(\times 10^{12}/\text{L})}$$

$$\text{MCHC (g/L)} = \frac{\text{Whole blood hemoglobin concentration (g/L)}}{\text{PCV(decimal fraction)}}$$

MCV varies widely between mammalian species, from ~15 fL in goats to ~90 fL in people. Avian and reptilian red cells are even larger, up to 300 fL. Nevertheless, MCHC varies little with species (or erythrocyte size), at ~330 g/L.

Several artifacts can cause significant and potentially misleading alterations to measured RBC parameters:

1. old samples cause RBCs to swell, thus increasing PCV and MCV and decreasing MCHC;
2. lipemia causes a falsely high Hgb reading, and hence a falsely high MCHC;
3. hemolysis causes PCV to decrease while Hgb remains unchanged, again leading to a falsely high MCHC;
4. underfilling of the tube causes RBCs to shrink, causing PCV and MCV to decrease and MCHC to increase;
5. autoagglutination causes a falsely low RBC count, and hence a falsely high MCV.

Visual description of RBC morphology on a Romanowsky stain also provides useful diagnostic information. The most common terms include

1. normocytic—cells are of normal size;
2. macrocytes—abnormally large cells, usually polychromatophilic;
3. microcytes—abnormally small cells, usually caused by a lack of hemoglobin precursors;
4. anisocytosis—variation in size of cells due to macrocytes, microcytes, or both;
5. normochromic—cells are of normal color;

6. polychromasia—variation in color of the cells, which usually describes the appearance of large, juvenile, bluish-staining polychromatophilic macrocytes (these broadly correspond to the "reticulocyte" seen with new methylene blue staining, in which the reticulum represents the remnants of the nucleus);
7. hypochromasia—decrease in staining density of the cells, usually due to a lack of hemoglobin precursors, especially iron; and
8. annulocyte—extreme form of hypochromic cell with only a thin rim of hemoglobin.

PCV is the variable usually used to assess the basic status of the erythron increased in polycythemia, decreased in anemia—although if a sample is too hemolyzed to allow measurement of PCV, a meaningful Hgb measurement may still be obtained. RBC count as such should not be interpreted clinically.

An abnormally high PCV (polycythemia) may be relative, due to a change in the proportion of circulating RBCs to blood plasma without any change in the size of the erythron, or absolute, due to a real increase in erythron size. Absolute polycythemia may be primary (eg, polycythemia vera or, rarely, erythropoietin-producing tumors) or secondary (a consequence of disease in another organ system).

Polycythemia vera and erythropoietin-producing tumors should be suspected only when PCV is very high, normally >0.7. The former is characterized by normal, mature RBCs and a normal (or low) erythropoietin concentration, whereas the latter may show a regenerative RBC picture with high erythropoietin concentration. Relative polycythemia may also be associated with very high PCV values, and normal, mature RBCs. Secondary polycythemia generally shows a more modest increase in PCV, often with evidence of regeneration (more so when the cause is pulmonary or cardiac, less so when the cause is hormonal). It is often possible to make the differential diagnosis of polycythemia on clinical grounds.

Abnormally low PCV (anemia) may be caused by loss of blood (hemorrhage), breakdown of RBCs in circulation (hemolysis), or lack of production of RBCs by the bone marrow (hypoplasia or aplasia). Presentation varies according to whether the condition is acute or chronic. Aplastic anemia is always chronic in onset, because anemia occurs gradually as existing cells reach the end of their lifespan.

In acute hemorrhagic anemia, external blood loss is easily appreciated clinically, but blood loss into a body cavity may be determined only on paracentesis. Initially, all hematologic parameters may be normal, because it may take 12 hr for fluid shifts to produce a decrease in the PCV. Within a few days, RBCs become regenerative, with juvenile forms appearing in circulation (except in horses, in which circulating evidence of regeneration is not readily appreciable). These consist of polychromatophilic macrocytes and normoblasts (nucleated RBCs). Late normoblasts have a small, nonviable nucleus and a moderate amount of cytoplasm colored similarly to that of the polychromatophilic macrocytes, whereas early normoblasts have a larger, viable nucleus and scanty cytoplasm. These are most easily distinguished from lymphocytes by their more densely staining nucleus.

If substantial amounts of blood have been lost from the body, the RBC picture may become hypochromic. Thus, this type of anemia shows an increase in MCV and a decrease in MCHC. If bleeding is into a body cavity, hypochromasia may not be evident because hemoglobin precursors will be recycled. However, slight jaundice may be seen as the sequestered cells are broken down. Some sequestered cells may also be returned to the circulation intact, if somewhat misshapen.

In acute hemolytic anemia, PCV will decrease immediately, and in the early stages some jaundice will be evident. In the very early stages, even a sample collected with extreme care may be markedly hemolyzed. As with hemorrhagic anemia, the RBCs will become regenerative within a few days, with polychromatophilic macrocytes and nucleated RBCs evident. Because hemoglobin precursors are not lost from the body, true hypochromasia is not seen.

Chronic hemorrhagic anemia may be difficult to appreciate if blood is lost in the feces or urine, or due to bloodsucking ectoparasites. Anemia may be severe, and the RBC picture will be regenerative on presentation. Hypochromasia is usually very marked. In very longstanding conditions, depletion of iron and other hemoglobin precursors can become so marked that most of the cells are microcytic, and MCV may paradoxically decrease. Intermittent intra-abdominal hemorrhage leads to a somewhat different picture, because blood shed into the peritoneal cavity can be returned to the circulation. PCV may therefore recover quickly (until the next episode), and signs of depletion of hemoglobin constituents do not emerge.

In chronic hemolytic anemia, RBCs are regenerative on presentation, except that some cases of autoimmune hemolytic anemia (AIHA) paradoxically show little or no regeneration until treatment has been initiated. Hypochromasia is less marked than in hemorrhagic conditions, and misshapen RBCs (including target cells and folded cells) are more common. The spherocyte, in which the erythrocyte loses its classic biconcave shape, is essentially pathognomonic for AIHA. Jaundice may be absent, because the products of the destruction of the RBCs may be cleared by the reticuloendothelial system and the liver as quickly as they are formed.

Hypoplastic and aplastic anemia may be mild if RBC production is merely depressed secondary to some other disease. Protein, mineral, or vitamin deficiencies may cause hypoplastic anemia, but these are more likely to be secondary to another disease (eg, chronic hemorrhage or malabsorption) than simple dietary deficiency. Other diseases may cause depression of erythropoietin production, eg, renal failure, deficiencies of hormones that usually stimulate erythropoietin production (eg, hypothyroidism, hyperadrenocorticism), and chronic, debilitating conditions (eg, chronic infections, chronic parasitism, and neoplasia). RBC morphology is nonregenerative and may be hypochromic if a deficiency state is involved. Paradoxically, vitamin B12 and/or folic acid deficiency produces a macrocytic RBC picture due to early maturation arrest of the erythrocytes. Neoplasia of the bone marrow may cause severe anemia as erythropoietic elements are crowded out, but some regeneration may be seen as the remaining bone marrow attempts to compensate. In this case, other bone marrow cell lines will also be affected.

True aplastic anemia refers to a failure of the entire bone marrow. The shorter-lived granulocytes and platelets decrease first, followed by a progressively severe anemia that is normocytic and normochromic.

White Blood Cells

The WBCs consist of the granulocytes (neutrophils in most mammals, called heterophils in rabbits, reptiles, and birds (and these look like eosinophils in smears)-; eosinophils; and basophils) and the agranulocytes (lymphocytes and monocytes). Although each type is traditionally counted by determination of its percentage of the total WBC population, meaningful interpretation requires that the absolute number of each type be calculated by multiplying the total WBC by the fraction attributable to the individual cell type. Percentages of each cell type alone are not helpful. An increased percentage that is due to an absolute decrease in another cell type is not an increase at all.

Mature neutrophils have a lobulated nucleus, but when demand is high, immature cells with an unlobulated band nucleus (no constriction of the nucleus is more than half the width of the nucleus) may be released into circulation. They function as phagocytes and are important in infectious conditions and in inflammation. Increased neutrophil counts (neutrophilia) are caused by inflammation, bacterial infection, acute stress, steroid effects, and neoplasia of the granulocytic cell line (granulocytic leukemia can be difficult to differentiate from a simple neutrophilia without special stains or bone marrow biopsy). Decreased neutrophil counts (neutropenia) are caused by viral infections, toxin exposure (including foodborne toxins), certain drugs (eg, carbimazole and methimazole), autoimmune destruction of neutrophils, bone marrow neoplasia not involving the granulocytes, and bone marrow aplasia.

Eosinophils are characterized by prominent pink-staining granules on a Romanowsky stain. They inactivate histamine and inhibit edema formation. Increased eosinophil counts (eosinophilia) are caused by allergic/hypersensitivity reactions, parasitism, tissue injury, mast cell tumors, estrus, and pregnancy or parturition in the bitch. Some large dog breeds (eg, German and Belgian Shepherds, Rottweilers) normally have a relatively high eosinophil count. Extremely high eosinophil counts (hypereosinophilic syndrome), possibly due to an out-of-control hypersensitivity reaction, and eosinophil leukemia (a form of chronic myeloid leukemia) are also described. Decreased eosinophil count (eosinopenia) is almost always caused by the action of glucocorticoids, either endogenous or therapeutic.

Basophils are rare in most species and are characterized by blue-staining granules on a Romanowsky stain. They are more easily seen in cattle. They are closely related to mast cells and, like them, initiate the inflammatory response by releasing histamine. An increased basophil count (basophilia) accompanies eosinophilia in some species as part of the hypersensitivity reaction. Monocytes are large cells with blue-gray cytoplasm, which may be vacuolated, and a kidney bean-shaped or lobulated nucleus. Their main function is phagocytosis, and they are essentially identical to tissue macrophages. An increased monocyte count (monocytosis) may occur in any chronic disease, especially chronic inflammation, and may be very marked in neoplasia. Monocytes also increase as part of the steroid response in dogs.

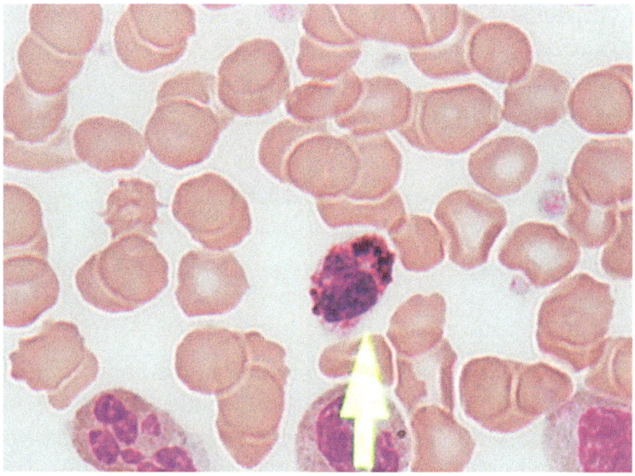

Lymphocytes mainly develop outside the bone marrow in the lymph nodes, spleen, and gut-associated lymphoid tissue. They are the smallest of the WBCs, with a round, evenly staining nucleus and sparse cytoplasm. Larger, reactive lymphocytes can be seen after antigenic stimulation, and care must be taken to differentiate them from neoplastic lymphocytes. Their primary function is immunologic, including both antibody production and cell-mediated immune responses. Some survive only a few days, but many are long-lived. The number in circulation is a balance between populations in the blood, lymph, lymph nodes, and splenic follicles and does not necessarily reflect changes in lymphopoiesis. An increased lymphocyte count (lymphocytosis) may occur for physiologic reasons, especially in cats, but significant increases usually indicate leukemia. Immature or bizarre cells may also be recognized. Decreased lymphocyte counts (lymphopenia) are usually due to an effect of corticosteroids, either endogenous (stress or Cushing disease) or therapeutic, and may also accompany neutropenia in some viral infections, especially the parvoviruses. Lymphopenia may also be a feature of solid-organ lymphosarcomas, when leukemia is absent.

Platelets

Mammalian platelets are pale blue granular fragments (much smaller than RBCs) shed from multinucleate megakaryocytes in the bone marrow; avian and reptilian platelets are true cells with nuclei. They maintain the integrity of the endothelium and act as part of the clotting process to repair damaged endothelium, where they ensure mechanical strength of the clot.

Increased platelet counts (thrombocytosis) occur as a reaction to consumption after injury, when large juvenile platelets may also appear; after splenectomy, as splenic stores are liberated to the circulation; after vincristine treatment, which increases platelet shedding from megakaryocytes; and in megakaryocytic leukemia.

Decreased platelet counts (thrombocytopenia) are caused by autoimmune reactions, thrombotic/thrombocytopenic purpura, bone marrow suppression and aplasia, bone marrow neoplasia, and equine infectious anemia. Signs are petechiation and ecchymosis more than frank hemorrhage, and little may be seen until the platelet count is $<20 \times$

10^9/L. Platelet functional abnormalities present similarly, but platelet numbers and morphology are normal.

Applications of Hematology

The main area of study in hematology is the blood, so hematology research focuses on the substance itself, organs that form blood, diseases involving blood, and blood-forming organs. Most hematology applications are thus found in the medical field. Hematopathologists, for example, work to diagnose and treat blood disorders. Similar applications include transfusions and stem cell transplants. Blood studies can also further understanding of body organs and body processes.

Blood is a carrier of many substances throughout the body. In many respects, it is the messenger between not only various parts of the body, but between the body and the outside world. Blood supplies nutrients and other substances. Scientists may therefore use blood's unique standing to deliver medicines and other substances in a quick and valuable fashion.

Hematologists have uncovered several diverse components that sustain blood. Each of these components can be studied to better understand the human body's function. Platelets, for example, help medical professionals understand the process of clotting and therefore develop aids for this process. White blood cells and red blood cells tell scientists much about the body's disease-fighting capabilities and its subsequent vulnerabilities to disease.

Due to the complexities of the blood, it is susceptible to a wide range of threats. Through hematology, researchers better understand the workings of blood diseases like anemia or leukemia. With this understanding comes greater hope for treatments and cures.

Aided by their clinical laboratory work, hematologists also offer important insights into some non-blood specific conditions as well. For example, these researchers often work hand-in-hand with oncologists to explore the complexities and potential treatments for cancers. The use of bone marrow due to its blood-cell generating capacities also introduces promising research into stem cells. Unmarked stem cells hold the potential for treatments for a wide variety of ailments

In addition, hematology plays an important role in blood transfusions, or the exchange of blood between two organisms. Several factors must be considered in this process, from determining the health of the donor blood to matching blood types between donors and recipients. All such concerns may be addressed by a hematologist.

Since blood is plays such a prominent bodily role, it can also increase knowledge of organs, particularly the heart and the blood vessels. Diseases involving these bodily systems are among the most prevalent and the most fatal in many regions. Recognizing how factors like diet and exercise impact the cardiovascular system helps medical professionals, government officials, and society as a whole develop programs and raise awareness to promote a healthy and balanced body.

1
CHAPTER

THE OLD AND THE NEW CONCEPTS OF HISTOCHEMISTRY

Giuseppe Musumeci

Keywords: Histochemistry, cytochemistry, autoradiographic, histology

EDITORIAL

Histochemistry

Histochemistry has an interesting history, extending back to ancient times when researchers had a desire to understand the functions of the human body and the roles that various "humors" or chemicals have in those processes [1]. Histochemistry is the study of the distribution of chemical compounds within and between biological cells using histological techniques such as histology stains (Table 1), through various colorants (Table 2) and observed under light (optical) and electron microscopy [2]. This science provides information on the content and the nature of the chemicals in biological tissues examined, rather than on morphological appearance of the preparation. To highlight a particular functional group or a particular ion present in various tissues and cells, scientists perform one or more chemical reactions, stoichiometrically exact and specific. The colored precipitates obtained will be analyzed by the optical microscope, or, in the case of fluorophores, fluorescence microscopy.

Citation: Musumeci G. The old and the new concepts of histochemistry. J Histol Histopathol. 2015; 2:10. http://dx.doi.org/10.7243/2055-091X-2-10.

Table 1: Colorants commonly used

Name	Type	Affinity
Eosin	Basic	Stain the nucleus light pink
Hematoxylin	Acid	Stain the cytoplasm blue-violet
Toluidine blue	Amphoteric	Stain the nucleus blue-violetStain nucleic acids blue-violetStain the cytoplasm blue-violetStain some polysaccharides red
Fuchsin acid	Acid	Stain erythrocytes orange
Methyl violet	Acid	Stain amyloid purple
Green light	Basic	Stain collagen fibers green
Alcian blue	Basic	Stain some mucosubstances (glycosaminoglycans) blue
Congo red	Amphoteric	Stain nuclei blueStain amyloid redStain connective red

Table 2: Some widely used histochemical staining

Hematoxylin and eosin
Ziehl-Neelsen
PAS reaction
Prussian reaction
Feulgen reaction
Hillarp reaction
Mallory's trichrome
Masson's trichrome
van Gieson's trichrome
Gomori trichrome
Goldner trichrome
Trichrome Heidenhain (Mallory-Azan)
Nissl method
Azan
Orcein
Ignesti
Iron Hematoxylin (hematoxylin Heidenhain)
Alcian Blue
Giemsa & Wright
Toluidine blue
Methyl green-pyronin
Sudan black/Osmium

Histochemistry took its first steps in the early 1950s but it was between the 1950s and the 1960s that discoveries in histochemistry, cytochemistry and autoradiography prospered. Enzyme histochemistry gained popularity with the development of new techniques and applications to localize enzymatic activities in cells and tissues, evolving into a major discipline in the life sciences and pathology [3]. The transmission electron microscope was introduced in the 1960s leading to significant discoveries in cell ultrastructure and functions of cell organelles, such as lysosomes and peroxisomes [4]. Autoradiography allows us to study dynamic aspects of cell biology, by both the light and electron microscope [5]. Histochemistry takes its origin from medical sciences such as biochemistry and histochemistry that have become so advanced that they have giving rise to specialist sub-disciplines. Those subjects are not usually debated in school or college-level courses, but they may address students to further scientific subjects at more advanced levels [6]. The histochemistry includes cytochemistry, immunohistochemistry and immunocytochemistry [7]. Cytochemistry is the study of the actions of chemical compounds within living cells. Immunohistochemistry allows us to detect antigens using antibodies binding to specific targets in sections of biological tissue, in which each cell is surrounded by the tissue structures and other cells normally found in the intact tissue. Immunocytochemistry uses antibodies to target specific peptides or protein antigens in cells that could have been grown within a culture, deposited from suspension, or taken from a smear. Indeed immunocytochemistry is different from immunohistochemistry because the tissues studied have their surrounding extracellular matrix removed [7]. The scope of histochemistry has expanded over the years in pathological diagnosis and research including new techniques involving specific antibodies, imaging, quantification, and in situ hybridization. The quantification of stained or immunolocalized images of specific colored reaction products is made by computerized image analysis systems (such as ImagePro® or analySIS®) and similar software packages [8] that measure and compare changes in the intensity of staining reactions. Several histochemical methodologies have risen and fallen during the last couple of decades, including the use of colloidal gold labeling at the ultrastructural level [4]. Transmission electron microscopy has been replaced in much histopathology diagnostics by novel light microscopy techniques including the use of specific monoclonal antibodies [6,9]. Light microscopy techniques are indeed experiencing a period of renaissance, with novel techniques using super-resolution microscopes and live cell imaging [10]. Confocal light fluorescence microscopy provided clear images of the morphology of cells. Autoradiographic methods lost their role as a result of safety issues and special requirements of radiation safety officers in dealing with radioactive compounds, especially because alternative methodologies are often available [8]. The recent molecular biological techniques allow us to correlate quantitative data to the microscope images using histochemical, cytochemical and tissue microarrays techniques [11]. We are also seeing the increasing use of histochemical research in this extremely fertile period of cell biology which has led to the establishment of new scientific journals devoted specifically to histochemistry and cytochemistry (Table 3).

Table 3: Some Scientific histochemistry and cytochemistry journals

Histochemistry and cell biology
European Journal of Histochemistry
Journal of Histochemistry & Cytochemistry
Biotechnic & Histochemistry
Progress in Histochemistry and Cytochemistry
Acta Histochemica
Journal of Molecular Histology
Journal of Histology & Histopathology
Applied Immunohistochemistry and Molecular Morphology
Chinese Journal of Histochemistry and Cytochemistry
Histology & Histopathology
Histopathology
Journal of Cytology & Histology

CONCLUSION

In its long history, histochemistry had many connections with the other life sciences. It is now one of the most objective methods in biology and medicine, used in a variety of clinical differential diagnostic settings. The rapidity, reproducibility, and relatively low costs related to this technique, allow it to maintain its value after nearly 200 years of existence. With this editorial I want to remind us of the evolution of this investigative and diagnostic discipline that began from the efforts of medicinal chemists and then rose to be at the basis of current practice of anatomical pathology, combining histology and biochemistry. In conclusion, I can hypothesize that the use of histochemistry is currently widespread and very important both for scientific research and for clinical diagnostics, without which we would not be able to evaluate some morphological alterations of both cells and tissue.

ACKNOWLEDGEMENT

I thank Professor Gaetano Magro from Department of Medical and Surgical Sciences and Advanced Technologies, G.F. Ingrassia, Azienda Ospedaliero-Universitaria "Policlinico-Vittorio Emanuele", Anatomic Pathology Section, University of Catania, Catania, Italy, for his kind support.

REFERENCES

1. Wick MR. Histochemistry as a tool in morphological analysis: a historical review. *Ann Diagn Pathol.*2012; 16:71-8.
2. Titford M. Progress in the development of microscopical techniques for diagnostic pathology. *J Histotechnol.* 2009; 32:9-19.

3. Coleman R. The impact of histochemistry--a historical perspective. *Acta Histochem.* 2000; 102:5-14.

4. Coleman R. Professor Moshe Wolman: pioneer in histochemistry. *Acta Histochem.* 2002; 104:117-21.

5. Ostrowski A, Nordmeyer D, Boreham A, Holzhausen C, Mundhenk L, Graf C, Meinke MC, Vogt A, Hadam S, Lademann J, Ruhl E, Alexiev U and Gruber AD. Overview about the localization of nanoparticles in tissue and cellular context by different imaging techniques. *Beilstein J Nanotechnol.* 2015; 6:263-80.

6. Coleman R. The long-term contribution of dyes and stains to histology and histopathology. *Acta Histochem.* 2006; 108:81-3.

7. Musumeci G, Castrogiovanni P, Mazzone V, Szychlinska MA, Castorina S and Loreto C. Histochemistry as a unique approach for investigating normal and osteoarthritic cartilage. *Eur J Histochem.* 2014;58:2371.

8. Coleman R. Acta Histochemica celebrates 60 years of publication (1954-2014). *Acta Histochem.* 2014;116:1-4.

9. Musumeci G. Past, present and future: overview on histology and histopathology. *J Histol Histopathol.*2014; 1:5.

10. Coleman R. Eponyms in histology and histochemistry: do they still serve a purpose, or should they be abandoned in favor of standard non-eponymous terminology? *Acta Histochem.* 2006; 108:241-2.

11. Coleman R. The Kyoto Protocol: beyond the limit of histochemistry. *Acta Histochem.* 2013; 115:1-2.

2
CHAPTER

DETACHMENT OF METHACRYLATE-EMBEDDED SECTIONS FROM MICROSCOPE SLIDES CAN BE PREVENTED BY HEATING ON HOTPLATE

Yu Xiang and Zheng-Wei Yang

Keywords: Detachment of sections, glycol methacrylate, histological structures, thickness of sections

INTRODUCTION

Glycol methacrylate (GMA), a resin or plastic also called 2-hydroxyethyl methacrylate, has been used for embedding and then sectioning of biological specimens for light microscopy since 1970s, yielding semi-thin sections morphologically superior to paraffin embedded sections [1,2]. Besides, GMA embedded sections have negligible or much less distortion or shrinkage of the tissue embedded, especially useful for quantitative (morphometric or stereological) study of histological structures [3]. With the necessity of thick sections for sampling or counting particles (e.g., nuclei or nucleoli) according to the method of optical disector in stereology [4], thick (e.g., 20-25 μm in thickness) GMA-embedded sections have become an essential part of contemporary stereological tools [3]. However, thick GMA sections were liable to detaching from microscope slides during staining. In managing to solve problems arising from our recent work with thick GMA sections [5], we found, to our surprise, that heating of the sections at a high temperature could prevent the detachment. A series of experiments were therefore designed and conducted in this study, using GMA-embedded testicular

Citation: Xiang Y and Yang Z-W. Detachment of methacrylate-embedded sections from microscope slides can be prevented by heating on hotplate. J Histol Histopathol. 2014; 1:10. http://dx.doi.org/10.7243/2055-091X-1-10.

sections available in our laboratory, to confirm the finding and determine a heating temperature that would not only prevent section detachment but also maintain section quality.

MATERIALS AND METHODS

10 testicular tissue blocks of similar sizes, obtained from normal male Sprague-Dawley rats (age 8 weeks), were embedded in GMA (Historesin by Leica Microsystems Nussloch GmbH, Germany); 10–30 sections were cut from each block at a set thickness of 10 or 20 μm using a microtome (RM2235, Leica Biosystems Nussloch GmbH), with the average areas of the tissue sections and the entire sections (including the tissue and the GMA around the tissue) being approximately 24 and 64 mm^2, respectively. The sections were randomly assigned to different experiments with different treatments such as different temperatures (90-290°C) of heating of sections, different slides (conventional slides, and adhesive slides with positively charged surface produced by Yifan Experiment, China), and different procedures of staining, see Tables 1 and 2.

Table 1: Number of sections detached after heating at different temperatures

	Experiment 1				Experiment 2	
	Staining without 70% ethanol		Staining with 70% ethanol		Staining with 70% ethanol	
	Not detached	Detached	Not detached	Detached	Not detached	Detached
90°C	5[a]	5[a]	0[a]	10[a]	-	-
140°C	10[b]	0[b]	6[b]	4[b]	14	6
190°C	5	0	5	0	6	0
240°C	5	0	5	0	6	0
290°C	-	-	-	-	6	0

In Experiments 1 and 2, glycol methacrylate embedded testicular sections (cut at a set thickness of 20 μm and mounted onto conventional slides) were placed on a hotplate at 90-290°C for 30 minutes before staining (periodic acid-Schiff's reagent and hematoxylin), which was not or was followed by dehydration in 70% ethanol for 2 minutes. $P \leq 0.05$ for the contingency table data a or b (Fisher exact test).

Table 2: Number of sections detached in experiment 3

	Not detached	Detached
90°C, conventional slides, 10 μm [a]	13	7
90°C, conventional slides, 20 μm[b]	2	18
90°C, adhesive slides, 20 μm[c]	4	16
115°C, conventional slides, 10 μm[d]	20	0
115°C, conventional slides, 20 μm[e]	15	5
115°C, adhesive slides, 20 μm[f]	14	6

Our protocol of sections staining was as follows: 30 minutes in 1% periodic acid, 1×3 minutes (i.e., 1 minute for 3 times) in distilled water, 50 minutes in Schiff's reagent, 10 minutes in running tap water, 1 minute in distilled water, 30 minutes in hematoxylin, a few seconds in running tap water, 10 minutes in tap water, 1 minute in distilled water, 2 minutes in 70% ethanol (this step of dehydration was omitted in 1 experiment, see Table 1), 2 minutes in 95% ethanol, 2×2 minutes in absolute ethanol, and 2×2 minutes in xylene. Before staining, sections were heated on a hotplate (H17.5D, Ingenieurbüro, M. Zipperer GmbH, Germany) for 30 minutes. Care was taken to ensure that the bottom surface of the glass (slide), not the upper surface on which the section was mounted, was put on the surface of the hotplate. After staining, they were mounted with a neutral balsam.

Detachment of a section was defined in this study as fully detaching of the section from the glass slide on which the section was mounted, i.e., the section fell off (or became separated from) the slide during staining.

Thickness of some sections (Tables 1 and 3) were measured after staining. As we previously described [6], the section was observed on a computer screen (final magnification×2240), using a×100 oil lens (UPlanSApo, NA 1.40, Olympus, Japan) on an Olympus BX51 microscope equipped with a stereology image system (Visiopharm, Denmark); 10 fields (distance between fields 1000 μm) were sampled per section in a systematic random manner; a frame (35 μm×26 μm) was superimposed at the center of each field; the upper surface of the section was first brought into focus within the frame area, and then the bottom surface was focused within the frame area; the distance between the 2 focal planes, which was measured by a microcater (Dr. Johannes Heidenhain GmbH, Germany) and shown on the screen, was a thickness of the section at the frame area. For thickness measurement of the thinner stained section (Table 3), the bottom surface in focus was the bottom surface of the stained structures (especially nuclei) whose shapes could be clearly seen, not the bottom surface of the embedding medium.

Table 3: Thickness (μm, X±SD, median, range) of sections after heating at different temperatures

	GMA sections	Thinner stained sections
90°C	19.8±0.6, 19.6, 18.7–20.9 (n=10)	-(n'=0)
140°C	19.8±1.1, 19.7, 18.4–22.6 (n=10)	18.2±1.5, 17.8, 16.3–21.4 (n'=10)*
190°C	19.0±0.7, 19.0, 17.4–20.1 (n=11)	13.2±2.0, 12.7, 10.9–17.1 (n'=11)#*
240°C	18.6±0.7, 18.7, 17.3–19.4 (n=11)#	5.4±6.0, 4.8, 0.0–17.2 (n'=11)#*
290°C	12.9±4.5, 12.1, 8.7–18.5 (n=6)#	0.1±0.4, 0.0, 0.0–0.9 (n'=6)#*

RESULTS

With heating of sections (thickness 20 μm) at 90°C, half (without dehydration in 70% ethanol after staining) or all (with dehydration in 70% ethanol) of the sections detached from slides before mounting (Table 1). When the heating temperature increased to 115°C or 140°C, no sections (without dehydration in 70% ethanol) or less than half of the sections (with dehydration in 70% ethanol) detached (Tables 1 and 2). At 190°C or higher heating temperatures, detachment of sections was completely prevented (Table 1).

Detachment occurred in fewer thinner sections (thickness 10 μm) compared to thicker ones (thickness 20 μm), and none of the thinner sections detached after heating at temperature 115°C (Table 2). In contrast, the use of adhesive slides did not show significant effect on the prevention of sections detachment (Table 2).

Detachment of sections occurred after staining with periodic acid-Schiff›s reagent (PAS) and hematoxylin. For more than 80% of the sections detached, it occurred at the step of dehydration in 70% ethanol (if there was this step in the staining) or in 95% ethanol (if there was not the step of dehydration in 70% ethanol).

In regard to the microscopic effect or quality, staining followed by dehydration in 70% ethanol, in comparison with staining without this step of dehydration, appeared to offer a slightly clearer section image. With increasing heating temperatures, the sections were stained increasingly lighter (Figure 1); at 290°C, only the shade of the structures was seen. In parallel, the embedding medium and, in particular, the tissue section embedded in the medium became thinner and thinner beyond 140°C; at 290°C, almost no structures were stained (Table 3). Poor staining of the tissue section started from its bottom surface on the slide. That is, the burning effect on the upper part of the section happened later. However, heating of sections up to even 240°C did not appear to induce appreciable changes in the size or shape of structures (nuclei or tissues) that were stained and seen.

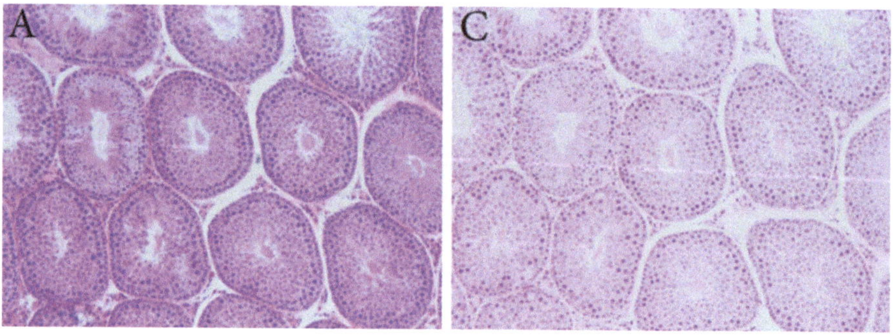

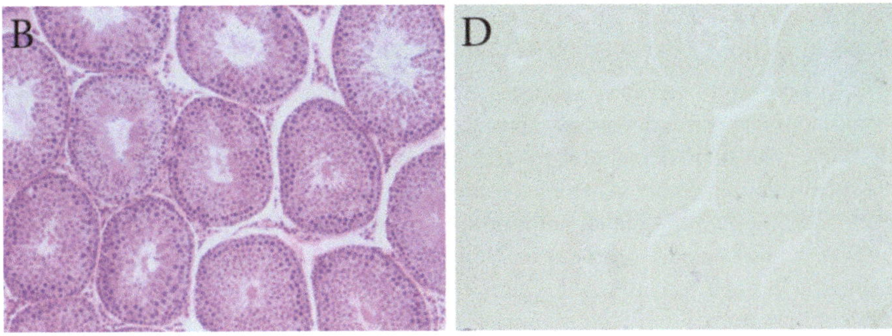

Figure 1 : Testicular micrographs (each with width 870 μm) taken from the focal plane at the upper surface of 20 μm thick GMA sections, which were heated, before staining with periodic acid-Schiff 's reagent and hematoxylin followed by dehydration in 70% ethanol, at 90°C (**A**), 140°C (**B**), 190°C (**C**) and 240°C (**D**) for 30 minutes, respectively.

DISCUSSION

GMA sections, often obtained with semi-thin thickness (e.g., 1–2 μm), were usually left to dry up, e.g., at room temperature overnight [7] or at 50–70°C for 1–4 hours [8,9], to ensure their adhesion to slides. But for thick GMA sections, their detachment from slides is a common problem. We have found in this study that this problem can be effectively solved by heating them on a hotplate at higher temperatures.

Based on the limited experiments in the current study, we recommend a heating temperature of 115–140°C (for 30 minutes) for detachment prevention of thick (10–20 μm) GMA sections (Tables 1 and 2). For sections less than 10 μm in thickness, 90°C (30 minutes) may be enough. Importantly, the morphology of the tissue structures or the thickness of the tissue sections (Table 3) was essentially unaffected by heating at these temperatures, suggesting that the embedding medium GMA, which was not dissolved or removed during staining, served as a good protection for the tissue embedded.

Apart from GMA-embedded testicular sections used in this study, as shown in our recent experience, the heating method also applies to GMA-embedded sections of the rat eye, seminal vesicle and spinal cord for effective prevention of section detachment. Whether the immunohistochemical staining will be affected by the heating, however, remains to be further studied. The study of paraffin sections (see below) suggests that it may be affected.

The experimental designs in the current study did not demonstrate a significant effect of adhesive slides on the affixing of GMA sections to slides (see Table 2). Although this does not necessarily mean that adhesive slides have no use for GMA sections, we can rest assured that the use of adhesive slides is not as effective as the heating of slides for the prevention of GMA sections detachment.

According to our years of experience, as also shown in the current study, detachment of GMA sections occurs frequently at the step of dehydration in 70% ethanol after staining. This procedure was designed in this study in order to obtain contrasting results.

As expected, we obtained efficient results with statistical significance using limited numbers of sections and experiments (Tables 1 and 2).

With respect to paraffin sections, according to our additional study (data not reported), heating (after dewaxing) of paraffin embedded renal and spinal cord sections at 90-140°C prevented detachment of sections, but resulted in not only marked reduction of the section thickness but also marked damage to the sections, including disappearance or poor staining of some nuclei, and more non-specific immunohistochemical staining and fewer immuno-positive structures. Similarly, decreased intensity of immunostaining was previously reported after heating at 80°C for 16 hours [10]. Thus the implication is that the high temperature heating method does not apply to paraffin sections.

AUTHORS' CONTRIBUTIONS

Authors' contributions	YX	ZWY
Research concept and design	--	√
Collection and/or assembly of data	√	--
Data analysis and interpretation	--	√
Writing the article	--	√
Critical revision of the article	--	√
Final approval of article	--	√
Statistical analysis	--	√

ACKNOWLEDGEMENT AND FUNDING

This study was supported by a grant from the Research Development Program of North Sichuan Medical College (CBY13-A-QN35).

REFERENCES

1. Bennett HS, Wyrick AD, Lee SW and McNeil JH. **Science and art in preparing tissues embedded in** plastic for light microscopy, with special reference to glycol methacrylate, glass knives and simple stains. *Stain Technol.* 1976; 51:71-97.
2. Litwin JA. Light microscopic histochemistry on plastic sections. *Prog Histochem Cytochem.* 1985; 16:1-84.
3. Yang ZW. Essential Tools for Morphometric Studies of Biological Tissues: Practical Stereological Methods. *Beijing: Science Press.* 2012.
4. Gundersen HJ, Bagger P, Bendtsen TF, Evans SM, Korbo L, Marcussen N, Moller A, Nielsen K, Nyengaard JR, Pakkenberg B and et al. The new stereological tools: disector, fractionator, nucleator and point sampled intercepts and their use in pathological research and diagnosis. *APMIS.* 1988; 96:857-81.
5. Yang ZW, Xiang Y, Guo Y, Peng B, Bai GQ, Dong XT, Huang XL, Ma L, Chen J, Du X and Zhang SH.Moistening in a wet box of embedded tissue blocks stored

for long can prevent or reduce tissue section breaking. *Journal of North Sichuan Medical College*. 2014; **29**:492-493.

6. Peng B, Chen MS, Li H and Yang ZW. Comparison of the compressions of paraffin-embedded sections from different organs. *Chinese Journal of Stereology and Image Analysis*. 2012; 17:219-225.
7. Casey TT, Cousar JB and Collins RD. A simplified plastic embedding and immunohistologic technique for immunophenotypic analysis of human hematopoietic and lymphoid tissues. *Am J Pathol.* 1988;131:183-9.
8. Dancey JT, Deubelbeiss KA, Harker LA and Greenaway J. Section preparation of human marrow for light microscopy. *J Clin Pathol.* 1976; 29:704-10.
9. Mason M and Mackie RM. Comparative study of three methods of plastic embedding in diagnostic dermatopathology. *J Clin Pathol.* 1985; 38:1397-9.
10. Jones WT, Stockard CR and Grizzle WE. Effects of time and temperature during attachment of sections to microscope slides on immunohistochemical detection of antigens. *Biotech Histochem.* 2001; 76:55-8.

3
CHAPTER

GROSS PATHOLOGY, BIOCHEMISTRY AND HISTOPATHOLOGY OF SELECTED ORGANS OF CAMELS SUFFERING FROM SUSPECTED MONENSIN TOXICOSIS IN AUSTRALIA

Al Jassim RAM, Shahsavari A, Owen H, and Khamas W

Keywords: Camels, Monensin toxicosis, Blood profile, Histopathology

INTRODUCTION

The rumen modifier monensin is a polyether ionophore antibiotic produced by the soil bacterium *Streptomyces cinnamonensis* [1]. It is widely used in Australian and US cattle production systems [2]. In addition to its anti-coccidial action, monensin improves energy efficiency and nitrogen metabolism in rumen bacteria, and reduces the incidence of metabolic disorders such as acidosis and bloat [3]. Monensin induces pH change within the cell, which can lead to a reduction in the secretion and/or transport of the chemicals important for the proper functioning of the cell. Monensin also affects the processes involved in formation of external structures on the cell surface and their growth by reducing the secretion of necessary substances [1]. It has been demonstrated that the cellular effects of monensin depend on the body size subjected to its action, the route of administration, and the dose of this antibiotic [1].

The mode of action of monensin is well established [4]. It forms a complex with extracellular Na^+, dissolves into the bilayer membrane of bacteria and protozoa causing total intracellular Na^+ to increase and total K^+ to decrease. In doing so, it disrupts the Na^+-K^+ pumps and kills bacteria and protozoa. While monensin is considered safe for

Citation: Al Jassim RAM, Shahsavari A, Owen H, Khamas W (2016) Gross Pathology, Biochemistry and Histopathology of Selected Organs of Camels Suffering from Suspected Monensin Toxicosis in Australia. J Veterinar Sci Techno 7:315. doi:10.4172/2157-7579.1000315.

cattle, swine and poultry, it is extremely toxic to horses [5] and incidents of toxicity have also been reported in several animal species in Egyptian camels [6]; in a group of bulls [7]; in two sheep flocks [8]; in a dairy herd [9] and an ostrich [10]. The blood profiles and histopathology in a camel herd, following suspected monensin toxicosis will be presented in this study.

In conclusion, the camel appears not to be in the same category of intermediate sensitivity like the cattle and therefore feeding them cattle ration supplemented with monensin is likely to result in morbidity or mortality.

MATERIALS AND METHODS

A group of Arabian camels (*Camelus dromedarius*) ranging in age from one to eight years were co-grazed with cattle in a paddock with native grass and different types of pine and eucalyptus trees and shrubs. They had access to varying levels of monensin for a period of approximately 4 weeks due to receiving a cattle breeder supplement containing the ionophore antibiotic feed additive monensin (250 mg/ kg). Thirteen camels out of a small herd of 40 camels showed clinical signs of monensin toxicity of variable severity. Blood samples were collected from these camels for blood profiling. Deaths of four camels were reported and two of these camels were necropsied on site immediately after their sudden death. Blood samples were also collected from twelve healthy camels that had no exposure to monensin and used as controls. Sera were separated by centrifugation and biochemical analysis was performed using an Olympus blood analyzer (Olympus Life and Material Science Europa GmbH, Hamburg, Germany). Tissues were collected during the post mortem for histological examination. Specimens (forestomach, colon, liver, heart and spleen) were preserved in 10% neutral buffered formalin solution, embedded in paraffin, sectioned at 5 μm and routinely stained with haematoxylin and eosin (H&E). Finally, the stained sections were examined under a light microscope for further evaluation and histological studies.

RESULTS

Clinical observation

Toxicity signs demonstrated by several camels ranged from depression and muscular weakness to inability to stand. Among the four dead, a 13 month old camel was presented with a history of "not doing well", being recumbent and not able to get up and having cyanotic mucus membrane. This animal died with torticollis (Figure 1). Post mortem and histological observations from the two dead camels are as follows: several litres of clear peritoneal fluid were present in the abdominal cavity (Figure 2). Furthermore, fluid was found to be in large quantity within the omentum/mesentery and inside the pericardial sac while the heart was found to be within normal shape (Figures 3 and 4).

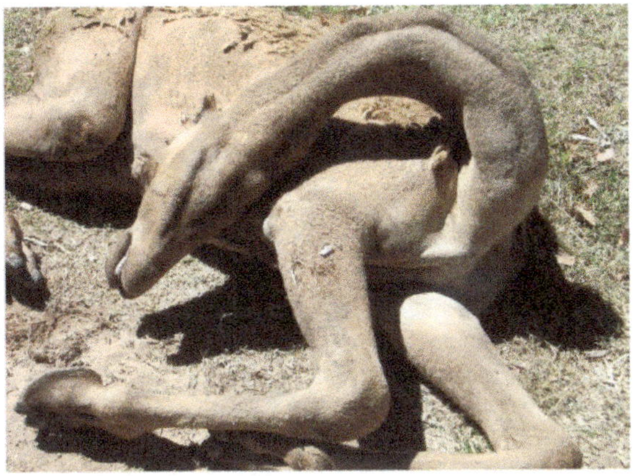

Figure 1: Torticollis, irreversible position of the neck before death of 13 month old camel.

Histopathology findings

Myocardial necrosis, a feature of ionophore toxicity in other species was not noted in the sections examined. Microscopically, the only change observed was occasional nuclear rowing in the cardiomyocytes. No oedema or alveolar macrophages containing hemosiderin that might suggest congestive heart failure were noted in the sections of the lung examined. Moderate to severe oedema was detected in the submucosa of the forestomaches. Oedema in the colon was transmural. Within the colonic lamina propria, there was an equivocal increase in lymphocytes and plasma cells and multifocal, small, dense aggregates of eosinophils. No changes of significance were noted in other tissues. Skeletal muscle was not collected.

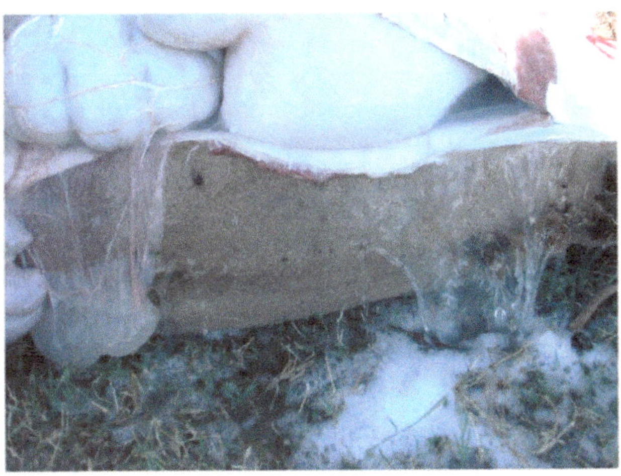

Figure 2: Severe oedema in a camel exposed to four-week monensin toxicity with large amount of clear peritoneal fluid inside the abdominal cavity.

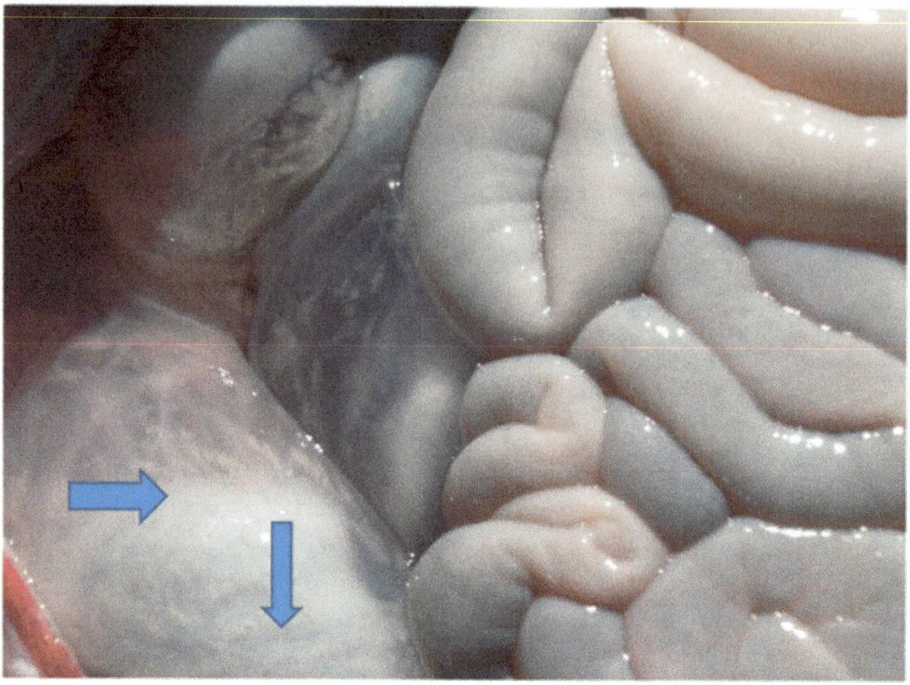

Figure 3: Peritoneal fluid below the omentum of 13 month camel (Arrows).

Blood chemistry profile

Blood profile showed an increase in alkaline phosphates (ALP), Lactate dehydrogenase (LDH) and creatine phosphokinase (CPK) when compared to physiologically normal healthy camels (Table 1) and reference ranges were reported in one study [11]. In comparison to the normal camels and published reference ranges, the average values from the exposed camels demonstrated marked hypoalbuminaemia($P<0.0001$), associated hypocalcaemia ($P<0.001$) and hyperphosphataemia ($P<0.01$) were detected but other parameters (Na, Cl, Anion Gap, Cholesterol, Creatinine, gamma-glutamyl transferase (GGT), Globulin, HCO_3 and Urea) in the blood profile remained unchanged ($P>0.05$). Camels exposed to monensin had a tendency toward higher levels of ALP (147.4 vs 93.8) but the statistical difference was not highly significant ($P>0.05$).

Table 1: Blood chemistry profile of camels suspected with monensin toxicity (n=13) compared to normal healthy camels (n=12). [a,b]Different superscripts denote significant statistical difference between groups while identical superscripts denote no statistical difference

Test	Monensin Toxicity (n=13, exposed camels)		Normal Range (n=12, non-exposed domesticated camels)		SI Unit	P value
	(Mean ± SE)	Range	(Mean ± SE)	Range		
Sodium	$146.3^{a} \pm 1.3$	134-154	$155.5^{b} \pm 0.38$	154-158	mmol/L	0.000
Na/K ratio	$25.4^{a} \pm 0.9$	17.4-29.0	$31.56^{a} \pm 0.36$	26.3-30.4		
Potassium	$5.9^{a} \pm 0.2$	5.1-7.7	$4.93^{a} \pm 0.05$	4.7-5.2	mmol/L	0.001
Chloride	$104.5^{a} \pm 7.4$	17-119	$119.5^{a} \pm 0.42$	117-122	mmol/L	0.065
Bicarbonate	$24.8^{a} \pm 1.0$	18-33	$22.17^{a} \pm 0.85$	16-25	mmol/L	0.060
Ca/P ratio	$0.74^{a} \pm 0.1$	0.32-1.03	$1.18^{a} \pm 0.03$	1.25-1.15		
Calcium	$1.81^{a} \pm 0.1$	1.44 -2.59	$2.17^{b} \pm 0.02$	2.09-2.27	mmol/L	0.000
Anion Gap	$22.85^{a} \pm 7.5$	11-111.4	$18.77^{a} \pm 1.12$	25.7-16.2	mEq/L	0.608
Magnesium	$1.0^{a} \pm 0.03$	0.78-1.2	$0.86^{a} \pm 0.01$	0.79-0.91	mmol/L	0.008
Phosphorus	$2.67^{a} \pm 0.2$	1.75-4.54	$1.85^{b} \pm 0.03$	1.67-1.98	mmol/L	0.003
AST (Alanine transaminase)	$202.5^{a} \pm 45.1$	110-604	$97.00^{b} \pm 3.37$	82-112	U/l@37°C	0.035
ALP (Alkaline Phosphatase)	$147.4^{a} \pm 41.7$	54-605	$93.83^{b} \pm 5.76$	65-122	U/l@37°C	0.234
LDH (GLDH) (Glutamate dehydrogenase)	$891.2^{a} \pm 120.1$	496-1981	$5.32^{b} \pm 0.40$	3.2-7.2	U/l@37°C	0.000
CPK (Creatine phosphokinase)	$293.0^{a} \pm 49.7$	130-789	$143.3^{b} \pm 17.02$	83-268	U/l@37°C	0.010
GGT (Gama glutamyl transferase)	$18.5^{a} \pm 6.0$	8-90	$12.43^{a} \pm 0.81$	8 - 16	U/l@37°C	0.343
Protein	$48.2^{a} \pm 2.5$	25-61	$59.0^{a} \pm 1.11$	54-64	g/L	0.001
Albumin	$17.3^{a} \pm 1.9$	6-34	$29.83^{b} \pm 0.76$	26-34	g/L	0.000
Globulin	$30.8^{a} \pm 1.5$	19-40	$29.26^{a} \pm 0.73$	24.5-32.4	g/L	0.369
A/G Albumin/Globulin	$0.58^{a} \pm 0.1$	0.32-1.48	$1.03^{a} \pm 0.04$	1.06-1.05		0.000
Urea	$4.18^{a} \pm 0.5$	2.5-9.5	$3.59^{a} \pm 0.19$	2.5-4.3	mmol/L	0.286
Creatinine	$102.8^{a} \pm 7.4$	81-171	$110.4^{a} \pm 5.51$	88-135	µmol/L	0.424
Cholesterol	$0.88^{a} \pm 0.3$	0.2-3.9	$0.84^{a} \pm 0.07$	0.5-1.2	mmol/L	0.902
Triglycerides	$0.34^{a} \pm 0.05$	0.05-0.6	$0.5^{a} \pm 0.0$	0.5-0.5	mmol/L	0.005
Total Bilirubin	$2.17^{a} \pm 0.1$	1.2-3.1	$2.93^{a} \pm 0.07$	2.5-3.3	µmol/L	0.000
Glucose	$5.49^{a} \pm 0.5$	0.6-9.8	$6.94^{a} \pm 0.29$	5.8 -8.3	mmol/L	0.030

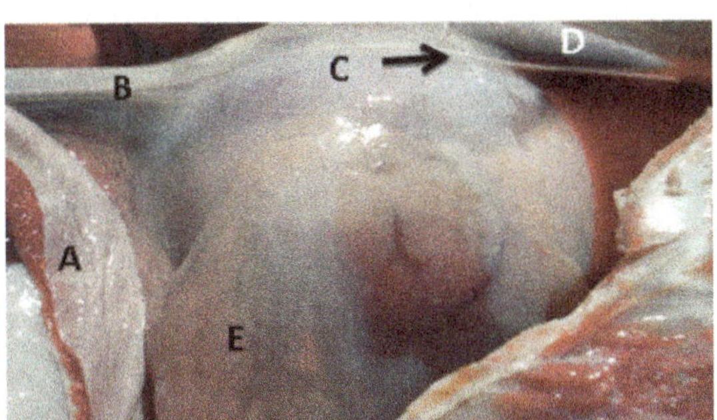

Figure 4: Increase pericardial fluid in 13 month old camel. Diaphragm (A); caudal vena cava (B); phrenic nerve (C); cranial vena cava (D); pericardial fluid (E).

DISCUSSION

Food mixing errors have been documented in the literature in diverse animal species. The suspected camel herd monensin toxicity reported in this article was due to this kind of error where cattle feed with monensin additives were offered to the camels without taking into consideration the camel's unknown sensitivity to this ionophore compound. LD_{50} of monensin was reported to be 1.4 mg/kg for horses [12] and 26.4 mg/kg in goats [13] while in broiler chickens; it was 214 mg/kg [14]. The most sensitive animal species was horses [1,12]. The toxicity of monensin for cattle and other species is well documented and is known to be dose dependent [15-18]. Unfortunately, no such data is available in the literature for camels.

No clear indication of extensive myocardial necrosis, a common feature of acute ionophore toxicity was observed or of myocardial fibre atrophy, indispersed with areas of myocardial hypertrophy and fibrosis which are features that have been described in cases of chronic ionophore toxicity in other species [17-18]. The only cardiac change observed was nuclear rowing which is an indication of early degeneration and regeneration initiation as reported by Mollenhauer et al. [19] in a Holstein heifer. The heart of this animal showed rare myocytes, characterized by rowing of nuclei and suggestive of attempted myofiber regeneration, with evidence of chronic yew toxicity in cattle. Some cases of chronic ionophore toxicity produce very localized or subtle cardiac lesions which may not be identified on limited sectioning of the heart. The severe ascites and visceral oedema could also be consistent with right sided congestive heart failure. Although the hypoalbuminaemia noted in the exposed animals may have been the cause of the ascites, it is possible that this hypoalbuminaemia was the result of rapidly developing congestive heart failure. This has been shown to occur in dogs and turkeys as a result of blood volume expansion, inanition and possibly loss of protein into the ascites fluid. An alternative explanation for the hypoalbuminaemia was not discovered, there was no histological or biochemical indication of extensive liver disease and protein-loss through the gut or kidney would be unlikely in multiple animals. A nutritional cause was also considered less likely as albumin concentrations in the control animals were substantially higher (29.83 vs 17.3, $P<0.0001$).

It is also possible that monensin toxicity in camels results in skeletal muscle necrosis while cardiac muscle cells show no clear changes of necrosis due to selective effect [20]. Serum CK, GLDH and AST activities were increased ($P<0.05$ and $P<0.0001$), a finding that could be consistent with skeletal muscle necrosis. Serum potassium concentration was also higher (5.85 vs 4.93, $P<0.001$) above normal. Myoglobinuria was not noted. Unfortunately skeletal muscle samples were not collected for histopathological examination.

Luckily, regardless of the exposure of meat animals to ionophores in feed, residues in the meat milk and its byproducts will have no potential effect on humans consuming these products [21].

In conclusion, the clinical signs associated with monensin toxicity in different animal species vary according to the dose and duration of exposure. In this case, no diarrhea was noted and histological evidence of extensive muscle damage was lacking.

Although no histopathological changes were observed in the cardiac muscles, cardiac damage can sometimes be localized and subtle and the severe ascites could be consistent with congestive heart failure.

From our observation, the camel is not in the same category of intermediate sensitivity like the cattle and therefore feeding them cattle ration supplemented with monensin is likely to result in mortality. Further observations of other possible cases of monensin toxicity or intoxication to clarify the rest of the unexplained changes in onehumped camels are very much needed if other cases arise.

REFERENCES

1. Lowicki D,Huczynski A (2013) Structure and Antimicrobial Properties of Monensin A and Its Derivatives: Summary of the Achievements. ,pp: 1-14.
2. Butaye P, Devriese LA, Haesebrouck F (2003) Antimicrobial growth promoters used in animal feed: effects of less well known antibiotics on gram-positive bacteria. ClinMicrobiol Rev 16: 175-188.
3. Lean IJ, Rabiee AR, Golder HM, Lloyd J (2011) Analysis of the potential to manipulate the rumen of northern beef cattle to improve performance. Meat & Livestock Australia.
4. Schelling GT (1984) Monensin mode of action in the rumen. J AnimSci 58: 1518-1527.
5. Roder JD (2011) Ionophore toxicity and tolerance. Vet Clin North Am Food AnimPract 27: 305-314.
6. Mousa HM, Elsheikh HA (1992) Monensin poisoning in dromedary camels. DtschTierarztlWochenschr 99: 464.
7. Janzen ED, Rodostits OM, Orr JP (1981) Possible monensin poisoning in a group of bulls. Can Vet J 22: 92-94.
8. Jones A (2001) Monensintoxicosis in 2 sheep flocks. Can Vet J 42: 135-136.
9. Gonzalez M, Barkema HW, Keefe GP (2005) Monensintoxicosis in a dairy herd. Can Vet J 46: 910-912.
10. Dedoussi A, Roubies N, Tserveni-Goussi A (2007) Monensin toxicity in ostriches on a farm in northern Greece. Vet Rec 161: 628-629.
11. Bogin E (2000) Clinical pathology of camelids: present and future. Revue MédVét 151: 563-568.
12. Matsuoka T, Novilla MN, Thomson TD, Donoho AL (1996) Review of monensintoxicosis in horses. JEVS 16: 8-15.
13. Deljou M, Aslani MR, Mohri M, Movassaghi AR, Heidarpour M (2014) Clinical, laboratory and pathological findings in sub-acute monensin intoxication in goats. Vet Res Forum 5: 161-167.
14. Sandercock DA, Mitchell MA (2004) The role of sodium ions in the pathogenesis of skeletal muscle damage in broiler chickens. PoultSci 83: 701-706.

15. Potter EL, VanDuyn RL, Cooley CO (1984) Monensin toxicity in cattle. J AnimSci 58: 1499-1511.

16. Van Vleet JF, Ferrans VJ (1983) Ultrastructural myocardial alterations in monensintoxicosis of cattle. Am J Vet Res 44: 1629-1636.

17. Bastianello SS, McGregor HL, Penrith ML, Fourie N (1996) A chronic cardiomyopathy in feedlot cattle attributed to toxic levels of salinomycin in the feed. J S Afr Vet Assoc 67: 38-41.

18. Peek SF, Marques FD, Morgan J, Steinberg H, Zoromski DW, et al. (2004) Atypical acute monensintoxicosis and delayed cardiomyopathy in belgian draft horses. J Vet Intern Med 18: 761-764.

19. Mollenhauer HH, Morre DJ, Rowe LD (1990) Alteration of intracellular traffic by monensin; mechanism, specificity and relationship to toxicity. Biochimica et BiophysicaActa 1031: 225–246.

20. Beasley V (1990) Organic compounds that affect the heart. In: Beasley V (Ed), Veterinary Toxicology, Ithaca, USA. Int Vet Information, pp: 618-620.

21. Novallis MN (2004) Expert report on the safety file for monensin sodium. Submitted to the Europian Medicines Agency CVM by Elanco Animal Health Division of Eli Lilly and company Indianapolis, IN, USA.

4
CHAPTER

DETECTION OF ANIMAL PRODUCTS IN RUMINANT FEEDS BY MICROSCOPY AND REAL TIME PCR

Luciana Pacheco Golinelli, Joab Trajano Silva, Ana Carolina Carvalho and Vânia Margaret Flosi Paschoalin

Keywords: Feeds for ruminants, Meat-and-bone meal, Mammalian and avian species-specific identification, Microscopic analysis, Realtime PCR tests

INTRODUCTION

Brazil is a major producer and exporter of many agricultural products (AAFM). According to the Brazilian Ministry of Agriculture, Livestock and Food Supply (MAPA), the cattle industry and its derivatives are a major component of world agribusiness. During the twenty-first century, Brazil has become the largest exporter, secondlargest producer, and third-largest consumer of beef [1]. The country has the second largest herd, with over 212 million cattle heads, and, in 2004, Brazil took the lead in meat export, since one-fifth of the meat sold to over 180 countries in international markets originated from Brazil [2,3].

In Brazil, pastures are the most economical source of food for feeding beef and dairy cattle, and 88% of the beef produced is grass-fed [4]. During the dry season the significant reduction in production and nutritional value of pasturage causes animal weight loss or low milk production, so confinement may be an option to provide a more balanced diet, using a supplement for ruminant feed [5]. Use of commercial feed is advisable if the increased production increases profitability, that is, when the increased cost of commercial feed is offset by increased profits [6].

Citation: Golinelli LP, Silva JT, Carvalho AC, Paschoalin VMF (2016) Detection of Animal Products in Ruminant Feeds by Microscopy and Real Time PCR. J Veterinar Sci Techno 7:316. doi:10.4172/2157-7579.1000316.

Two aspects of sanitation restrictions are important for Brazilian beef exports: foot and mouth disease (FMD) and bovine spongiform encephalopathy (BSE, or mad cow disease) [7]. Transmissible spongiform encephalopathies (TSEs) are a group of rare degenerative brain diseases, usually fatal in humans and animals, with a long incubation period; currently no treatment for any of these diseases exists. TSEs in animals include scrapie in sheep and goats, bovine spongiform encephalopathy (BSE), feline spongiform encephalopathy (FSE), transmissible mink encephalopathy (TME) and chronic wasting disease (CWD) found in deer, elk and moose populations. In humans, the most commonly known TSE is Creutzfeldt-Jakob Disease (CJD) [8,9]. A new variant of Creutzfeldt-Jakob disease (vCJD) that affects young individuals may be caused by transmission of BSE to humans through consumption of infected beef [10] he occurrence of BSE in cattle and its transmissibility to humans has become an international concern and requires global strategies to reduce human exposure to the disease through appropriate food quality control practices [8]. The World Health Organization (WHO), the World Organization for Animal Health (OIE) and the United Nations Food and Agriculture Organization (FAO) have recommended protective measures such as: (i) all animals at risk must be culled and disposed of, as well as products derived from these animals; (ii) the removal of specified risk material (SRM) from cattle, sheep and goats, to prevent the material from entering the food and feed chain; (iii) a ban on the use of processed animal protein (PAPs) in feed for farm animals; (iv) the establishment of procedures for surveillance and notification of BSE occurrences to health authorities in all countries [11].

According to the OIE, Brazil is a member of the "Negligible" risk group for BSE, the safest category [12]. Brazilian Ministry of Agriculture, Livestock and Food Supply (MAPA), allows the marketing of calcined bone (without proteins and fats), milk and milk products, and gelatin and collagen, prepared exclusively from hides and skins [13]. The banned animal materials can be detected by various analytical methods, such as microscopy capillary isoelectric focusing [14], enzyme-linked immunosorbent assays and near-infrared microscopy (NIRM) [15,16], as well as the identification of species-specific central nervous tissue by gas chromatography-mass spectrometry (GC-MS) [17]. Microscopic analysis is the official method for the detection and characterization of PAPs in feedstuffs, as established by the European Union (Commission Regulation EC/ 152/2009), which includes both the observation of morphological conformation of rough fragments with a stereomicroscope and the examination of histological structures of fine particles with a light microscope [18].

Molecular assays, such as conventional PCR and real-time quantitative PCR (qPCR), are more sensitive, specific and reproducible, and the latter allows for the semi-quantification of nucleic acids, especially when a fluorescent probe is used for detection of a specific PCR product, such as TaqMan qPCR, an automated technology with lower turnaround times [15,19,20].

The present study investigated the presence of prohibited animal products in commercial feeds obtained in the retail market of two Brazilian regions traditionally involved in livestock activities. Twentynine samples of commercial bovine feeds were evaluated by two methodologies: microscopy analysis and qPCR assays for the speciesspecific detection of ruminant, porcine and avian (chicken) mitochondrial DNA in bovine feeds.

MATERIALS AND METHODS

Reference sample Preparation and Samples Control

Reference samples free of animal material or meat-and-bone meal (MBM) were formulated at the laboratory. Fifteen grams and reference feeds were processed and homogenized by the paper cone riffler splitting method. The macroscopic and microscopic aspects of each feed and bovine MBM reference samples were evaluated. MBM-free feeds were spiked with increasing proportions of MBM, from 0.0125, 0.025, 0.05, 0.10, 0.20, 0.40 to 0.80% w/w, to obtain feeds with known amounts of animal-derived products. Three samples of each spiked feed were prepared as described by Sanches et al. and were tested in a blind analysis, where the spiked-feeds were coded and randomly distributed during assays [21].

Blood samples from cow, goat, sheep, pig and chicken were used as species-specific controls. Corn (maize) and soybean grains were used as endogenous controls, since Brazilian animal feeds are composed mainly of these grains.

Microscopic Analysis and Confirmatory Tests

Animal materials were detected by microscopy as described previously by the Brazilian Ministry of Agriculture, Livestock and Food Supply (MAPA), based on the morphological characteristics of different animal tissues, including bones (after rendering 133°C and 3 bars for 20 min for sterilization), muscle fibers, cartilage, and ligaments [2]. Parts of organs, skin, and other soft tissues are generally absent, or if present, barely detectable [22]. Qualitative chemical analyses were performed as confirmatory tests [23-25].

DNA Extraction and Quantification

Total genomic DNA was obtained from 100 mg of commercial, reference and spiked feeds from the blood of different vertebrate species, corn and soybean, and MBM-containing and MBM-free feeds. DNA templates were prepared using a DNeasy Blood and Tissue Kit (Qiagen, Hilden, Germany), according to the manufacturer's instructions. DNA concentrations were estimated by use of a Qubit fluorometer (Life Technologies-Invitrogen Corporation, Carlsbad, CA, USA).

Primers and Probes

The set of primers and probes used in this study are displayed in Table 1. The probes were labeled on the 5`-end with the fluorescent reporter dye 6-carboxyfluorescein (6-FAM) and on the 3`-end with a non-fluorescent quencher (NFQ) and a DNA minor groove binder (MGB). Primers and probes were synthesized by Life Technologies-Invitrogen Corporation, Carlsbad, CA- USA.

The specificity of each primer and probe set was tested against DNA templates targeting vertebrate species: cow, goat, sheep, pig and chicken. When the amplification plot did not cross the threshold and no Ct value was obtained ("undetermined"), a Ct value equal to 40 cycles was assumed for the assay [26].

Table 1: 6pecies-specific primer and probe sequences, targets and references used to Real-Time PCR assay

Species	Primers and probes	Sequences	Targets and references
Capra hircus	Forward Reverse	5′- 5′- AAAGGACTTGGCGGTGCTT- 3′	12S rRNA gene.
	TaqMan Probe	5′- 5′- TGACCTAACGTCTTTATGTGTGGTG-3′	
		5′- 5′- (FAM)-TAGAGGAGCCTGTTCTATAATCGATAAACCCCG-(TAMRA)-3′	
Sus scrofa	Forward	5′- CTTGCAAATCCTAACAGGCCTG-3′	Mithochondrial cytochrome b gene.
	Reverse	5′- CGTTTGCATGTAGATAGCGAATAAC-3′	
	TaqMan Probe	5′-(FAM)- ACAGCTTTCTCATCAGTTAC-(NFQ)(MGB)-3′	
Ovis aries	Forward	5′-CCTTATTACACCATTAAAGACATCCTAGGT-3′	
	Reverse	5′- GGGTCTCCGAGTAAGTCAGGC-3′	
	TaqMan Probe	5′-(FAM)- ACTAATCCTCATCCTCATGC-(NFQ)(MGB)-3′	
Bos taurus	Forward	5′-CCCGATTCTTCGCTTTCCAT-3′	
	Reverse	5′- CTACGTCTGAGGAAATTCCTGTTG-3	
	TaqMan Probe	5′-(FAM)- CATCATAGCAATTGCC-(NFQ)(MGB)-3′	
Gallus gallus	Forward	5′-GAAATCGGTAGACGCTACGGA- 3′	
	Reverse	5′-GAAATCGGTAGACGCTACGGA- 3′	
	TaqMan Probe	5′-(FAM)-CAAATTCAGAGAAACCCTGGAA(NFQ)MGB)- 3′	
Zea mays and Glycine max	Forward	5′-TCTGGGCTTAACTCTCATACTCACC-3′	Chloroplast trnLintron sequence Benedetto.
	Reverse	5′- GGTTACTAGTGGGTTTGCTGGG-3′	
	TaqMan Probe	5′-(FAM)-CATTCCTAACACTAGCCCTA-(MGB)-3′	

qPCR Test Conditions

The qPCR tests using the TaqMan PCR Master Mix reagent (Life Technologies - Invitrogen Corporation, Carlsbad, CA, USA) were performed in a volume of 25 µl in a 96-well reaction plate covered with Microamp (Life Technologies-Invitrogen Corporation, Carlsbad, CA, USA) using 900 nM of each primer, 300 nM of each probe and 10 ng of DNA template. Reactions were performed in a Step One Plus™ Real-Time PCR System (Life Technologies-Invitrogen Corporation, Carlsbad, CA, USA) starting at 50°C for 2 min and at 95°C for 10 min, followed by 40 cycles at 95°C for 15 s and annealing/elongation at 60°C for 1 min. All qPCR tests were run in the same conditions, in triplicate.

Sensitivity and Linearity

Calibration curves based on five points were constructed using measures in triplicate, corresponding to a 10-fold serial dilution (1, 1:10, 1:100, 1:1000 and 1:10000) of 50 ng/µl of DNA template for each ruminant species and endogenous control. The standard-curve slope of –3.32 indicates a PCR reaction with 100% efficiency [27].

RESULTS AND DISCUSSION

The specificity of primers and probes targeting porcine, bovine, caprine, ovine, and avian (chicken) material and endogenous controls was tested by screening the DNA templates from blood samples of each animal species and from corn and soybean against different animal species-specific qPCR systems. No cross-amplification was observed (Table 2).

Table 2: 6pecies-specific qPCR systems. &ross-amplification of DNA templates from each species was performed against others by using qPCR species-specific systems. Ct-values (mean and standard deviation) were obtained using 10 ng of each DNA template from animal blood and endogenous controls. Triplicate PCR reactions were run from each DNA template. ND- animal material not detected (no positive signal aier 40 qPCR cycles)

Species	Porcine- specific PCR system	Bovine- specific PCR system	Ovine- specific PCR system	Caprine specific PCR system	Avian (chicken)-specific PCR system	Endogenous control-specific PCR system
Capra hircus	ND	ND	ND	22.0± 0.0	ND	ND
Bos taurus	ND	23.0 ± 0.1	ND	ND	ND	ND
Ovis aries	ND	ND	22.0 ± 0.0	ND	ND	ND
Gallus gallus	ND	ND	ND	ND	21.4 ± 0.1	ND
Sus scrofa	17.8 ± 0.0	ND	ND	ND	ND	ND
Zea mays and Glycine max (endogenous controls)	ND	ND	ND	ND	ND	15.8 ± 0.0

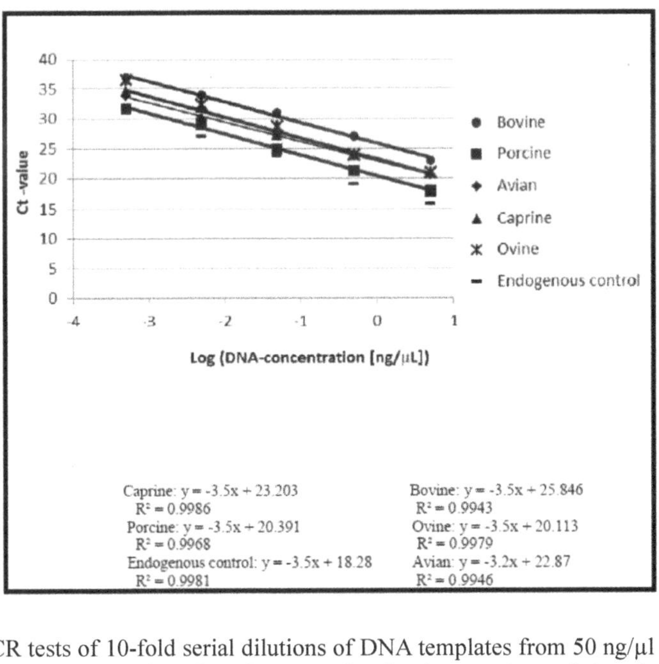

Figure 1: qPCR tests of 10-fold serial dilutions of DNA templates from 50 ng/µl (100%) to 0.5 pg obtained from blood samples of ruminant species (bovine, caprine and sheep), porcine, avian (chicken) and endogenous controls. Ct values obtained from reference samples of animal blood, corn and soybeans were plotted against the logarithm of DNA concentrations. He R-squared values and slopes were determined for each species.

TaqMan-qPCR tests were able to detect 500 pg of DNA templates from bovine, porcine, ovine, and caprine species and the endogenous controls, which corresponds to a 0.01% dilution from each DNA template. For the avian (chicken) sample, the minimum sensitivity was 50 pg, which corresponds to a 0.001% dilution of the DNA template. A test to determine whether a linear correlation between the amount of DNA template and the Ct was present was performed using DNA templates from corn and from the blood of each animal species. A plot test of the linearity Ct-values versus the logarithm of the DNA template amount indicated (Figure 1) a linear correlation for all species over four orders of magnitude. All curves showed a slope of - 3.5 except the curve for chicken, which presented a slope of - 3.2, very close to the theoretical value of -3.32. All species had R-squared values of 0.99, indicating that accurate results and comparable efficiencies of 90%, 92%, 92%, 92%, 104% and 91% for the cow, pig, sheep, goat, and chicken samples and the endogenous controls, respectively, were obtained.

Animal material-free feeds spiked with different amounts of MBM were tested by qPCR. The results were compared to those obtained by microscopic analysis, which is the official method used by Brazilian and European Union regulatory agencies. Samples spiked with 0.0125% (w/w) MBM w/w (Ct value 38.03 ± 0.90) or superior amounts were detected as positive by qPCR tests. When MBM concentrations from 0.20 to 0.40 were added, microscopy analysis was able to detect steamed bone and collagen; whereas if 0.8% (w/w) MBM was added, steamed bone, collagen and hair could be detected. The qPCR tests showed linear signals for detection of spiked samples with increasing MBM concentrations. Proportional Ct values of 38.03 ± 0.90, 37.13 ± 0.0, 34.34 ± 0.28, 33.16 ± 0.70, 30.20 ± 0.10, 29.68 ± 0.17 and 27.89 ± 0.08 were obtained for 0.0125%, 0.025%, 0.05%, 0.10%, 0.20%, 0.40% and 0.80% w/w MBM, respectively. The Ct values in concentrations above 0.20% were within the expected value for optimal amplification, generating Ct values from 20 to 30. The qPCR tests showed better performance than microscopic analysis in detecting the smallest amount of 0.0125% (w/w) MBM, confirming the difficulty in identifying low concentrations of animal-derived materials in complex feed matrices (Table 3).

Regulation (EC) 999/2001 of the European Parliament and of the Council of 22 May 2001 established rules for the prevention, control and eradication of certain transmissible spongiform encephalopathies [28]. Article 7 of Commission Regulation (EC) 999/2001 prohibits the feeding of certain categories of animal protein to certain categories of animals, and prohibits the inclusion of protein derived from mammals in feeds for ruminants. PAP produced from ruminant carcasses, some of which were infected, was assumed to be the transmission route of BSE. Based on these findings, a ban on the use of processed mammalian protein for feeding cattle, sheep and goats was initiated in July 1994.

Table 3: Comparative detection of MBM in spiked feeds free of animal material by qPCR tests and microscopic analysis. Feedstuﬀ samples free of animal material were spiked with increasing concentrations of MBM, from 0.0125 to 0.80% w/w. He Ct-values (mean and standard deviation) were obtained in triplicate PCR reactions from each DNA extraction. ND - animal material not detected

Spiked feeds Concentration of MBM (%) w/w added	qPCR tests for bovine material (Ct-value)	Microscopic analysis
0.0125	38.03 ± 0.90	ND
0.025	37.13 ± 0.0	Steamed bone
0.05	34.34 ± 0.28	Steamed bone
0.10	33.16 ± 0.70	Steamed bone
0.20	30.20 ±0.10	Steamed bone and collagen
0.40	29.68 ± 0.17	Steamed bone and collagen
0.80	27.89± 0.08	Steamed bone, collagen and hair

The ban was expanded in January 2001, prohibiting the feeding of any processed animal protein to all farm animals, with certain limited exceptions. This is to ensure that no cross-contamination occurs between feed containing PAP intended for species other than ruminants and feed intended for ruminants. A Brazilian regulation (Normative Instruction 8, MAPA, promulgated on March 25, 2004) bans the use of products containing proteins and fats of animal origin, including steamed bone, in ruminant feeds [29]. The poorly controlled manufacturing of MBM, as well as low quality control, especially in the Brazilian countryside, could eventually endanger the health of the national herd, which may affect meat exports and be a source of several diseases, such as botulism and BSE [30,31].

The use of MBM, a low-cost alternative supplement of ruminant feed, is widespread among producers, as a source of phosphorus for farm animals that are raised on pastures with mineral-deficient soil. The calcined bones are sterilized at temperatures above 600°C [32].

Steamed bone is the dried and ground product obtained from undecomposed bones that are heat-treated by autoclaving at temperatures above 140°C and pressures greater than 7.0 bar for a minimum of three hours. According to Brazilian regulations, fat and protein residues may or may not be removed during this process [33]. Microscopic analysis is currently the only validated method for detecting animal proteins in feed, including calcined and steamed bones. The discrepancy found between the detection of calcined bones by the qPCR tests and microscopy can be explained by an incomplete calcination process that left biological residues in a sub-product used to supplement feeds with a source of mineral elements.

The microscopic analysis method is able to distinguish the presence of animal-derived constituents, but is unable to quantify constituents of animal origin added to feed or to identify the contaminant species. Several analytical methods including electrophoretic, chromatographic and immunological assays can be used to determine the animal species in a wide array of degraded and processed substrates. Although these methods can identify the origin of species present in raw meats, they are significantly less sensitive in heat-treated materials due to proteolysis and/or alteration of the specific epitopes [34].

The amplification of a specific DNA sequence by PCR provides a rapid, sensitive and specific method for the detection of animal tissues in food and feed [35]. However, many PCR-based methods cannot be used for the detection of MBM, since the high temperatures used in the standard rendering process cause DNA fragmentation, leading to difficulty in obtaining reliable results [36]. The qPCR test used for the detection of species-specific DNA sequences can detect the smallest amounts of even highly degraded DNA. In this study, a qPCR test based on a TaqMan probe was used to detect very small amounts of degraded DNA from five animal species (cow, goat, sheep, pig and chicken). For this purpose, the mitochondrial genome was targeted [37], since it is a robust multi-copy DNA and is still present in meat meals treated at extremely high temperatures.

The present study used soybean and corn seeds as endogenous controls, since these grains usually comprise the major source of protein added to animal feedstuffs. Only sequences of multiple-copies genes were selected. For the analyses involving different vertebrate species, two mitochondrial genes were used: 12S rRNA caprine speciespecific and cytochrome b for bovine, ovine, porcine and avian material (chicken). For the endogenous control the tRNA leucine gene was analyzed, which is a sequence present in the chloroplast genome [35].

The material from bovine, ovine and caprine species showed sensitivity equal to or less than 500 pg DNA, which corresponds to 0.01% w/w; while for avian (chicken)-derived material the sensitivity was 50 pg, which corresponds to 0.001% w/w. The precision of the measurement decreased with the number of copies of the target sequence in the genome and harsher conditions during the processing of meat-and-bone meal, which lead to highly fragmented DNA. An alternative is to evaluate the mass concentrated from serial dilutions of each DNA template to establish the method sensitivity, as was conducted in this study [38].

The linearity of DNA detection for all species performed well, with R-squared values of 0.99 and slopes close to the theoretical optimum. This indicates that the results for the quantification of the bovine, porcine, caprine, ovine and avian (chicken) species and also the endogenous controls were reliable. However, these calculations are very challenging, since the amount of DNA per gram of tissue can differ in the reference and sample materials (e.g., tissue, processing, etc.), and the ingredients could be processed in different ways (e.g., cooked meat, but unprocessed fat, etc.), and consequently the response (Ct-values) of one species is not consistent and cannot be compared with those of other species.

In addition, the results of the present study can be carefully extended to different MBM samples and feed materials, since different kind of MBMs could generate a great variation in Ct values from those reported by this study at the same spike level (w/w) in feed samples. It is known that the mitochondrial DNA (mtDNA) is a variable and multicopy target (mitochondrial density can vary significantly between different kind of tissues, and, consequently, between derived MBMs).

The microscopy method is able to detect the presence of constituents of animal origin in feed at the level of 1 g/kg with hardly any false negatives. Nevertheless, microscopy cannot determine the species of animal matter and requires a skilled operator [22]. Moreover the lower limit of detection of MBM in feeds by microscopic analysis, as mentioned previously, was 0.025% w/w; already an interlaboratory study by the European Union reached an upper limit of 0.1% w/w [39]. A study by Sanches and collaborators [21] on the detection and identification of animal-derived material in ruminant feedstuffs found a detection limit of 0.05% w/w for MBM. The detection limit of 0.0125% achieved by qPCR tests for bovine-derived material, as shown in the present study, is similar to the limit described by Jonker and collaborators, using a different food matrix. These authors presented a method based on qPCR tests for identification of beef, pork, horse, mutton, chicken and turkey materials in processed meat products at the level of 0.01% w/w, using a set of primers and species-specific probes. However, the performance of the qPCR tests used in the present study was superior when compared to the results of several other studies in this field. Prado et al. carried out an inter-laboratory study using the TaqMan-qPCR system, which detected the amount of 0.1% w/w bovine MBM or mixtures with different raw materials of animal origin in ruminant feedstuffs, which corresponds to the same detection limit found herein [40]. Brodmann and Moor, compared the sensitivity of TaqMan-qPCR to microscopic analysis in detecting MBM, and concluded that qPCR tests cannot compete with the microscopic method [38]. A detection limit around 1% in meat and bone-meal samples may be insufficient to eradicate BSE. To improve the detection limit, further investigation of the DNA extraction method is needed. Martín et al. using a real-time PCR approach with the SYBR Green targeting the mitochondrial 12S rRNA gene for the analysis of experimental bovine tissues in feeds, demonstrated that the assay can detect 0.1% w/w bovine DNA, even after severe heat treatment (up to 133°C for 20 min at 300 kPa) of the bovine-derived material [41]. Additionally, Cawthraw et al. using feed free from animal material and spiked with MBM generated by a commercial rendering process, showed that 0.1% w/w MBM could be detected using species-specific real-time PCR assays targeting for 16S rDNA [42].

As the production of ruminant feeds involves heat treatment that denatures proteins and DNA, the techniques based on DNA analysis, combined or not with a fluorescent probe (real-time PCR), in addition to requiring undamaged DNA, cannot distinguish different kinds of tissues, since each cell of every tissue in an advanced organism has identical DNA [39]. Although microscopic methods have difficulty in distinguishing mammal from poultry bones and the success in identifying animal structures depends on the expertise of the analyst, this technique is the only test that the Commission of the European Communities endorses [25]. In addition, there are many advantages in detecting animal meals in feed by microscopy: the method is unaffected by sample heat treatment, and has accepted detection limits, low cost, simplicity and speed when the operator has experience in identifying animal structures.

Prions are responsible for transmissible spongiform encephalopathies (TSEs) [43]. The infective dose of prions in animal material is another point to consider when analyzing feedstuffs intended for ruminants. Fryer and McLean studied the data and mathematical models that describe scrapie infections in mice following an experimental challenge over a broad range of doses [44]. These authors analyzed data from 4,338 mice inoculated at doses ranging over ten orders of magnitude. These data were compared to the results from a within-host model in which prions accumulate according to a stochastic birth-death process. Crucially, this model assumes no threshold for the dose required to produce infection. The data revealed that even a 1000-fold dilution of the initial dose was capable of causing a prion infection in half of the challenged animals (ID50). These findings imply that there is no safe dose to prevent a prion infection, and, thus, assessments regarding the risk from a low-dose exposure can correctly assume a linear relationship between the dose and the probability of infection.

The results of this study indicate that, because of their efficiency, represented by specificity and sensitivity, qPCR tests should be included in routine evaluation of feeds in Brazil. Classical microscopic analysis will probably remain the first-line monitoring method, but the qPCR technique should be implemented in the future and could be legally accepted as a complementary method. The combined use of microscopy and qPCR can be important in the discrimination of potential false positive and/or false negative results. The speciesspecific qPCR assays evaluated herein demonstrate potential for use in the rapid and routine detection of the presence of bovine, caprine, ovine, porcine and avian (chicken) MBM in feedstuffs, in order.

ACKNOWLEDGEMENTS

This paper is dedicated to the memory of Professor D. S. Joab Trajano Silva, with gratitude for his guidance, friendship and dedication during the investigation. We thank the Laboratório Nacional Agropecuário de Minas Gerais (LANAGRO)-National Agriculture and Livestock Laboratories for aiding with the microscopic analysis and for kindly providing the bovine MBM reference samples. We also thank Dr. Cecília Ribeiro from the Fluminense Federal University, Niterói, Brazil for providing the animal blood samples. CAPES and FAPERJ provided financial support.

REFERENCES

1. Ribeiro RF (2012) The Ox from the Four Corners of the World: The Historic Origins of the Brazilian Beef Industry. Agrarian South: Journal of Political Economy 3: 315-340.
2. Brasil (2003) Ministry of Agriculture, Livestock and Supply. Approves the standardization of methodology for Byproducts Detection of Animal ingredients in mixtures for Power Ruminants by microscopy.
3. ABIEC (2012) AssociaçãoBrasileira das IndústriasExportadoras de Carne. Brazilian beef profile.
4. Estanislau M, CançadoJr (2000) Economic aspects of beef cattle, Magazine Tell Agriculture 21: 5-16.
5. Tamminga S (1996) A review on environmental impacts of nutritional strategies in ruminants. J AnimSci 74: 3112-3124.
6. Schoenian S (2014) Small Ruminant Info Sheet. The truth about grain: feeding grain to small ruminants.
7. Sumption K (2007) Epidemiological Events in 2005–2006. FAO EMPRES (Emergency Prevention System) Focus-On 1: 1-11.

8. Dormont D (2002) Prions, BSE and food.Int J Food Microbiol 78: 181-189.
9. Concepcion GP, Padlan EA (2003) Are humans getting 'mad-cow disease' from eating beef, or something else. Med Hypotheses 60: 699-701.
10. Plews M, Lamoureux L, Simon SL, Graham C, Ruddat V, et al. (2011) Factors affecting the accuracy of urine-based biomarkers of BSE. Proteome Sci 9: 6.
11. World Health Organization (1996) Report of a WHO consultation on public health issues related to human and animal transmissible spongiform encephalopathies with the participation of FAO and OIE, Geneva. World Health Organization.
12. Mathews KH, Vandeveer M, Gustafson RA (2006) An Economic Chronology of Bovine Spongiform Encephalopathy in North America/ LDP-M-143-01 Washington, DC: Economic Research Service/ USDA, Electronic outlook report from the economic researchService/USDA.
13. Brasil (2008) Ministry of Agriculture, Livestock and Supply. Approves the Technical Regulation of Sanitary Hygienic Inspection and Technology of Animal Waste Processing and Model Waste Animal Transport Document in Annexes I and II, respectively.
14. Winterø AK, Thomsen PD, Davies W (1990) A comparison of DNA-hybridization, immunodiffusion, countercurrent immunoelectrophoresis and isoelectric focusing for detecting the admixture of pork to beef. Meat Sci 27: 75-85.
15. Fumière O, Dubois M, Baeten V, von Holst C, Berben G (2006) Effective PCR detection of animal species in highly processed animal byproducts and compound feeds. Anal BioanalChem 385: 1045-1054.
16. Van Raamsdonk LWD (2007) New developments in the detection and identification of processed animal proteins in feeds. Anim Feed SciTechnol 133: 63-83.
17. Niederer M, Bollhalder R (2001) Identification of species specific central nervous tissue by gas chromatography–mass spectrometry (GC–MS) A possible method for supervision of meat products and cosmetics. MitteilungenausdemGebiete der Lebensmitteluntersuchung und Hygiene 92: 133-144.
18. AOAC (1998) Association of Official Analytical Chemists, Official method. Microscopy of animal feed, Gaithersburg, MD.
19. Arya M, Shergill IS, Williamson M, Gommersall L, Arya N, et al. (2005) Basic principles of real-time quantitative PCR. Expert Rev MolDiagn 5: 209-219.
20. Prado M, Fumière O, Boix A, Marien A, Berben G, et al. (2009) Novel approach for interlaboratory transfer of real-time PCR methods: detecting bovine meat and bone meal in feed. Anal BioanalChem 394: 1423-1431.
21. Sanches RL, Alkmin-Filho JF, De Souza SVC, Junqueira RG (2006) In-house validation of a method for detection of animal meals in ruminant feeds by microscopy, Food Control 17: 85–92.
22. Liu X, Han L, Veys P, Baeten V, Jiang X, et al. (2011) An overview of the legislation and light microscopy for detection of processed animal proteins in feeds. Microsc Res Tech 74: 735-743.

23. Huss W (1975) Microscopy and quality control in the manufacture of animal feeds. Hohenheim: Roche.
24. AAFM (1992) American Association of Feed Microscopists. Manual of microscopic analysis of feedstuffs pp: 113- 145.
25. Comission of the European Communities (1998) Commission Directive 98/99/EC of 13 November 1998 establishing guidelines for the microscopic identification and estimation of constituents of animal origin for the official control of feedingstuffs, Official Journal of the European Communities318: 0045–0050.
26. Juusola J, Ballantyne J (2007) mRNA profiling for body fluid identification by multiplex quantitative RT-PCR.J Forensic Sci 52: 1252-1262.
27. RadoniÄ‡ A, Thulke S, Mackay IM, Landt O, Siegert W, et al. (2004) Guideline to reference gene selection for quantitative real-time PCR. BiochemBiophys Res Commun 313: 856-862.
28. Commission Regulation (EC) (2001) Laying down rules for the prevention, control and eradication of certain transmissible spongiform encephalopathies. Pp: 147: 1-40.
29. Brasil (2004) Ministry of Agriculture, Livestock and Supply Regulatory Instruction No. 7 of 17 March 2004 prohibits the importation of ruminants, their products and by-products for any purposes, and products for veterinary use which contain in their composition inputs derived from ruminants in originating in or coming from high-risk countries by SDA. Official Gazette of the Union Brasilia.
30. Döbereiner J, Tokarnia CH, Langenegger J, Dutra IS (1992) Epizootic botulism of cattle in Brazil.DtschTierarztlWochenschr 99: 188-190.
31. Bliska FMM (2001) Considerations Bovine Spongiform Encephalopathy and Brazilian beef exports. National Beef Magazine 288: 100.
32. Ooi CY, Hamdi M, Ramesh S (2007) Properties of hydroxyapatite produced by annealing of bovine bone. Ceram Int 33: 1171-1177.
33. Brasil (2007) Ministry of Agriculture, Livestock and Supply. Instruction No. 5 of 23 February 2007 approves the definitions and rules on the specifications and warranties, tolerances, registration, packaging and labeling of mineral fertilizers used in agriculture, Official Gazette of Brasilia Union, DF.
34. Hofmann K (1996) Proof of proper heating of meat and bone meals, Fleischwirtschafte, 76: 1037–1039.
35. Benedetto A, Abete MC, Squadrone S (2011) Towards a quantitative application of real-time PCR technique for fish DNA detection in feedstuffs. Food Chem 126: 1436-1442.
36. Colgan S (2001) Development of a DNA-based assay for species identification in meat and bone meal. Food Res Int 34: 409–414.
37. Dalmasso A, Fontanella E, Piatti P, Civera T, Rosati S, et al. (2004) A multiplex PCR assay for the identification of animal species in feedstuffs. Mol Cell Probes 18: 81-87.

38. Brodmann PD, Moor D (2003) Sensitive and semi-quantitative TaqManâ„¢ real-time polymerase chain reaction systems for the detection of beef (Bostaurus) and the detection of the family Mammalia in food and feed.Meat Sci 65: 599-607.

39. Momcilovic D, Rasooly A (2000) Detection and analysis of animal materials in food and feed.J Food Prot 63: 1602-1609.

40. Prado M, Berben G, Fumière O, van Duijn G, Mensinga-Kruize J, et al. (2007) Detection of ruminant meat and bone meals in animal feed by real-time polymerase chain reaction: result of an interlaboratory study.J Agric Food Chem 55: 7495-7501.

41. Martín I, García T, Fajardo V, Rojas M, Hernández PE, et al. (2008) Real-time PCR for quantitative detection of bovine tissues in food and feed.J Food Prot 71: 564-572.

42. Cawthraw S, Saunders GC, Martin TC, Sawyer J, Windl O, et al. (2009) Real-time PCR detection and identification of prohibited mammalian and avian material in animal feeds.J Food Prot 72: 1055-1062.

43. Curcio L (2015) PRNP polymorphisms in four Italian sheep breeds. Livest Prod Sci 181: 38-42.

44. Fryer HR, McLean AR (2011) There is no safe dose of prions.PLoS One 6: e23664.

5

CHAPTER

KIDNEY ISCHAEMIA REPERFUSION INJURY IN THE RAT: THE EGTI SCORING SYSTEM AS A VALID AND RELIABLE TOOL FOR HISTOLOGICAL ASSESSMENT

Usman Khalid, Gilda Pino-Chavez, Prabhu Nesargikar, Robert H. Jenkins, Timothy Bowen, Donald J. Fraser and Rafael Chavez

Keywords: Ischaemia reperfusion injury (IRI), histology scoring system, EGTI scoring system, jablonski score

INTRODUCTION

Ischaemia reperfusion injury (IRI) is a complex pathological process characterized by initial restriction of blood supply to the organ followed by subsequent restoration of blood flow and oxygenation, and is an inevitable consequence of organ transplantation, causing significant morbidity and mortality. In kidney transplantation, IRI manifests as primary non-function and delayed graft function, leading to an increased risk of complications, acute allograft rejection and poorer long-term outcomes [1-3]. Due to the increasing donor shortage problem, expanded criteria donor organs' with the additional risk of increased IRI, are now increasingly used [4].

The pathophysiological processes involved in IRI are complex and include interactions between the endothelium, components of the immune system and cell death programs [3]. Briefly, ischaemia and resultant hypoxia cause an increase in vascular permeability and impaired endothelial cell barrier function. Cell death programs that consist of cell apoptosis, phagocytosis, and necrosis are activated. Apoptosis causes nuclear fragmentation, loss of mitochondrial integrity and cell shrinkage. Activation of the innate and adaptive components of the immune system, such as complement, contributes significantly to injury [3,5].

Citation: Khalid U, Pino-Chavez G, Nesargikar P, Jenkins RH, Bowen T, Fraser DJ and Chavez R.Kidney ischaemia reperfusion injury in the rat: the EGTI scoring system as a valid and reliable tool for histological assessment. J Histol Histopathol. 2016; 3:1. http://dx.doi.org/10.7243/2055-091X-3-1.

In renal IRI, endothelial damage is the result of the initial ischaemia and hypoxia leading to impaired cell barrier function. This causes endothelial swelling and disruption, eventually leading to loss of endothelial integrity [6,7]. Tubular injury is a characteristic feature of kidney IRI since the tubules are most prone to ischaemic damage, and therefore potentially reversible acute tubular necrosis is a hallmark of kidney injury. Specifically, in IRI, hypoxia results in formation of plasma membrane blebs and loss of brush border membrane leading to loss of polarity and integrity of tight junctions. Cast formation occurs secondary to cell death and sloughing. As a result, cast formation and other debris lead to tubular obstruction. These changes, along with tubular necrosis, signify extensive tubular damage [8]. Interstitial damage is also seen in acute kidney injury, but may also result from chronic and progressive damage of varied aetiology. Inflammation, haemorrhage and necrosis are the hallmarks of acute ischaemic damage to the tubulo-interstitium [9]. Thickening of Bowman's capsule, retraction of the glomerular tuft and, in severe cases, glomerular fibrosis are the histological features of ischaemic glomerular damage [10].

Full and comprehensive documentation of these complex features of acute kidney injury is important, to facilitate determination of prognosis following biopsy, and to enable mechanistic studies in this area. The widely adopted 'gold standard' scoring system for reporting histological damage in kidney injury is the Jablonski scoring system [11]. This simple system is designed to give a rapid and objective assessment of kidney injury. In reality, however, it provides a limited score documenting predominantly the degree of necrosis within tubular cells only, ranging from 0 signifying 'no damage', to 4 'necrosis affecting all 3 segments of the proximal convoluted tubule'. It does not provide an assessment of the damage seen within the other cellular components, such as endothelial and glomerular cells. The Jablonski scoring system was originally described following a prolonged recovery period after ischaemic injury, and includes features of recovery (e.g., Tubular cell mitoses) that may not be evident in the typical recovery periods used experimentally, or in clinical samples.

The damage seen in IRI is not limited to tubular cells and includes also endothelial, glomerular and interstitial changes. Exclusive focus on the proximal tubule removes the possibility of detection of varied propensity for injury in these compartments, depending on clinical context and/or experimental therapeutic approach applied. There is a need, therefore, to develop a more detailed scoring system that is simple, reliable and more informative regarding the degree of tissue damage to the various cellular components of the kidney.

Here, we present the EGTI (Endothelial, Glomerular, Tubular, Interstitial) scoring system, and its analyisis in rat models of acute IRI, in comparison with the Jablonski scoring system. In addition, scores were correlated with established acute kidney injury markers neutrophil gelatinase-associated lipocalin (NGAL) and kidney injury molecule 1 (KIM-1), together with serum creatinine as a measure of excretory kidney function, in order to establish their inter-relationships in this model.

METHODS

Rat models of IRI

Adult (8 to 12 week old) male Lewis rats weighing 180-220g were used (Harlan Laboratories, UK). The rats were given a 7-day period of acclimatisation to their new environment and were housed and handled according to the local institutional policies and procedures licenced by the Home Office. Analgesia was provided 24 hours pre-op throughout until the time of retrieval in the form of 200mcg of buprenorphine dissolved in 500ml of drinking water. The animals were anaesthetized using Isoflurane and midline laparotomy incisions were made.

Two rat models were used: unilateral IRI and bilateral IRI. In the unilateral model, the left renal pedicle was identified and clamped for 45 minutes using a vascular clip (IRI group). In the bilateral model, both kidneys were identified and their pediclessimultaneously clamped for 45 minutes using vascular clips (IRI group). In both models, the kidneys were visually assessed for both ischaemia upon clamping and subsequent reperfusion upon release of the clamp. Sham controls underwent the same operation without the renal pedicle clamping. During the ischaemic period the abdominal cavity was covered with saline-soaked gauze. The kidneys were retrieved at 48 hours following terminal anaesthesia.

Histology

Kidney tissue was embedded in paraffin and 5 μm tissue sections obtained for Haemotoxylin and Eosin (H&E) staining. Histological damage was assessed by an experienced histopathologist blinded as to group allocation (sham versus IRI) and quantified using the EGTI scoring system devised specifically for animal research on kidney tissue in the context of injury (Table 1). The scoring system consists of histological damage in 4 individual components: Endothelial, Glomerular, Tubular, and Interstitial. The scoring was performed in both the preserved and damaged parts of the renal cortex. The Jablonski scorewas also recorded.

Table 1: The EGTI histology scoring system

Tissue type	Damage	Score
Tubular	No damage	0
	Loss of Brush Border (BB) in less than 25% of tubular cells. Integrity of basal membrane.	1
	Loss of BB in more than 25% of tubular cells, Thickened basal membrane	2
	(Plus) Inflammation, Cast formation, Necrosis up to 60% of tubular cells	3
	(Plus) Necrosis in more than 60% of tubular cells	4
Endothelial	No damage	0
	Endothelial swelling	1
	Endothelial disruption	2
	Endothelial loss	3
Glomerular	No damage	0
	Thickening of Bowman capsule	1
	Retraction of glomerular tuft	2
	Glomerular fibrosis	3
Tubulo/ Interstitial	No damage	0
	Inflammation, haemorrhage in less than 25% of tissue	1
	(Plus) necrosis in less than 25% of tissue	2
	Necrosis up to 60%	3
	Necrosis more than 60%	4

RT-qPCR

Total RNA was extracted using TRIzol reagent (Life technologies) according to manufacturer's instructions. Generation of cDNA was carried out using the High Capacity Reverse Transcription Kit (Life Technologies) with random primers, and RT-qPCR was performed on a ViiA7 Fast Real-Time PCR System (Life Technologies). NGAL and KIM-1 were quantified using the POWER SYBR® GREEN PCR Master Mix (Life technologies) with gene-specific primers and normalized to house keeping gene GAPDH. Changes in gene expression were analysed usingthe 2-DDCT method [12].

Primers› sequences used were:

GAPDH (forward, 5›-CCTCTGACTTCAACAGCGACAC-3′; reverse, 5′-TGTCATACCAGGAAATGAGCTTGA-3′)

NGAL (forward, 5›-GGGCTGTCCGATGAACTGAA-3›; reverse, 5›-CATTGGTCGGTGGGAACAGA-3›),

KIM-1 (forward, 5›-CGGCTAACCAGAGTGACTTGT-3›; reverse, 5›-TACAGAGCCTGGAAGAAGCAG-3›)

Serum Creatinine

Serum creatinine in mmol/l was measured using the Jaffe reaction before operation and at time of retrieval in the bilateral IRI model.

Statistical Analysis

Statistical analyses were performed using GraphPad Prism v6 software. Data were expressed as mean±SEM or median (and range) and assessed for statistical significance by unpaired Student's t test or Mann Whitney U test. The EGTI Histology score and the Jablonski score were correlated with serum ceatinine, NGAL and KIM-1. Correlation analysis was reported with significance levels as indicated, where appropriate, in the figures provided: *$p<0.05$, **$p<0.01$, ***$p<0.001$.

RESULTS

Histology

Ten rats were used for the unilateral model (5 IRI, 5 sham) and 17 for the bilateral model (9 IRI and 8 sham). Forty-five minutes of unilateral and bilateral IRI in the rat caused marked histological damage at 48 hours when compared with sham controls.

Figures 1A-1C show normal appearance of the renal cortex in a Sham rat. Figure 1A shows that the brush border of the tubular cells is intact with no thickening of the basal membrane. No inflammation or necrosis is seen (Tubular score 0). There is no visible interstitium signifying no damage/abnormality within the interstitial compartment (Interstitial score 0). Figure 1B shows a uniform endothelium with no swelling or disruption of the endothelial cells (Endothelial score 0). Figure 1C shows an intact glomerulus with thin walled Bowman's capsule and no tuft retraction (Glomerular score 0).

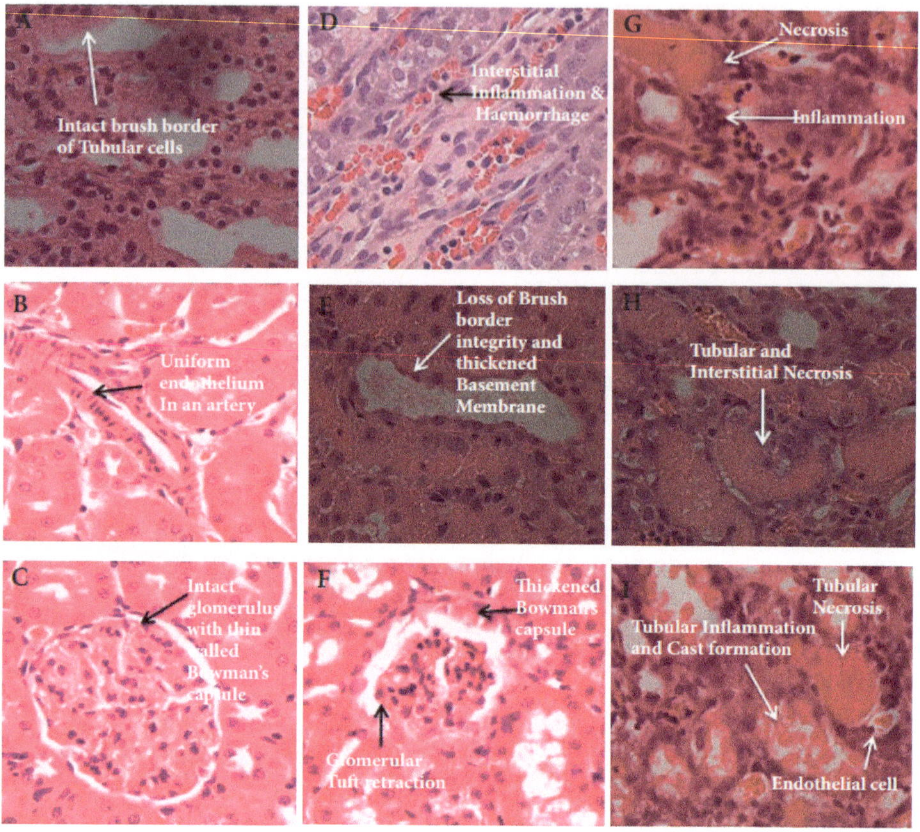

Figure 1: Histological images of rat renal cortex sections. Renal cortex H&E (x400) paraffin sections, from sham and 45-minute IRI in rats, at 48 hours after reperfusion (Bilateral sham n=8, Bilateral IRI n=9, Unilateral sham n=5, Unilateral IRI n=5) were assessed for Endothelial, Tubular, Glomerular and Interstitial cell damage. (A-C) Normal appearance of renal cortex ina sham rat. (D-F) Mild to moderate damage of the renal cortex in 45-minute bilateral IRI rats. (G-I) Moderate to significant damage of the renal cortex in unilateral 45-minute IRI rats.

Figures 1D-1F show varying degrees of damage of the renal cortex in 45-minute bilateral IRI rats. Figure 1D shows inflammation and haemorrhage within the interstitium which is present in less than 25% of the tissue without any evidence of necrosis (Interstitial score 1). Figure 1E shows thickened basal membrane of the tubular cells with loss of the brush border in more than 25% of the tubular cells, without the presence of cast formation or necrosis (Tubular score 2). Figure 1F shows a glomerulus with evidence of thickened Bowman's capsule (Glomerular score 1), and glomerular tuft retraction (Glomerular score 2).

Figures 1G-1I show varying degrees of damage of the renal cortex in 45-minute unilateral IRI rats. Figure 1G shows inflammation and haemorrhage within the interstitial compartment, with necrosis in up to 60% of the cells (Interstitial score

3). Figure 1H shows complete necrosis in tubular and interstitial cellular compartments (Tubular score 4, Interstitial score 4). Figure 1I shows evidence of inflammation and cast formation within the tubules with evidence of necrosis in up to 60% of tubular cells (Tubular score 3), and endothelial cell disruption and loss (Endothelial score 3).

Figure 2 shows mild damage of the renal cortex in a 45-minute bilateral IRI rat. There is endothelial swelling of the capillaries (A) and the vessel (B) without any disruption (Endothelial score 1).

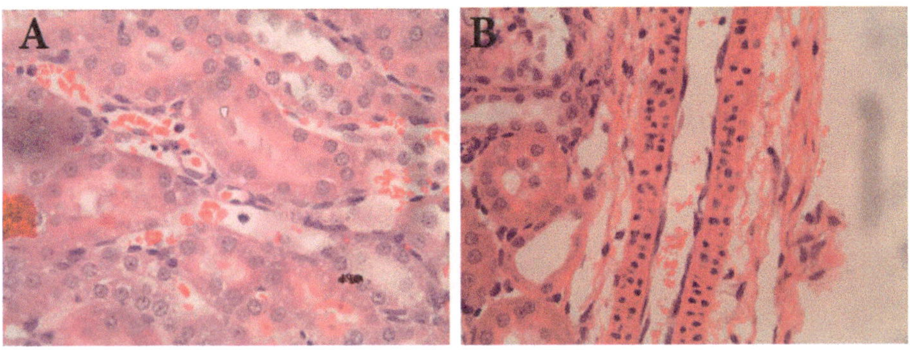

Figure 2: Histological images of endothelial cell swelling in rat renal cortex sections.

Renal cortex H&E (x400) paraffin sections, from sham and 45-minute IRI in rats, at 48 hours after reperfusion (Bilateral sham n=8, Bilateral IRI n=9, Unilateral sham n=5, Unilateral IRI n=5) were assessed for Endothelial, Tubular, Glomerular and Interstitial cell damage. Mild damage of the renal cortex in a 45-minute IRI rat

Unilateral IRI

The median (and range) EGTI histology score was 10 (8-11) in the IRI group compared to 0 (0-1) in the sham group ($p=0.0079$). The mRNA expression of KIM-1 and NGAL was increased 300-fold and 30-fold in the IRI group respectively compared to sham group ($p<0.0001$) [13].

Bilateral IRI

The median (and range) EGTI histology score was 8 (6-9) in the IRI group compared to 0 (0-2) in the sham group ($p<0.0001$). Mean serum creatinine at 48 hours was 76.63(±13.36) mmol/l in the IRI group compared with 31.90(±0.25) mmol/l in the sham group ($p=0.0067$). The mRNA expression of KIM-1 and NGAL was increased 150-fold and 14-fold in the IRI group respectively ($p<0.0001$) (Figure 3). The individual components of the EGTI score were also significantly higher in the IRI group compared with sham (Figure 4).

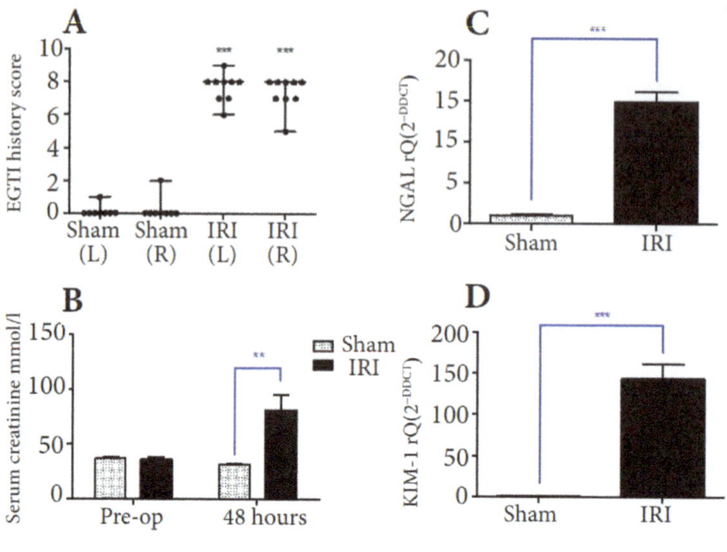

Figure 3: Effect of bilateral IRI on EGTI score, serum creatinine and expression of NGAL and KIM-1.

(A) Renal cortex sections from sham and 45-minute bilateral IRI in rats at 48 hours after reperfusion were stained with H&E and assessed using a comprehensive scoring system comprising of Endothelial, Glomerular, Tubular, and Interstitial cell damage (Sham n=8, IRI n=9). Histology scores are plotted as median and range, ***p<0.0001.

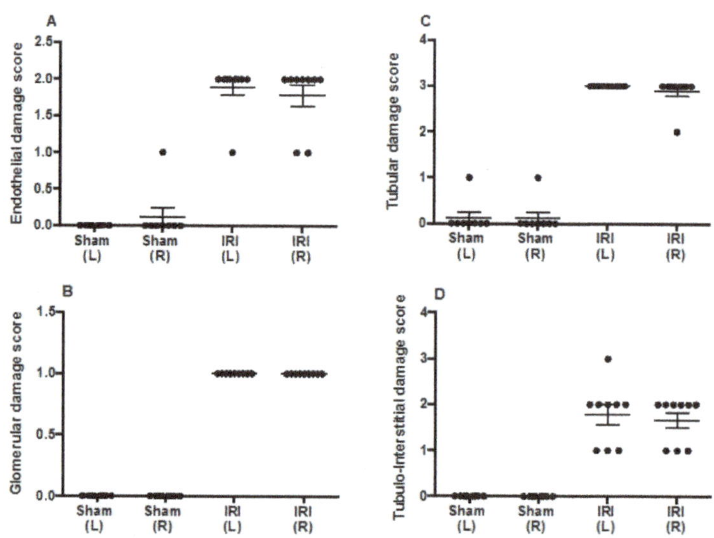

Figure 4: Effect of bilateral IRI on Endothelial, Tubular, Glomerular and Tubulo-Interstitial damages scores.

Renal cortex sections from sham and 45-minute bilateral IRI in rats at 48 hours after reperfusion were stained with H&E and assessed using a comprehensive scoring system comprising of Endothelial, Glomerular, Tubular, and Interstitial cell damage (Sham n=8, IRI n=9). Individual cellular component scores are plotted as median and range for Tubular (A), Endothelial (B), Glomerular (C) TubuloInterstitial (D) components.

Correlation of EGTI Histology Scores and Jablonski Scores with Serum Creatinine, and AKI Markers

The EGTI and Jablonski scores both correlated significantly with serum creatinine at 48 hours, and expression of NGAL and KIM-1 (Figure 5). This suggests that both the EGTI score and the Jablonski score are highly predictive of kidney function and structural damage.

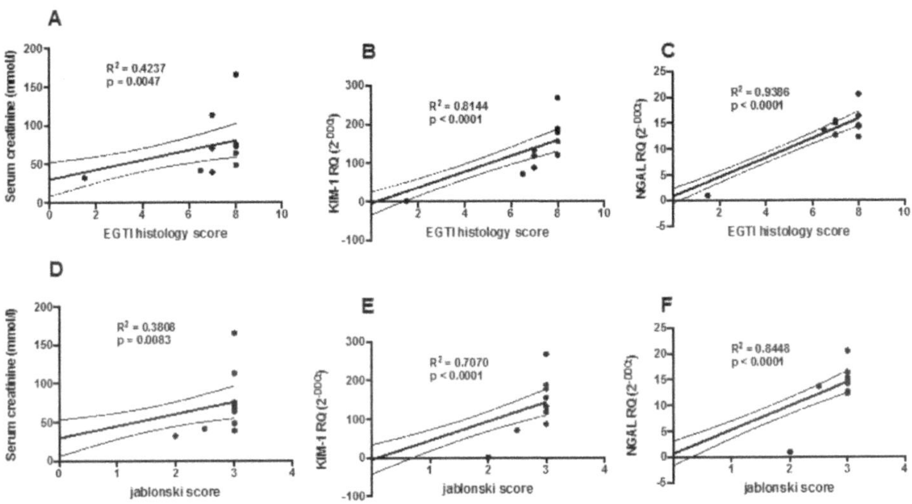

Figure 5 : Correlation of EGTI and Jablonski scores with serum creatinine, NGAL and KIM-1.

Renal cortex sections from sham and 45-minute bilateral IRI in rats at 48 hours after reperfusion (Sham n=8, IRI n=9) were stained with H&E and scored using a comprehensive scoring system comprising of Endothelial, Glomerular, Tubular, and Interstitial cell damage, in addition to the Jablonski histology score. Serum creatinine was measured at 48 hours and RT-qPCR analysis of KIM-1 and NGAL was performed, with expression normalized to GAPDH. EGTI and Jablonski scores were both plotted and correlated with serum creatinine (A and D), KIM-1 (B and E), and NGAL (C and F).

In addition to this, the association between each component on the EGTI histology scoring system and serum creatinine at 48 hours, and expression of NGAL and KIM-1 was examined using univariate logistic regression analyses. Tubular, endothelial, glomerular, and tubulo-interstitial components were independently associated with serum creatinine at 48 hours ($p<0.05$), and NGAL and KIM-1 ($p<0.0001$).

DISCUSSION

This study used rat models of acute IRI to evaluate a new scoring system todocumentchanges in the histological architecture of the renal cortex, established acute kidney injury markers and renal function.

The rat models used in this study are well-established *in vivo* models of acute kidney injury [14,15]. Adult male rats are known to be more susceptible to injury, and so consistent sex selection is an important component [16]. The 45-minutes of cross-clamping of the renal pedicle produces significant but non-fatal, and potentially reversible, injury. The 48-hour reperfusion period is ample to assess the effects of a treatment modality on injury in the acute setting [17], and previous reports have shown that the 45-minute model of IRIused here allows robust and reproducible evaluation of treatment effects on IRI [18,19]. In kidney transplantation most damage occurs in the acute setting, therefore the model used in this study was chosen to reflect this. To ensure that the newly developed scoring system was robust in the presence of functional as well as structural changes as a consequence of IRI, bilateral as well as unilateral IRI models were employed.

The majority of studies investigating kidney IRI report the histological damage according to Jablonski›s acute tubular necrosis score [11]. This score is based solely on damage within the tubular cells. It does not document any damage seen to the other cellular components within the renal cortex. Tubular injury is arguably the most characteristic feature of kidney IRI but damage to other structural renal components is also important. The Jablonski scoring system is designed to give a rapid and objective assessment of kidney tubular injury, and is relatively straightforward to use. This system was originally described in a rat model of ischaemia followed by 7 or 14 days of reperfusion [11]. Such a prolonged reperfusion period results in the development of time-dependent morphological features in kidney tissue. For example, a score of ‹1› includes reference to the presence of mitoses. Mitoses are evident in the presence of tubular cell regeneration, which does not occur in acute models of IRI such as those used in the present study. For acute IRI models, the Jablonski scoring system must therefore be modified to exclude this mitotic criterion. Another significant limitation of the Jablonski system is the absence of brush border observations. One of the first tubular cell changes seen following iscahemic injury is loss of the brush border membrane, prior to cast formation or necrosis.

Kidney IRI is a complex pathophysiological process that causes structural damage to tubular, endothelial, glomerular and tubulo-interstitial cells. Loss of endothelial cell integrity, acute tubular necrosis, tubulo-interstitial damage and glomerular ischaemic damage are all hallmarks of kidney IRI thatare important to document fully and comprehensively. It is evident from Figures 1B-1D that there is some variation in IRI animals in terms of the damage to various cellular components. This supportsfurther the need for a histology scoring system that reports damage to all of these cellular components.

KIM-1 and NGAL were selected as accurate, robust and reliable biomarkers of acute kidney injury [14,20,21]. It is evident from the histological and acute kidney injury marker changes that the models of IRI used in this study led to significant injury to the kidney. Serum creatinine was selected as a marker of kidney function in the bilateral IRI model. It is the most widely usedmarker of excretory kidney function, reliablyestimating glomerular filtration rate in clinical practice [22]. In this study,changes in serum creatinine between bilateral sham and bilateral IRI rats suggest that this model of acute injury is robust.

The EGTI histology scoring system proposed in this study correlated significantly with established AKI markers and serum creatinine, demonstrating itsvalidity, reliability and sensitivity. Moreover, by reporting changes seen within all of the cellular components of the renal cortex, our new system offers a greater insight into the severity and range of damage than the Jablonski system. Similarly to the EGTI scores, the Jablonski scores correlated significantly with serum creatinine, NGAL, and KIM-1, although the correlation was slightly less pronounced.

CONCLUSION

The EGTI histology scoring system described in this paper is a reliable, sensitive and validtool to assess the degree of damage observed in kidney IRI. It is also more comprehensive than the widely used Jablonski scoring system.

AUTHORS' CONTRIBUTIONS

Authors' contributions	**UK**	**GPC**	**PN**	**RJ**	**TB**	**DF**	**RC**
Research concept and design	√	√	√	--	--	√	√
Collection and/or assembly of data	√	√	√	√	--	--	--
Data analysis and interpretation	√	√	√	√	√	√	√
Writing the article	√	--	--	--	--	--	--
Critical revision of the article	√	√	√	√	√	√	√
Final approval of article	√	√	√	√	√	√	√
Statistical analysis	√	--	--	√	--	--	--

ACKNOWLEDGEMENT AND FUNDING

We would like to thank Kidney Wales Foundation grant (for funding this project) and Department of Pathology, University Hospital of Wales, Cardiff (for their help with processing of kidney tissue specimens in formalin).

REFERENCES

1. Ojo AO, Wolfe RA, Held PJ, Port FK and Schmouder RL. **Delayed graft function: risk factors and implications for renal allograft survival**. *Transplantation*. 1997; 63:968-74.

2. Perico N, Cattaneo D, Sayegh MH and Remuzzi G. **Delayed graft function in kidney transplantation**.*Lancet*. 2004; 364:1814-27.
3. Eltzschig HK and Eckle T. **Ischemia and reperfusion--from mechanism to translation**. *Nat Med*. 2011;17:1391-401.
4. Transplant NBa. NHS Blood and Transplant Organ Donation and Transplantation Activity Report in the UK. 2014-15.
5. Godwin JG, Ge X, Stephan K, Jurisch A, Tullius SG and Iacomini J. **Identification of a microRNA signature of renal ischemia reperfusion injury**. *Proc Natl Acad Sci U S A*. 2010; 107:14339-44.
6. Bonventre JV and Yang L. **Cellular pathophysiology of ischemic acute kidney injury**. *J Clin Invest*. 2011; 121:4210-21.
7. Rabelink TJ, de Boer HC and van Zonneveld AJ. **Endothelial activation and circulating markers of endothelial activation in kidney disease**. *Nat Rev Nephrol*. 2010; 6:404-14.
8. Patschan D, Patschan S and Muller GA. **Inflammation and microvasculopathy in renal ischemia reperfusion injury**. *J Transplant*. 2012; 2012:764154.
9. Bonventre JV and Weinberg JM. **Recent advances in the pathophysiology of ischemic acute renal failure**. *J Am Soc Nephrol*. 2003; 14:2199-210.
10. Munshi R, Hsu C and Himmelfarb J. **Advances in understanding ischemic acute kidney injury**. *BMC Med*. 2011; 9:11.
11. Jablonski P, Howden BO, Rae DA, Birrell CS, Marshall VC and Tange J. **An experimental model for assessment of renal recovery from warm ischemia**. *Transplantation*. 1983; 35:198-204.
12. Livak KJ and Schmittgen TD. **Analysis of relative gene expression data using real-time quantitative PCR and the 2(-Delta Delta C(T)) Method**. *Methods*. 2001; 25:402-8.
13. Khalid U, Jenkins R, Pino-Chavez G, Bowen T, Fraser D and Chavez R. A Localized Ischemic Preconditioning Regimen Increases Tumor Necrosis α Expression in a Rat Model of Kidney Ischemia-Reperfusion Injury. *Experimental and Clinical Transplantation*. 2015.
14. Mishra J, Ma Q, Prada A, Mitsnefes M, Zahedi K, Yang J, Barasch J and Devarajan P. **Identification of neutrophil gelatinase-associated lipocalin as a novel early urinary biomarker for ischemic renal injury**. *J Am Soc Nephrol*. 2003; 14:2534-43.
15. Kato J, Nakayama M, Zhu WJ, Yokoo T and Ito S. **Ischemia/reperfusion of unilateral kidney exaggerates aging-induced damage to the heart and contralateral kidney**. *Nephron Exp Nephrol*. 2014; 126:183-90.
16. Park KM, Kim JI, Ahn Y, Bonventre AJ and Bonventre JV. **Testosterone is responsible for enhanced susceptibility of males to ischemic renal injury**. *J Biol Chem*. 2004; 279:52282-92.
17. Dokuyucu R, Demir T, Yumrutas O, Erbagci AB, Orkmez M, Bahar AY, Bayraktar

R, Bozgeyik I, Kaplan DS, Cengiz B and Bagci BC. **The role of hepcidin and its related genes (BMP6, GDF-15, and HJV) in rats exposed to ischemia and reperfusion.** *Turk J Med Sci.* 2014; 44:576-81.

18. Delbridge MS, Shrestha BM, Raftery AT, El Nahas AM and Haylor JL. **The effect of body temperature in a rat model of renal ischemia-reperfusion injury.** *Transplant Proc.* 2007; 39:2983-5.
19. Wystrychowski W, Wystrychowski G, Zukowska-Szczechowska E, Obuchowicz E, Grzeszczak W, Wiecek A and Wystrychowski A. **Nephroprotective effect of pentoxifylline in renal ischemia-reperfusion in rat depends on the timing of its administration.** *Transplant Proc.* 2014; 46:2555-7.
20. Vaidya VS, Ozer JS, Dieterle F, Collings FB, Ramirez V, Troth S, Muniappa N, Thudium D, Gerhold D, Holder DJ, Bobadilla NA, Marrer E, Perentes E, Cordier A, Vonderscher J, Maurer G, Goering PL, Sistare FD and Bonventre JV. **Kidney injury molecule-1 outperforms traditional biomarkers of kidney injury in preclinical biomarker qualification studies.** *Nat Biotechnol.* 2010; 28:478-85.
21. Mishra J, Dent C, Tarabishi R, Mitsnefes MM, Ma Q, Kelly C, Ruff SM, Zahedi K, Shao M, Bean J, Mori K, Barasch J and Devarajan P. **Neutrophil gelatinase-associated lipocalin (NGAL) as a biomarker for acute renal injury after cardiac surgery.** *Lancet.* 2005; 365:1231-8.
22. Suzuki Y, Matsushita K, Yoshida T, Sawabe Y and Nomura F. **[Clinical validity of renal function markers including serum cystatin C on chronic kidney disease classification].** *Rinsho Byori.* 2011; 59:345-51.

6
CHAPTER

HISTOLOGICAL EFFECT OF OVARIECTOMY AND ESTROGEN REPLACEMENT ON PAROTID GLAND OF ADULT ALBINO RAT

Dalia A. Mohamed, Heba M. Elnegris and Rania A. Wahdan

Keywords: Parotid gland, ovariectomy, ultrastructure, estrogen replacement

INTRODUCTION

The average woman lives about one-third of her life beyond menopause and many undergo hormonal replacement therapy to relieve menopausal symptoms. Oral discomfort is a common symptom in these women and may be documented as one of the systemic aspects of menopause [1].

In postmenopausal period the endogenic estrogen level decreases. This is a primary change provides for many characteristic alterations in almost all the body. Estrogen acts through two intracellular receptor proteins called estrogen receptors (ER) [2]. It was reported that ER present in oral buccal mucosa, minor salivary glands, parotid and submandibular glands [3].

The most important and annoying oral affections in menopause are alteration in taste and burning mouth syndrome (BMS). BMS refers to a chronic orofacial pain disorder that occurs in about 1.3 million American women in the postmenopausal period. Hormonal changes may affect the composition or the rate of saliva [4].

Streckfus et al., [5] reported that there was reduction in the salivary flow of submandibular and sublingual glands with the increase in age and reduction in the levels of estrogen production. The ovarian hormones act on the oral mucosa by specific

Citation: Mohamed DA, Elnegris HM and Wahdan RA. Histological effect of ovariectomy and estrogen replacement on parotid gland of adult albino rat. J Histol Histopathol. 2015; 2:23. http://dx.doi.org/10.7243/2055-091X-2-23.

receptors, which select, recognize, and bind the hormone to the cell cytoplasm or nucleus. The deficiency of these hormones (estrogen) possibly causes changes in the oral mucosa at the tissue level, because these hormones influence the proliferation, differentiation, and keratinization of the gingival epithelium and stimulate the proliferation of fibroblasts [6].

Sex steroid hormones are known to regulate cell growth, differentiation and function in reproductive as well as nonreproductive tissues [7]. Also, these hormones appear to play a significant role in the physiology of the human oral cavity. A number of studies suggest that oral soft tissues are sensitive to changes in female sex steroid blood levels. So, some diseases and disorders of the oral cavity, show a prediction for women [8], supporting a role for estrogen in disease etiology.

Additionally, it was reported that estrogens are known to modulate epithelial maturation in classic target organs, and similarly, the decrease in estrogen levels during menopause is thought to affect the oral epithelial maturation process, leading to thin and atrophic epithelium prone to inflammatory changes [7].

Oral dryness can lead to considerable difficulty in speaking, eating and tasting, and predispose mucosa to wounds, abrasion and infection. A number of studies have shown that hormone replacement therapy (HRT) can relieve this oral discomfort in postmenopausal women, further suggesting a role for female sex hormones in the maintenance of oral tissues [9,10].

Apoptosis, i.e., programmed cell death, plays an important role in homeostasis of the body. Previously, it was reported that a reduction of estrogen (belongs to female hormones) could have influence on age-related histological changes in the female rat parotids induced by apoptosis .One component of inducing apoptosis is free radical. Recently, it have been noticed that free radical has an effect on aging.

A living body has superoxide dismutase (SOD), which can eliminate free radical. SOD decreases with aging progress [11].

Together, these observations suggest that estrogens may play an important role in oral mucosal and salivary gland physiology. Even though the salivary glands are not classical targets of female sexual hormones, this study was performed to analyze the influence of the sex hormones on these glands as little is known about this relation.

MATERIALS AND METHODS

Thirty Female Sprague–Dawley rats, 3 months in age and approximately 120 g in weight, were used. The animals were housed in individual cages and received a standard diet and tap water ad libitum. The room temperature and humidity were maintained at 23°C and 60%, respectively. The light cycle was fixed at 12 h. They were equally divided into three groups; I, II and III.

Group I: was the control (C) that was subdivided into two subgroups; Ca (sham-operated) and Cb (vehicle-treated) groups received daily SC injections of sesame oil (0.1ml /day).

Group II: was the experimentally induced ovariectomy (OVX).

Group III: was the experimentally induced ovariectomy and received immediate daily subcutaneous (SC) injections of 17-estradiol (E2) dissolved in sesame oil (Teikoku Hormone Mfg. Co., Ltd., Tokyo, Japan) (50 mg per day) consecutively for 14 days (treated) [11].

After 1 week acclimatization in the animal house, each group (10 animals) underwent an operation. The animals were anesthetized with intraperitoneal injection of pentobarbital sodium (15 mg/kg body weight) for the surgical procedure. In the ovariectomized group, small incisions were made on each flank. The ovaries and their surrounding fat were externalized and after ligation of the ovarian arteries the ovaries were removed. The distal ends of each uterine horn were then returned to the peritoneal cavity and the incisions were closed with 4-0 nylon sutures. Each rat received an intramuscular injection of 0.1 ml PenicillinG procaine (300,000 unit ml-1, Phoenix Pharmaceutical Inc., St. Joseph, MO) as a prophylactic measure. The sham-operated group underwent a similar surgical procedure, exposing the ovaries but replacing them in the same position.

The animals were sacrificed two weeks after the operation and specimens from right parotid of each animal were fixed in 10 % neutral formol saline for 24 hours and were processed to prepare 5 μm thick paraffin sections for haematoxylin and eosin stain and Mallory trichrom stains [12] Also, parts of the same specimens were processed for electron microscope examination [13].

Quantitative Morphometric Measurements

Serial sections stained with H&E and Mallory's trichrome were morphometrically analyzed for detection of diameter of the parotid ducts; area % of blue stained collagen fibers in the septa, around duct and blood vessels using Leica Qwin 500 image analyzer computer system (Cambridge, England) at Pathology Department, Faculty of Dentistry, Cairo University. The image analyzer consisted of a colored video camera, colored monitor, hard disc of IBM personal computer connected to the Olympus microscope (CX 41) and controlled by Leica Qwin 500 software. The image analyzer was first calibrated automatically to convert the measurement units (pixels) produced by the image analyzer program into actual micrometer units. The measuring frame of a standard area is equal to 7286, 78μm^2. For each parameter ten different non overlapping fields from ten different specimens were examined in each group.

Cu, Zn-SOD (cupper, zinc Superoxide Dismutase) Immunohistochemical study

Deparaffinized sections were incubated in 0.3% H2O2 in methanol for 30 min at room temperature to inhibit endogenous peroxidase activity. The avidin–biotin–peroxidase complex method [14] was performed as follows. The sections were treated in 10% normal goat serum for 30 min, and incubatedb in anti-Cu, Zn-SOD anti-serum (1.5 mg/ml, Sterssgen) of a dilution of 1:200 for overnight at 4°C, and then incubated in biotinylated anti-rabbit IgG solution for 30 min at room temperature and the avidin–biotin–peroxidase complex solution of a Vectastain ABC Kit (Vector Laboratories Inc) for

1 h at room temperature. All the antibody solutions were diluted with 0.01 M phosphate buffer saline (pH 7.4). All the sections were then stained with 3.3 diaminobenzidine containing 0.03% H2O2. We used fixed reaction times for the processing in all cases. Positive staining was clearly cytoplamic reactivity

Statistical Analysis

The obtained data from morphometrical analysis were subjected to one way analysis of variance (ANOVA) and post hoc test using Statistical Package for the Social Sciences (SPSS) version 11. The P value <0.05, <0.001 and >0.05 were considered significant, highly significant and non significant respectively.

RESULTS

Light microscopic results

Examination of H&E stained sections showed that control groups (Ca&Cb) had the same structures. The parenchyma of parotid gland was formed of serous acini and duct system. The acini appeared rounded with secretory cells and narrow lumima. They had basal basophilic nuclei and apical acidophilia. The intralobular duct had normal structure. Thin connective tissues appeared around ducts, blood vessels and inbetween the lobules (Figure 1A). Examination of H&E stained sections of operated group (II) revealed that most of the acini appeared irregular with darkly stained nuclei and many vacuoles in their cytoplasm. They were separated by thickened septa containing cellular infiltration. Homogenous acidophilic material was also seen (Figure 1B). The interelobular ducts were dilated and lined by stratified epithelium. Congested blood vessels were also found (Figure 1C). Examination of H&E stained sections of treated group (III) showed apparent normal appearance of serous acini and ducts (Figure 1D).

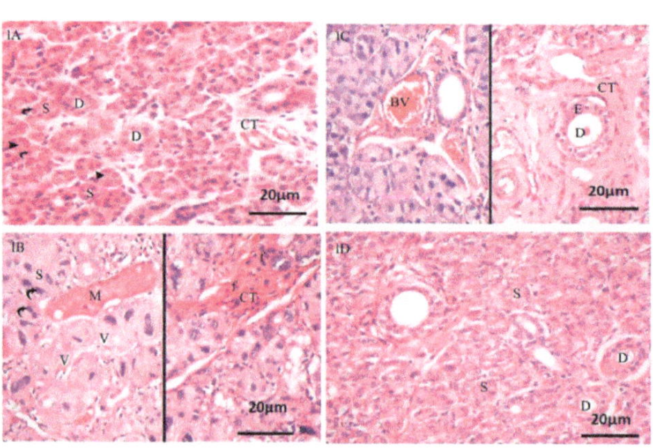

Figure 1: H&E stained sections.

(A): Control group showing rounded serous acini (S) with narrow luminae. They have basal basophilic nuclei (curved arrow) and apical acidophilia (arrowhead). Note, normal appearance of intralobular ducts (D) and thin septa (CT). (B): Operated group showing irregular acini (S) with darkly stained nuclei (curved arrow) and cytoplasmic vacuolations (V). Cellular infiltration (f) inside thick connective tissue (CT) septa is also seen. Notice, homogenous acidophilic material (M). (C): Showing dilated interlobular ducts (D) with stratified epithelial lining (E); prominent thick septa (CT) are also seen. Congestion of blood vessels (BV) is also seen. (D): Treated group showing apparently normal serous acini (S) and intralobular ducts (D) of parotid gland. (Scale bar=20μm).

Mallory's trichrome stained sections clarified the occurrence of little collagen fibers inbetween the lobules, around interlobular ducts and blood vessels in parotid gland of group I (Figure 2A). While in group II, collagen fibers of extensive amount appeared in between the lobules and around blood vessels (Figure 2B). Group III revealed moderate amount of collagen fibers (Figure 2C).

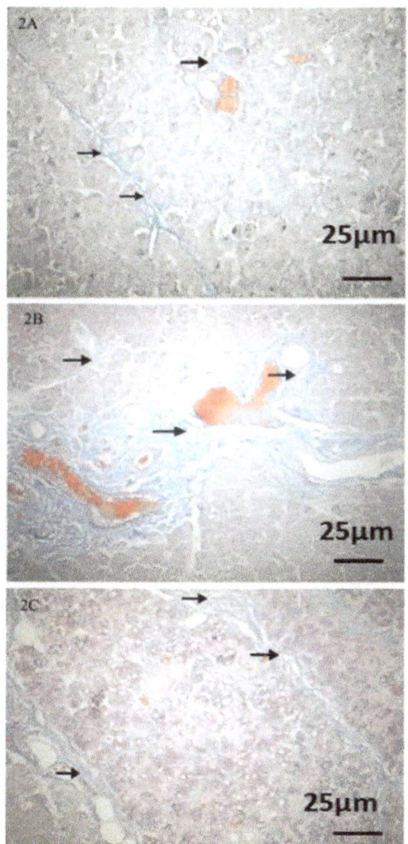

Figure 2: Mallory's trichrome sections.

(A): Control group showing little collagen fibers (arrow) in between the lobules, around interlobular ducts and blood vessels. (B): Operated group showing increased collagen fibers (arrow) in between the lobules, and around blood vessels. (C): Treated group showing moderate amount of collagen fibers (arrows) in between the lobules. (Scale bar=25μm).

Examination of the semithin section of group I revealed the normal appearance of the acini and intrelobular ducts of the gland. The acini were lined by pyramidal cells that had basal vesicular nuclei and apical secretory granules. In between the lobules, the ducts appeared with normal structure (Figure 3A). While examination of group II showed irregular acini with variable sizes. They had apoptotic nuclei and many vacuoles in their cytoplasm. The acini separated by thick connective tissue septa containing dilated interlobular ducts. Some of the epithelial lining of the ducts appeared with darkly stained nuclei (Figure 3B). Treated group examination showed apparent normal serous and interlobular ducts of parotid gland (Figure 3C). Immunohistochemical stained sections of control group (I) showed positive cytoplasmic reaction for CU,Zn-SOD (Figure 4A). This reaction decreased in ovariectomized group (II) (Figure 4B) and became stronger in treated group (III) (Figure 4C).

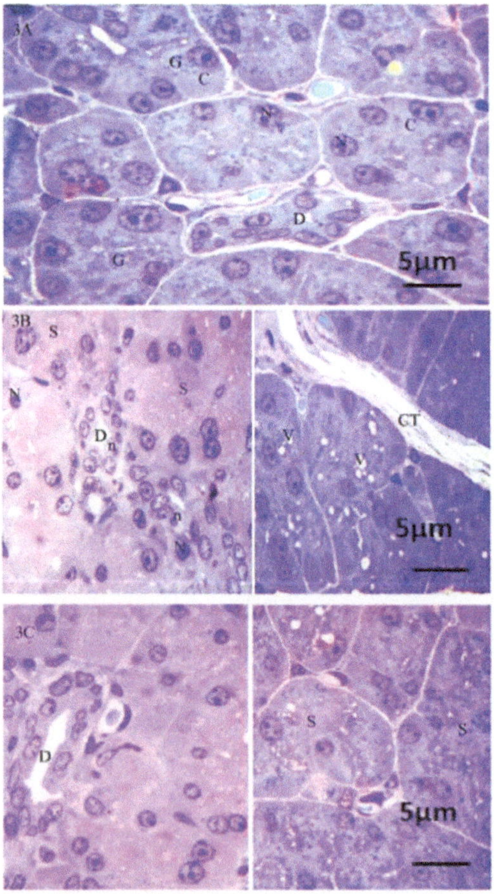

Figure 3: Semithin sections stained with Toulidine blue.

(A): Control group showing normal serous acini lined by pyramidal cells (C). They have basal vesicular nuclei (N) and apical secretory granules (G). Note, interlobular duct (D) in between the lobules have normal structure. (B): Operated group showing irregular variable sized acini (S).They have apoptotic nuclei (N) and vacuolated cytoplasm (V). Thick connective tissue septa are also seen (CT). The interlobular duct (D) has some darkely stained nuclei (n). (C): Treated group showing apparent normal serous acini (S) and interlobular ducts (D) of parotid gland. (Scale bar=5μm).

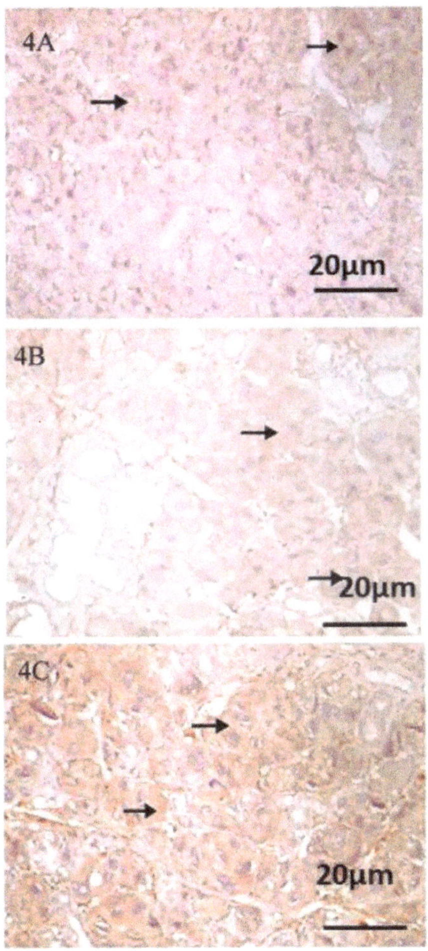

Figure 4: Immunohistochemical stained sections.

(A): control group showing moderate positive immunostaining reaction for Cu, Zn-SOD (arrow) in cytoplasm of acini. (B): Operated group showing mild positive immunostaining reaction for Cu, Zn-SOD (arrow) in acinar cell cytoplasm. (C): Section of treated group showing strong positive immunostaining reaction for Cu, Zn-SOD (arrow) in acinar cell cytoplasm. (Scale bar=20μm).

Electron Microscope Results

Examination of the ultrathin sections of control group (I) showed normal acinar cells with apical electron dense and electron lucent secretory granules, densly packed rough endoplasmic reticulum and mitochondria (Figure 5A). Secretory ducts lined mainly with cuboidal epithelium had rounded nuclei and cytoplasmic granules. They attached together with intercellular desmosomes (Figure 5B). While examination of operated group (II) clarified the presence of apoptotic acinar cells with irregular heterochromatic nuclei, dilated rarified rough endoplasmic reticulum, electron lucent and electron dense secretory granules. Other cells contained extensive vacuoles in their cytoplasm (Figure 5C). The ducts of same group contained apoptotic cells with irregular heterochromatic nuclei, many electron dense granules and intercellular desmosomes (Figure 5C). On the other hand examination o treated group (III) showed acinar cells with different affection; some appeared apoptotic with heterochromatic nuclei, and others appeared normal. Electron dense and electron lucent granules, rough endoplasmic reticulum were seen in their cytoplasm (Figure 5D). Dilated duct with apparently normal lining cells could be seen (Figure 5E).

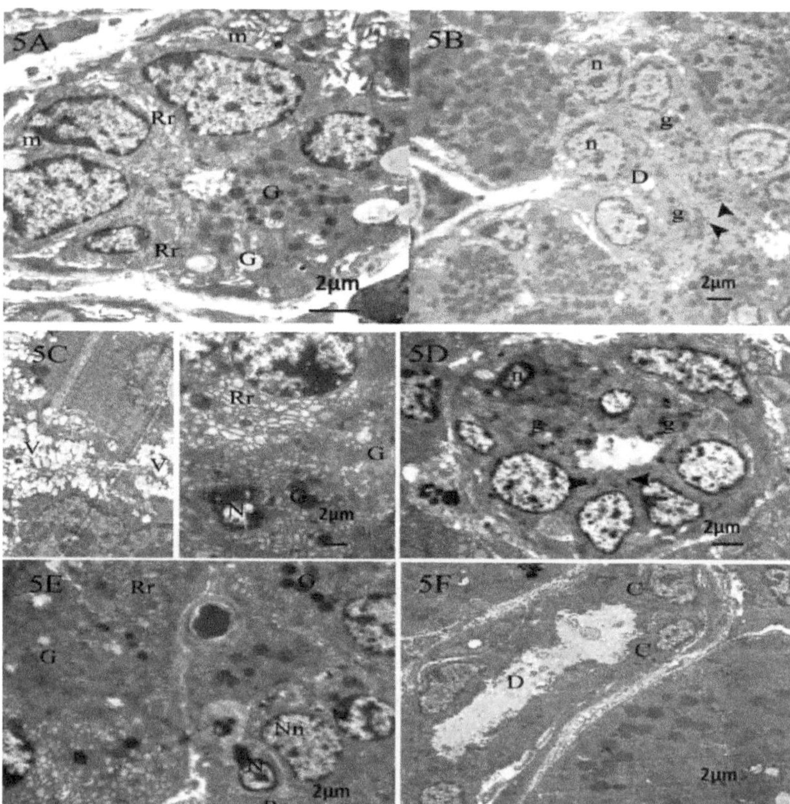

Figure 5: Ultrathin sections.

(A): Control group showing acinar cell with apical electron dense and electron lucent secretory granules (G), densely packed rough endoplasmic reticulum (Rr) and mitochondria(m). (B): Duct (D) is lined by rounded nuclei (n) and has cytoplasmic granules (g). Note, intercellular desmosome (arrowhead) inbtween the duct cells. (C): Operated group showing irregular heterochromatic nucleus (N), dilated rarified rough endoplasmic reticulum (Rr), electron dense secretory granules and electron lucent granules (G). Extensive cytoplasmic vacuolations (V) are seen in their cytoplasm. (D): Showing irregular heterochromatic nucleus (n) of lining epithelium of interlobular duct with many electron dense granules (g). Notice intercellular desmosomes (arrowhead). (E): Treated group showing some acini have heterochromatic nuclei (N), electron dense granules, electron lucent granules (G), and dilated rough endoplasmic reticulum (Rr). Other acinar cells have euchromatic nuclei (Nn). (F): Dialated duct (D) appears with apparently normal lining cells(C). (Scale bar=2μm).

Morphometrical Results

The duct diameter and the mean area % of collagen fiber for all groups were presented in (Table 1 and Figure 6): there was a significant increase ($P<0.05$) in collagen % of OVX group (II) compared with control group (I). While, there was a significant decrease in collagen fiber % in treated group (group III) as compared with OVX group (group II).

Table 1: Mean values of the area % of collagen fibers and the duct diameters in the different studied groups.

Groups	Area %of collagen fiber	Duct diameter
Control(I)	11.4 ± 2.24^{n}	33.3 ± 10.62^{n}
OVX group(II)	20.51 ± 4.6^{a}	65.07 ± 9.78^{a}
Treated group (III)	14.46 ± 3.79^{b}	40.44 ± 9.2^{b}

[n]non-significant difference with group I
[a]highly significant difference with group I
[b]highly significant difference with the group II

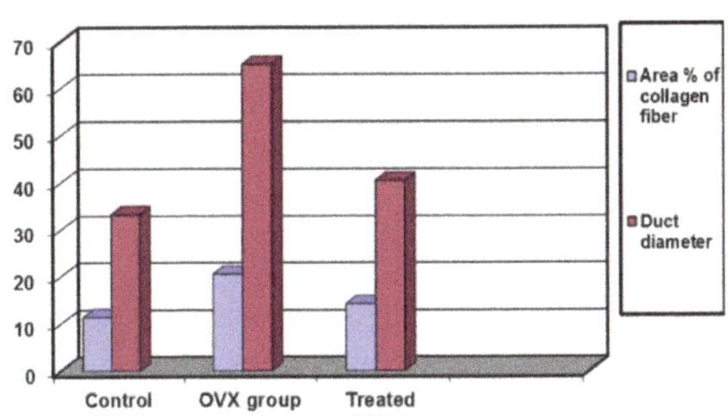

Figure 6 : Histogram showing the area % of collagen fibers and the duct diameters in the different studied groups.

DISCUSSION

Several aspects of menopause are universal: hot flashes, excessive transpiration, and vaginal atrophy, caused by estrogen deficiency and manifested in most women after menopause. The systemic aspects of menopause are well documented and include oral manifestations, such as changes in salivary secretion, gingivitis, bleeding, BMS and altered taste sensation [6].

Burning mouth syndrome (BMS) is a relatively common condition with prevalence between 0.7 and 4.6% of the general population. The etiology of this disorder is poorly understood even though new evidence for a possible neuropathic pathogenesis of idiopathic BMS is emerging [4].

Burning mouth syndrome may be primary (idiopathic) [14,15] or secondary condition. Secondary type may be caused by local or systemic disease, including nutritional deficiencies, hormonal changes associated with menopause, local oral infections, and denture-related lesions. Professional delay in diagnosing, referring, and appropriately managing of BMS patients occurs frequently. Treatment should be tailored to each patient to avoid this condition [16-18].

Female sex steroids may have a beneficial effect on the salivary glands [19] and some studies, Hietala [20] & Laine [21] demonstrate increased saliva flow rate after hormone treatment. During pregnancy, Hormone-related changes of the composition could affect saliva function, increase the severity of gingival inflammation [22] and lead to development of gingival pyogenic granuloma [23].

The results of the present work provide evidence that ovariectomy induces different forms of degenerative changes in parotid gland of group II. Most of the acini appeared irregular with darkly stained nuclei and many vacuoles in their cytoplasm. They were separated by thickened septa containing cellular infiltration. Homogenous acidophilic material was also seen. The interalobular ducts were dilated and lined by stratified epithelium. Congested blood vessels were also found.

These changes were reported by several studies younis [24] & Stramandinoli-Zanicott et al., [25] who referred them either to denervation of the gland or Hypocellularity, hypovascularity and hypoxia.

Degenerated structures were replaced with homogenous acidophilic areas which detected in gland. These amorphous acidophilic areas were described as hyaline degeneration of duct cells [26] Also, El-Sakhawy& Saeid [27] reported the same histological changes in parotid gland. Estrogen regulates the balance between endothelial dependent vasoconstrictor and vasodilator influences, possibly via estrogen-specific actions on nitric oxide and prostaglandin (PG2)-dependent pathways. This leads to vasodiltataion of blood vessels and edema [28]. Edema manifested by cellular infilteration within thickened CT septa and blood vessels congestion [27].

Also, significant dilatation of the parotid ducts was evident by morphometrical analysis of diameters of operated group. Affection of the parotid ducts is related to accumulation of ROS in their lining cells [29]. Collagen fibers appeared in extensive amount in between the lobules and around blood vessels in the same group. Estrogen is antioxidant hormone and acts as radical scavengers and inhibits lipid peroxidation in vivo and in vitro. So, low level of this hormone could lead to oxidative stress in overiectomized rats [30]. RamosDeconte et al., [31] reported that oxidative stress caused increase in collagen fiber in parotid of diabetic rats.

In current work, operated group revealed mild positivity for Cu, Zn-SOD while this immunoreaction became stronger in treated group. These results in accordance with Kusunoki et al [11]. They reported that administration of estrogen to postmenopausal women will be useful for preventing senile disturbances as osteoporosis, atherosclerosis, Alzheimer;s, etc. Urabe [32], Mortel et al., [33] and Honjo [34] mentioned that estrogen could suppress apoptosis in rat cranial nerve cells [11]. Also some researchers Oztekin et al., [35] reported that estradiol supplementation to ovariectomized rats decreased lipid peroxidation in liver tissue.

Ultrastructurally, parotid gland of operated group (II) clarified the presence of apoptotic acinar cells with irregular heterochromatic nuclei, dilated rarified rough endoplasmic reticulum, electron lucent and electron dense secretory granules. Extensive cytoplasmic vacuoles and apoptotic cells lining their ducts were also found. These results were in accordance with younis [24] and Omar [36] who concluded that generation of large number of free radicals (nitrogen &oxygen) could damage cellular proteins. Oxidative stress caused by estrogen deficiency in this group is the major factor that induced cellular damage. This damage might trigger the process of apoptosis [30]. Steven and Lowe [37] concluded that, the stagnant secretion in the excretory ducts might be due to mitochondrial affections. This mitochondrial affection lead to depletion of ATP with failure of biosynthesis and membrane pumps and as a result, the cells had no energy for the process of secretion transport.

Moreover, researchers Tirapelli et al., [38] detected these ultrastructural alterations in the parotid glands of alcoholic animals. They explained the presence of cytoplasmic vesicles by the great penetration of fluids in the cytoplasm of the acinar cells. Dilatation of rough endoplasmic reticulum was found in the acinar cells due to alterations in the cytoplasm of the striated ducts [39].

In the current work, examination of treated group (III) showed apparent normal appearance of serous acini and ducts and moderate amount of collagen fibers. The acinar cells appeared with different affection; some appeared apoptotic with heterochromatic nuclei, and others appeared normal. Electron dense and electron lucent granules, rough endoplasmic reticulum were seen in their cytoplasm. Dilated duct with apparently normal lining cells could be also seen.

To prove the role of a hormone in the pathogenesis of any disease, firstly, hormone must first exist in the target tissue. Second, the hormone's specific receptor must reside in the target tissue. Third, the absence of the hormone in the target tissue should contribute to the onset of the disease. Finally, the replacement of the hormone should induce the response. It is known that sex steroids exist in saliva [40].

Ovaries are the main source of natural estrogens. Their dysfunction decreases oestradiol level in blood and at the same time its stimulatory function in target tissues. Presence of estrogen receptors in cells of soft tissues causes changes evoked by lack of natural estrogen [41,42]. Drugs used in the prevention of postmenopausal osteoporosis and protect body against alterations caused by hypoestrogenism. Prevention of postmenopausal hypoestrogeny can be based not only on simple supplementation with missing hormone, but also drugs modulating estrogen receptors can be used, e.g. raloxifene [43,44]. Changes caused by estrogen deficiency are manifested in the vascular, urogenital and skeletal systems. There are many studies about structural and functional changes in the urogenital system in women.

Postmenopausal women frequently use hormonal therapy which elevate estrogen in serum and affect the saliva composition of protein and carbohydrate structure [1]. It was mentioned that a tissue-specific estrogen receptor is widely expressed in both oral epithelium and the salivary glands. Consequently, sex steroid hormone (estrogen) appears to play an important and complex role in the regulation of salivary glands especially ductal cells [7].

It was reported that low estrogen after ovariectomy reflects trophical changes in many organs including salivary glands. Oral discomfort in postmenopausal women may be improved with replacement therapy. Also, this therapy leads to apparent normalizing of oral salivary gland structure. Rahnama et al., [3] and Kusunoki et al., [11] suggested that sex hormone could influence age related histological changes in the parotid gland induced by apoptosis. Recently, administration of estrogen to postmenopausal women reported to be useful for preventing multiple senile disturbances.

The previous results concluded that estrogen deficiency in postmenopausal women lead to variable degenerative changes in parotid salivary glands of adult female albino rats with relative limitation of these changes in estrogen supplemented group. This may constitute an argument for further more complex studies on biological and health consequences of ovariectomized women, to test the necessity to use hormonal replacement during menopause with special recommendation to use estrogen as a protective measure.

AUTHORS' CONTRIBUTIONS

AUTHORS' CONTRIBUTIONS	DAM	HME	RAW
RESEARCH CONCEPT AND DESIGN	√	√	√
COLLECTION AND/OR ASSEMBLY OF DATA	√	√	--
DATA ANALYSIS AND INTERPRETATION	√	--	--
WRITING THE ARTICLE	√	--	--
CRITICAL REVISION OF THE ARTICLE	--	√	√
FINAL APPROVAL OF ARTICLE	--	√	√
STATISTICAL ANALYSIS	--	--	--

ACKNOWLEDGEMENT

We would like to thank Dr. Mona El shwadfi for her aid in statistical results.

REFERENCES

1. Eliasson L, Carlen A, Laine M and Birkhed D. **Minor gland and whole saliva in postmenopausal women using a low potency oestrogen (oestriol).** *Arch Oral Biol.* 2003; 48:511-7.
2. Carlstedt-Duke J. **Cellular estrogen activity: implications for pulsed estrogen therapy**. *Maturitas*. 2001; 38 Suppl 1:S7-S13.
3. Rahnama M, Swiatkowski W, Lancut M and Wojcik A. **Influence of raloxifene and 17 B-oestradiol on rats' oral mucosal structure**. *Bull Vet. Inst. Pulawy*. 2004; 48:329-332.
4. Maltsman-Tseikhin A, Moricca P and Niv D. **Burning mouth syndrome: will better understanding yield better management?** *Pain Pract*. 2007; 7:151-62.
5. Streckfus CF, Baur U, Brown LJ, Bacal C, Metter J and Nick T. **Effects of estrogen status and aging on salivary flow rates in healthy Caucasian women**. *Gerontology*. 1998; 44:32-9.
6. Seko K, Kagami H, Senga K, Ozeki K, Mizutani H and Ueda M. **Effects of ovariectomy and estrogen replacement on rat oral mucosa**. *Maturitas*. 2005; 50:44-51.
7. Valimaa H, Savolainen S, Soukka T, Silvoniemi P, Makela S, Kujari H, Gustafsson JA and Laine M. **Estrogen receptor-beta is the predominant estrogen receptor subtype in human oral epithelium and salivary glands**. *J Endocrinol*. 2004; 180:55-62.
8. Yih WY, Richardson L, Kratochvil FJ, Avera SP and Zieper MB. **Expression of estrogen receptors in desquamative gingivitis**. *J Periodontol*. 2000; 71:482-7.
9. Forabosco A, Criscuolo M, Coukos G, Uccelli E, Weinstein R, Spinato S, Botticelli A and Volpe A. **Efficacy of hormone replacement therapy in postmenopausal women with oral discomfort**. *Oral Surg Oral Med Oral Pathol*. 1992; 73:570-4.
10. Eliasson L, Carlen A, Laine M and Birkhed D. **Minor gland and whole saliva in postmenopausal women using a low potency oestrogen (oestriol).** *Arch Oral Biol.* 2003; 48:511-7.
11. Kusunoki T, Shiraishi H, Murata K, Nishida N and Tomura T. **Apoptosis and estrogen on aging changes of female rat parotids**. *Aging cell Acta Med Kinki Univ.*, 2004; 29:27-30.
12. Bancroft JD and Gamble M. **Theory and Practice of Histological Techniques. 5th ed.**, Churchill Livingstone. New york, London, Philadelphia. 2002; 125-138.
13. Glauert AM and Lewis PR. Biological Specimen Preparation for Transmission Electron Microscopy. Portland press. London. 1998; 17.
14. Granot M and Nagler RM. **Association between regional idiopathic neuropathy and salivary involvement as the possible mechanism for oral sensory complaints.** *J Pain*. 2005; 6:581-7.
15. Nagler RM and Hershkovich O. **Sialochemical and gustatory analysis in patients with oral sensory complaints.** *J Pain*. 2004; 5:56-63.

16. Benzon HT, Raja SN and Molloy RE et al. **Cervicogenic headache and orofacial pain**. In: Phero JC, Bonzon H, ed. Essentials of Pain Medicine and Regional Anesthesia, 2nd ed. Philadelphia: Elsevier. 2005; 301-310.
17. Barker KE and Savage NW.(2005). Burning mouth syndrome: an update on recent Barker KE and Savage NW. **Burning mouth syndrome: an update on recent findings**. *Aust Dent J.* 2005; 50:220-3; quiz 288.
18. Brown RS, Farquharson AA, Sam FE and Reid E. **A retrospective evaluation of 56 patients with oral burning and limited clinical findings**. *Gen Dent.* 2006; 54:267-71.
19. Leimola-Virtanen R, Salo T, Toikkanen S, Pulkkinen J and Syrjanen S. **Expression of estrogen receptor (ER) in oral mucosa and salivary glands**. *Maturitas.* 2000; 36:131-7.
20. Hietala EL, Heikkinen J, Vaananen HK and Larmas M. **Effect of postmenopausal estrogen treatment on some diagnostic salivary variables**. *Ann N Y Acad Sci.* 1993; 694:286-8.
21. Laine M and Leimola-Virtanen R. **Effect of hormone replacement therapy on salivary flow rate, buffer effect and pH on perimenopausal and postmenopausal women**. *Arch Oral Biol.* 1996; 41:91-6.
22. Hugoson A. **Gingivitis in pregnant women. A longitudinal clinical study**. *Odontol Revy.* 1971; 22:65-84.
23. Daley TD, Nartey NO and Wysocki GP. **Pregnancy tumor: an analysis**. *Oral Surg Oral Med Oral Pathol.* 1991; 72:196-9.
24. Younis R, AbouElkhier M, Mourad M and Elnahas W. **Ultrastructural changes in the parotid gland of rats after intraglandular injection of botulinum toxin A**. *Annals of Oral &Maxillofacial Surgery.* 2013; 1-16.
25. Stramandinoli-Zanicotti RT, Sassi LM, Schussel JL, Torres MF, Funchal M, Smaniotto GH, Dissenha JL and Carvalho AL. **Effect of fractionated radiotherapy on the parotid gland: an experimental study in Brazilian minipigs**. *Int Arch Otorhinolaryngol.* 2013; 17:163-7.
26. Cawson RA, Gleeson MJ and Eveson JW. Sialadenitis In: Pathology and surgery of the salivary glands.*Oxford Edn Isis Medical Media.* 1997; 25-33.
27. El-Sakhawy M and Saeid S. Effect of long term adminsteration of aspartame on the parotid salivary glands of male albino rats. *Int. J. of Adv. Res.* 2014; 2:850-857.
28. Smith J, Lindsay M, Rahimian R and Anderson L. **The influence of estrogen and progesterone on parasympathetic vasodilatation in the rat submandibular gland**. *Auton Neurosci.* 2009; 146:87-94.
29. Wei PF, Ho KY, Ho YP, Wu YM, Yang YH and Tsai CC. **The investigation of glutathione peroxidase, lactoferrin, myeloperoxidase and interleukin-1beta in gingival crevicular fluid: implications for oxidative stress in human periodontal diseases**. *J Periodontal Res.* 2004; 39:287-93.

30. Kiray M, Ergur BU, Bagriyanik A, Pekcetin C, Aksu I and Buldan Z. **Suppression of apoptosis and oxidative stress by deprenyl and estradiol in aged rat liver**. *Acta Histochem*. 2007; 109:480-5.

31. Deconte SR, Oliveira RJ, Calabria LK, Oliveira VN, Gouveia NM, Moraes Ada S and Espindola FS. **Alterations of antioxidant biomarkers and type I collagen deposition in the parotid gland of streptozotocin-induced diabetic rats**. *Arch Oral Biol*. 2011; 56:744-51.

32. Urabe S. Estrogen and aging. *Adv Obstet Gynecol*. 1998; 50:161- 2.

33. Mortel KF and Meyer JS. **Lack of postmenopausal estrogen replacement therapy and the risk of dementia**. *J Neuropsychiatry Clin Neurosci*. 1995; 7:334-7.

34. Honjo H and Kikuchi N. **Estrogen and Alzheimer's disease**. *Geriatric Med*. 2000; 38:651-8.

35. Oztekin E, Baltaci A, Tiftik A and Mogulkoc R. **Lipid peroxidation in ovariectomized and pinealectomized rats: the effects of estradiol and progesterone supplementation**. *Cell Biochem Funct*. 2006.

36. Omar S.M.M. Effect of Aspartame on the Frontal Cortex of Adult Male Albino Rats. *A light and Electron Microscopic Study*. 2009; 32:346-357. | Pdf

37. Stevens A and Lowe J. Pathology.Firstedition, Alan Stevens/James Lowe Mosby, Baltimore, Philadelphia, Toronto. 1995; 23-33.

38. Tirapelli L, Tirapelli D and Schimming B. **Ultrastructural alterations of the parotid glands of rats (Rattus norvegicus) submitted to experimental chronic alcoholism**. *Rev. Chil. Anat*. 2001; 19. | Article

39. Sasahara M, Matsuo M, Kakizaki G, Aikawa T, Sato T, Uejima K, Yamada A, Saito M and Nakamura K. **The effect of long term ethanol intake on the parotid gland in rats**. *Tohoku J Exp Med*. 1990; 160:251-75.

40. Myers A and Naylor GD. **Glossodynia as an oral manifestation of sex hormone alterations**. *Ear Nose Throat J*. 1989; 68:786, 789-90.

41. Coleman H, Benghuzzi H, Tucci M and Cason Z. **The effects of thyroid and reproductive hormones on the viability of human buccal epithelium**. *Biomed Sci Instrum*. 2001; 37:143-8.

42. Leimola-Virtanen R, Pennanen R, Syrjanen K and Syrjanen S. **Estrogen response in buccal mucosa -- a cytological and immunohistological assay**. *Maturitas*. 1997; 27:41-5.

43. Frolik CA, Bryant HU, Black EC, Magee DE and Chandrasekhar S. **Time-dependent changes in biochemical bone markers and serum cholesterol in ovariectomized rats: effects of raloxifene HCl, tamoxifen, estrogen, and alendronate**. *Bone*. 1996; 18:621-7.

44. Delmas PD. **Treatment of postmenopausal osteoporosis**. *Lancet*. 2002; 359:2018-26.

7

CHAPTER

COMBINED TOXICITY OF ENDOSULFAN AND OCHRATOXIN-A IN RATS: HISTOPATHOLOGICAL CHANGES

Shashi Nandar Kumar, Banajit Bastia, Avinash Gopal Telang, Karam Pal Singh, Rambir Singh and Arun Kumar Jain

Keywords: Ochratoxin-A, endosulfan, toxicity, histopathology, liver, kidney

INTRODUCTION

Mycotoxins can be found in nearly all agricultural commodities, such as cereals (maize, wheat, oats and barley) and cereal by-products. Moulds or fungi and their associated mycotoxins have been shown to be present on all crops in varying amounts, depending on the climatic conditions. Correct storage of feeds and feedstuffs is critical in preventing mould growth. While improper storage of feed stuff may result in excessive mycotoxin contamination, current agricultural practices with emphasis on widespread use of pesticides may cause pesticide contamination of agricultural items which become toxic for consumption. These contaminations can cause serious problems, both for human health as well as for the economic value of crops.

Endosulfan is a persistent, toxic, broad-spectrum organochlorine insecticide and acaricide used on food and non-food crops. It has been enlisted as one of the persistent organic pollutants (POPs) that is largely used in agriculture, viticulture and horticulture [1]. Endosulfan contamination in blood, fat, milk, vegetables, cashew leaves, soil and water has been reported from Padre village of Kasargod district of Kerala, India [2,3]. It causes toxic effect on almost all the organs of both humans and animals including the liver, lung, central nervous system, genital system, pancreas etc [4]. Endosulfan acts

Citation: Kumar SN, Bastia B, Telang AG, Singh KP, Singh R and Jain AK. Combined toxicity of endosulfan and ochratoxin-A in rats: histopathological changes. J Histol Histopathol. 2015; 2:22. http://dx.doi.org/10.7243/2055-091X-2-22.

as an endocrine disruptor, causing reproductive and developmental damage; and has also been reported to cause immune suppression and cancer in experimental animals [1,5-10].

Ochratoxin-A (OTA) is one of most toxic mycotoxins produced by numerous varieties of *Aspergillus* and *Penicillium*[11,12]. Worldwide contamination of OTA has been reported in a wide range of foods, including cereals and peanuts [13], poultry feeds [14], feedstuffs [15], green coffee beans [16], cocoa beans [17], wine grapes ([18], dried vine fruits [19] and beer [20]. It is also reported toxic manifestations of OTA include nephrotoxicity, teratogenicity, immunotoxicity, carcinogenicity, and mutagenicity [21]. OTA is suspected to be responsible for human Balkan Endemic Nephropathy (BEN) [21,22]. Thus, kidney is considered to be one of the main target organs of OTA [23]. Due to its ubiquitous occurrence in a range of foodstuffs, the complete avoidance of OTA exposure is virtually impossible [23-25].

Further, in real life, organisms are concurrently exposed to several i.e., more than one pollutants or toxins. Therefore, the present study was aimed to examine the pathological changes in liver and kidney of adult male rats in case of combined exposure to OTA and Endosulfan.

MATERIALS AND METHODS

Production and analysis of OTA

Aspergillus ochraceus NRRL-3174 was initially procured from National Centre for Agriculture Utilization Research, Peoria, Illinois, USA. It was grown on sterilized maize as per the method described by Trenk and coworkers [26]. The extraction and clean up of the toxin sample were done by AOAC method [27] and quantification of OTA was done with the help of TLC scanner (CAMAG, Switzerland).

Preparation of toxicated feed

Cultured maize powder containing known amount of OTA was added to basal ration (which were tested negative for presence of contaminating mycotoxins) in such proportion that the final concentration of OTA was adjusted to 4 mg kg^{-1} feed. Aliquots were taken from the mixed diet and the toxin was further quantified to ensure proper mixing of the toxin.

Dosing of endosulfan

Endosulfan (>99.98% pure crystalline Technical grade Shriram Chemicals Ltd., India) was dissolved in corn oil (vehicle) at a concentration of 5 mg kg^{-1} body weight and oral gavage was given to male rats, daily for 30 days. Fresh solution of endosulfan was prepared on each day of treatment. Control animals received an equal volume of corn oil similar to those treated with endosulfan.

Experimental plan

Forty sexually mature male Wistar rats (Age: 7 to 8 weeks; weight:180±20 g), procured from the Laboratory Animal Resource (LAR) section of the Indian Veterinary Research Institute were maintained on standard feed and water available *ad libitum*. After 1 week of acclimatization period, the animals were randomly distributed in to 4 groups of ten rats each and treated for 30 days as follows: Group-I animals were given with a diet containing OTA at the level of 4 mg kg^{-1} feed; Group-II animals received endosulfan at a concentration of 5 mg kg^{-1} body weight by oral gavage; Group-III animals received both OTA (4 mg kg^{-1} feed) and endosulfan (5 mg kg^{-1} body weight) and Group-IV animals were fed a standard mycotoxins-free basal diet. All the experimental procedure and sacrifice of rats were carried out as per the approved guidelines of Institutional Animal Ethics Committee (IAEC) and Committee for the Purpose of Control and Supervision of Experiments on Animals (CPCSEA).

Pathological changes

The liver and kidney of all the groups were examined for gross morphological and pathological changes. Wet organ weights were recorded before collecting tissue samples for processing. Representative tissue samples were collected in 10% buffered formalin for histopathological studies. The tissues were properly processed and embedded in paraffin wax. The sections were stained with hematoxylin and eosin stain [28] and were then examined under light microscope.

Statistical analysis

Data generated during the study were suitably analyzed using student's 't'test to detect differences between means among groups. All analyses were performed with GraphPad InStat software (San Diago, USA). All the statements of significance were based on a probability level of $p<0.05$.

RESULTS

Gross Lesions and Relative Weight of Kidney And Liver

Macroscopic examination of rats fed with OTA or Endosulfan or their combination for 30 days, showed focal areas on liver surface. Liver was slightly pale and molted. There was a significant reduction in relative weight of kidney and liver in Group-I (OTA-treated) and Group-III (combination of OTA and endosulfan diet) as compared to those of controls (Table 1). The reduction was highly significant in Group-III.

Table 1: Effect of OTA and Endosulfan (ES) administered alone and in combination on relative weight of liver and kidney of adult male rats

Group →	Control	OTA	Endosulfan (ES)	Combination (OTA+ES)	Significance
Organs	**Organ weight (gm) expressed as mean± SE (n=10)**				
Liver	3.93 ± 0.24^{b}	3.27 ± 0.66^{a}	3.57 ± 0.18^{ab}	3.12 ± 0.11^{a}	$P<0.05$
Kidney	1.03 ± 0.07^{b}	0.79 ± 99^{a}	0.86 ± 0.04^{b}	0.70 ± 0.064	$P<0.05$

Ochratoxin A (OTA) treatment

Kidney

As compared to controls (Figure 1), the proximal convoluted tubules in OTA-treated animals showed degenerative changes along with the presence of pinkish homogenous mass in the lumen (Figure 2). Some of the tubules showed pyknotic and karyorrhectic nuclei. Vascular congestion was observed both in cortex and medulla. Several glomeruli showed widening of Bowman's space with deposition of proteinaceous mass. Tubular lumen was found to be obliterated due to degeneration and swelling of lining epithelial cells.

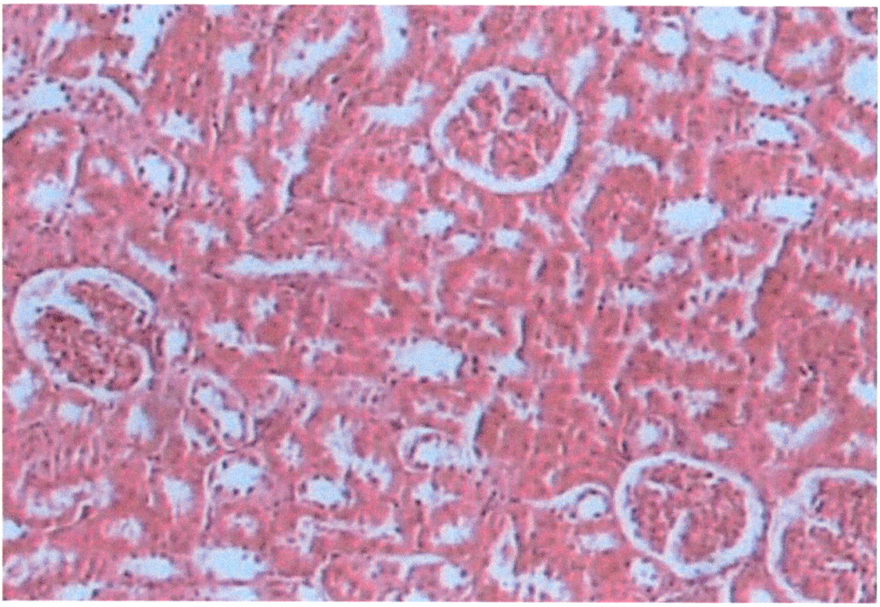

Figure 1: Kidney section showing normal glomeruli and proximal and distal convoluted tubules H&E×100.

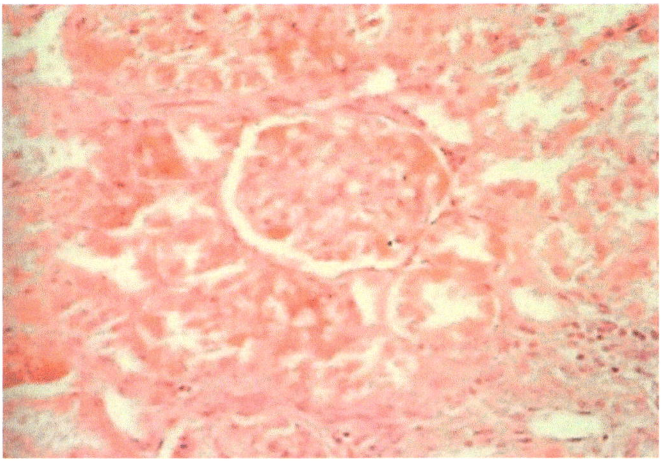

Figure 2: OTA-treated kidney: Marked necrotic and degenerative changes in proximal convoluted tubules.

Note the detachment of necrosed lining cells H&E×200.

Liver

Rats fed on toxin-free diet showed normal liver architecture (Figure 3). In comparison, hepatocytes in rats fed with OTA (Group-I) showed degenerative and necrotic changes with granular cytoplasm (Figure 4). Cytoplasm in most of the hepatocytes was pale or less stained. Hepatic sinusoids along with central and portal veins showed mild to moderate congestion. Mild to moderate fatty changes were observed in hepatocytes of centrilobular area (Figure 4).

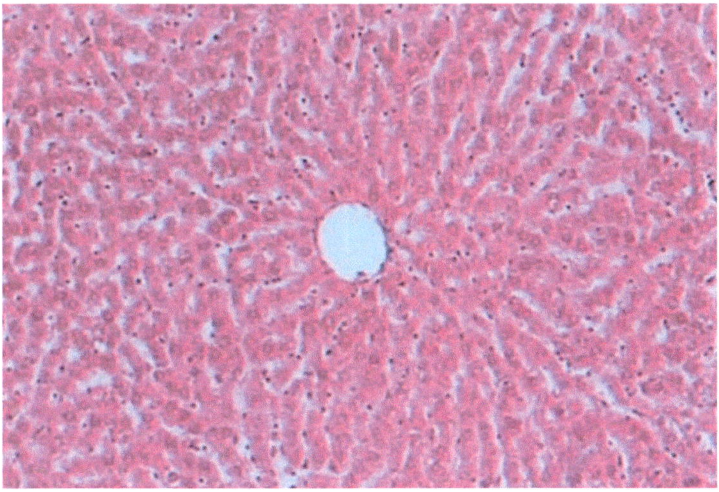

Figure 3 : Liver section showing normal architectural arrangement of hepatic cords.

The hepatocytes also appear normal with centrally placed nucleus and eosinophilic cytoplasm H&E×100.

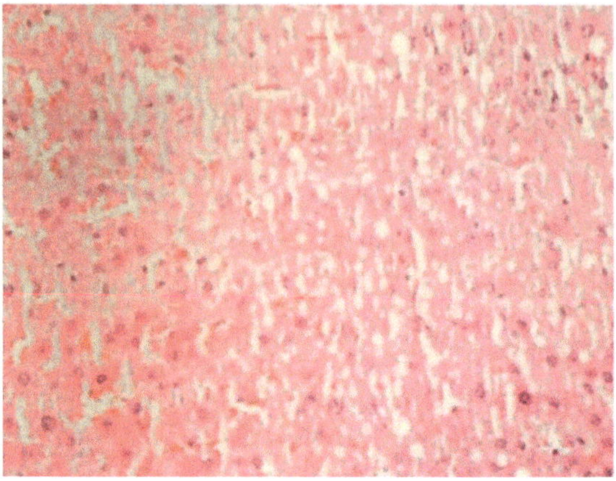

Figure 4 : OTA-treated liver: Marked fatty changes and degenerative changes in hepatic parenchyma H&E×200.

Endosulfan treatment

Kidney

Proximal convoluted tubules in group–II, revealed degeneration and necrosis of the lining cells. The tubular lumen showed presence of detached necrosed pinkish mass (Figure 5). Inter-tubular blood vessels were mildly congested.

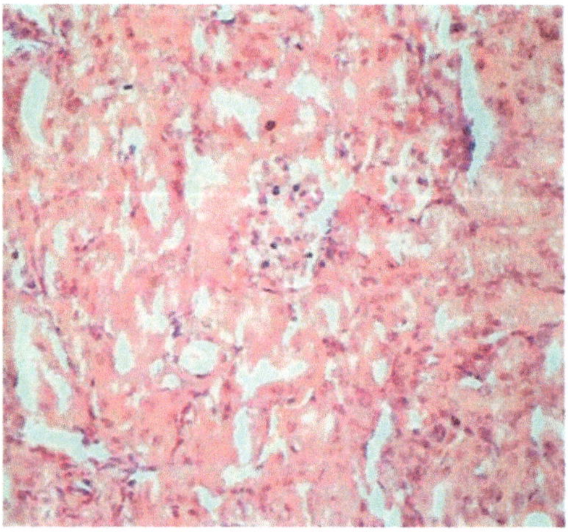

Figure 5 : Endosulfan-treated kidney: Marked necrotic changes in the proximal convoluted tubules.

Necrosed lining cells detached into the lumen H&E×200.

Liver

Hepatocytes in endosulfan-toxicated group-II rats, showed mild degeneration with granular cytoplasm in comparison to OTA alone (Figure 6).

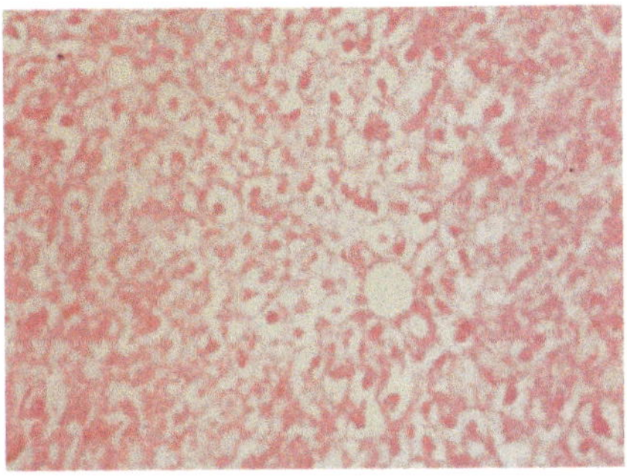

Figure 6 : Endosulfan-treated liver: Hepatocytes shows loss of cytoplasm, giving the appearance of emptiness H&E×200.

Endosulfan+OTA combination treatment

Kidney

In group-III, proximal convoluted tubules exhibited degenerative changes with pinkish granules in the cytoplasm and vacuolations in the lining of epithelial cells (Figure 7). The swelling of the cells resulted into the obstruction of the lumen. Some of the glomeruli showed presence of pinkish homogenous proteinaceous mass and vacuoles in the capillary tuft with increased Bowman's space (Figure 7). The inter-tubular blood vessels were occasionally congested.

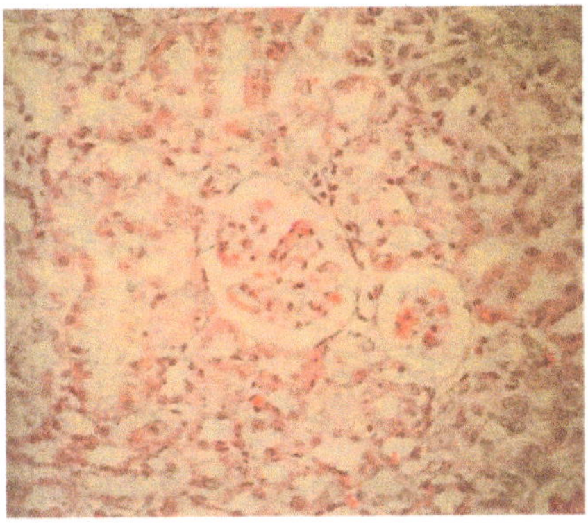

Figure 7: OTA and Endosulfan-treated kidney: Glomeruli with widened Bowman's space; degenerated convoluted tubules and presence of homogenous mass in the lumen. H&E×200.

Liver

Hepatic sinusoids and portal veins in group-III animals, showed mild to moderate vascular congestion. Swelling with fine granules in the cytoplasm and occasional double nuclei was observed in hepatocytes. Hepatic lobules revealed degeneration with presence of small to large fatty vacuoles in hepatocytes pushing the nucleus towards periphery (Figure 8). These fatty changes were mostly confined around the central vein. At places mononuclear cell reaction was noticed in the centre of the portal lobules around the portal triad. Focal areas of necrosis with isolated hepatocytes were seen in hepatic parenchyma at few places (Figure 8).

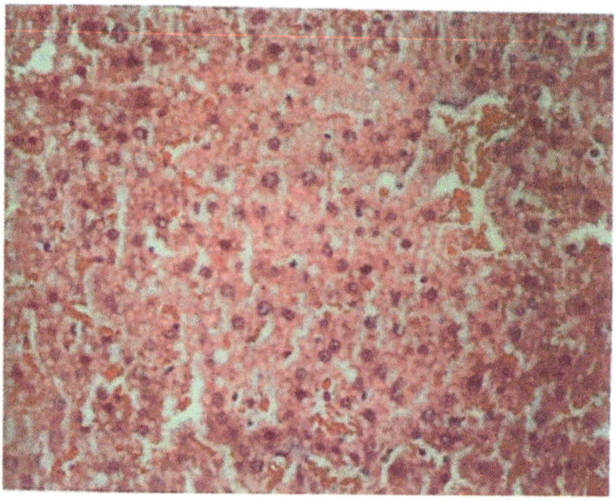

Figure 8: OTA and Endosulfan-treated liver: Hepatic parenchyma shows marked necrosis and fatty vacuoles in the hepatocytes with focal vascular congestion. H&E×200.

DISCUSSION

Gross lesion observed were swollen and slightly mottled liver and slightly pale kidneys. The relative weight to these organs was also found to be decreased. The changes in liver and kidneys were comparatively more intense in combination group as compared to OTA or Endosulfan alone. These observations were in accordance with the findings of earlier worker [29-31]. The absolute and relative organ weight of liver and kidney were in agreement with the observations of [32] in rats and [33] in chicks administered with Endosulfan. Contrary to our observations on organ weights, earlier workers [34-36] reported increased organ weight of liver and kidneys. These discrepancies could be due to many factors such as age, sex and strain of animals, the influence of the vehicle or difference in the administration regimen. OTA and Endosulfan alone caused pale discoloration of liver and kidneys, increased fragility of liver, which could be attributed to degenerative changes as detected on histopathological examination. OTA and Endosulfan are known to be hepatotoxic and nephrotoxic. These effects have been seen in our experimental animal rat. The changes in liver were of degenerative in nature including fatty changes and vascular congestion. Similar changes have also been reported by earlier workers in different species of animals i.e., rat [29,30,36], rabbits [31,37-39] and poultry [40]. The degenerative and vascular changes observed in kidney tubules and renal corpuscles were in consensus with the findings of earlier workers [29,36,40,41]. The gross or microscopic changes observed in the present study may be classified as mild, probably due to low dose of ochratoxin-A or endosulfan. The histopathological changes in kidneys explain, at least in parts, the functional alterations (increased level of creatinine and blood urea nitrogen) recorded in serum analysis of these experimental rats in a previous study [42]. From the present study it was concluded that OTA and Endosulfan are potentially toxic to liver and kidney in combination as compared to their toxic effects alone.

AUTHORS' CONTRIBUTIONS

Authors' contributions	SNK	BB	AGT	KPS	RS	AKJ
Research concept and design	√	--	√	--	√	--
Collection and/or assembly of data	√	--	--	√	--	--
Data analysis and interpretation	√	--	--	√	--	--
Writing the article	√	√	--	--	--	√
Critical revision of the article	--	--	--	--	--	√
Final approval of article	--	--	--	--	--	√
Statistical analysis	--	--	√	√	--	√

ACKNOWLEDGEMENT

The researchers would like to acknowledge the help extended by In-charge, Division of Pathology, Indian Veterinary Research Institute.

REFERENCES

1. Du H, Wang M, Dai H, Hong W, Wang J, Weng N, Nie Y and Xu A. **Endosulfan isomers and sulfate metabolite induced reproductive toxicity in Caenorhabditis elegans involves genotoxic response genes.***Environ Sci Technol.* 2015; 49:2460-8.
2. Omnipresent Poison. | Website
3. Ramesh A and Vijayalakshmi A. **Environmental exposure to residues after aerial spraying of endosulfan: residues in cow milk, fish, water, soil and cashew leaf in Kasargode, Kerala, India**. *Pest Manag Sci.* 2002;58:1048-54.
4. O. Ozmen. Pathology of Endosulfan. in *Pesticides in the Modern World - Effects of Pesticides Exposure*, M. Stoytcheva, Ed. InTech. 2011.
5. Gupta PK and Gupta RC. **Pharmacology, toxicology and degradation of endosulfan A review**. *Toxicology.* 1979; 13:115-30.
6. Sutherland TD, Home I, Weir KM, Russell RJ and Oakeshott JG. **Toxicity and**

residues of endosulfan isomers. *Rev Environ Contam Toxicol.* 2004; 183:99-113.

7. N.D.Singh, A.K.Sharma, P.Dwivedi, Kumar M and R.D.Patil. Immunosuppressive effect of combined citrinin and endosulfan toxicity in pregnant Wistar rats. *Vet. Arh.* 2011; 81.
8. Singh ND, Sharma AK, Dwivedi P, Patil RD and Kumar M. **Citrinin and endosulfan induced teratogenic effects in Wistar rats**. *J Appl Toxicol.* 2007; 27:143-51.
9. Singh ND, Sharma AK, Dwivedi P, Patil RD and Kumar M. **Citrinin and endosulfan induced maternal toxicity in pregnant Wistar rats: pathomorphological study**. *J Appl Toxicol.* 2007; 27:589-601.
10. S. N. Kumar A. G. Telang R. D. Patil A. K. Jain and K. P. Singh. Cytogenetic Effects of Combined Ochratoxin A and Endosulfan in Rats. *J. Environ. Anal. Toxicol.* 2014; 4:1.
11. Baudrimont I, Sostaric B, Yenot C, Betbeder AM, Dano-Djedje S, Sanni A, Steyn PS and Creppy EE.Aspartame prevents the karyomegaly induced by ochratoxin A in rat kidney. *Arch Toxicol.* 2001; 75:176-83.
12. Al-Anati L and Petzinger E. **Immunotoxic activity of ochratoxin A**. *J Vet Pharmacol Ther.* 2006; 29:79-90.
13. Magnoli C, Hallak C, Astoreca A, Ponsone L, Chiacchiera S and Dalcero AM. **Occurrence of ochratoxin A-producing fungi in commercial corn kernels in Argentina**. *Mycopathologia.* 2006; 161:53-8.
14. Rosa CA, Ribeiro JM, Fraga MJ, Gatti M, Cavaglieri LR, Magnoli CE, Dalcero AM and Lopes CW. **Mycoflora of poultry feeds and ochratoxin-producing ability of isolated Aspergillus and Penicillium species**. *Vet Microbiol.* 2006; 113:89-96.
15. Magnoli C, Hallak C, Astoreca A, Ponsone L, Chiacchiera SM, Palacio G and Dalcero A. **Surveillance of toxigenic fungi and ochratoxin A in feedstuffs from Cordoba Province, Argentina**. *Vet Res Commun.* 2005; 29:431-45.
16. Romani S, Sacchetti G, Chaves Lopez C, Pinnavaia GG and Dalla Rosa M. **Screening on the occurrence of ochratoxin A in green coffee beans of different origins and types**. *J Agric Food Chem.* 2000; 48:3616-9.
17. Serra Bonvehi J. **Occurrence of ochratoxin A in cocoa products and chocolate**. *J Agric Food Chem.* 2004;52:6347-52.
18. Magnoli C, Violante M, Combina M, Palacio G and Dalcero A. **Mycoflora and ochratoxin-producing strains of Aspergillus section Nigri in wine grapes in Argentina**. *Lett Appl Microbiol.* 2003; 37:179-84.
19. Magnoli C, Astoreca A, Ponsone L, Combina M, Palacio G, Rosa CA and Dalcero AM. **Survey of mycoflora and ochratoxin A in dried vine fruits from Argentina markets**. *Lett Appl Microbiol.* 2004; 39:326-31.
20. Medina A, Jimenez M, Gimeno-Adelantado JV, Valle-Algarra FM and Mateo R. **Determination of ochratoxin A in beer marketed in Spain by liquid**

chromatography with fluorescence detection using lead hydroxyacetate as a clean-up agent. *J Chromatogr A*. 2005; 1083:7-13.

21. Pfohl-Leszkowicz A and Manderville RA. **Ochratoxin A: An overview on toxicity and carcinogenicity in animals and humans**. *Mol Nutr Food Res*. 2007; 51:61-99.
22. Gekle M, Schwerdt G, Freudinger R, Mildenberger S, Wilflingseder D, Pollack V, Dander M and Schramek H.Ochratoxin A induces JNK activation and apoptosis in MDCK-C7 cells at nanomolar concentrations. *J Pharmacol Exp Ther*. 2000; 293:837-44.
23. Liang R, Shen XL, Zhang B, Li Y, Xu W, Zhao C, Luo Y and Huang K. **Apoptosis signal-regulating kinase 1 promotes Ochratoxin A-induced renal cytotoxicity**. *Sci Rep*. 2015; 5:8078.
24. Kuiper-Goodman T and Scott PM. **Risk assessment of the mycotoxin ochratoxin A**. *Biomed Environ Sci*. 1989; 2:179-248.
25. Simon P, Godin M and Fillastre JP. **Ochratoxin a: a new environmental factor which is toxic for the kidney?***Nephrol Dial Transplant*. 1996; 11:2389-91.
26. Trenk HL, Butz ME and Chu FS. **Production of ochratoxins in different cereal products by Aspergillus ochraceus**. *Appl Microbiol*. 1971; 21:1032-5.
27. P. Cunniff and Association of Official Analytical Chemists. *Official methods of analysis of the AOAC International*. Washington (D.C.): AOAC International. 1995.
28. L. G. Luna. Manual of histologic staining methods of the Armed Forces Institute of Pathology. 1968.
29. Choudhary N, Sharma M, Verma P and Joshi SC. **Hepato and nephrotoxicity in rat exposed to endosulfan**.*J Environ Biol*. 2003; 24:305-8.
30. K. Prasanna, A. K. Sharma, P. Dwivedi, C. C. Satheesh and A. G. Telang. Pathogenesis of ochratoxin A induced nephropathy in rats with special reference to oxidative damage, cytokine profile and ultrastructural changes. *Indian J. Vet. Pathol.* 2007; 31:1–10.
31. Wangikar PB, Dwivedi P, Sharma AK and Sinha N. **Effect in rats of simultaneous prenatal exposure to ochratoxin A and aflatoxin B1. II. Histopathological features of teratological anomalies induced in fetuses**. *Birth Defects Res B Dev Reprod Toxicol*. 2004; 71:352-8.
32. Dortant PM, Peters-Volleberg GW, Van Loveren H, Marquardt RR and Speijers GJ. **Age-related differences in the toxicity of ochratoxin A in female rats**. *Food Chem Toxicol*. 2001; 39:55-65.
33. N. V. Kurkure, A. G. Bhandarkar, M. V. Joshi, R. D. Sadekar and S. S. Bhagwat. Immunosuppressive and histotoxic effects of endosulphan in chicks. *Indian J. Anim. Sci. India*. 1993.
34. Munro IC, Moodie CA, Kuiper-Goodman T, Scott PM and Grice HC. **Toxicologic changes in rats fed graded dietary levels of ochratoxin A**. *Toxicol Appl Pharmacol*. 1974; 28:180-8.

35. Kiran R and Varma MN. **Biochemical studies on endosulfan toxicity in different age groups of rats**. *Toxicol Lett.* 1988; 44:247-52.

36. C. C. Satheesh, A. K. Sharma, K. Prasanna and P. Dwivedi. Ultrastructural changes in kidneys and liver in experimentally induced ochratoxicosis in wister rats. *Indian J. Vet. Pathol. India.* 2004.

37. M. S. Mir, P. Dwivedi and K. Charan. Ochratoxin A induced acute toxicity in rabbits. 1999.

38. M. S. Mir and P. Dwivedi. Clinical studies on experimental subacute ochratoxicosis in rabbits. *Indian J Vet Pathol.* 2000; 24:99-101.

39. Wangikar PB, Dwivedi P, Sinha N, Sharma AK and Telang AG. **Teratogenic effects in rabbits of simultaneous exposure to ochratoxin A and aflatoxin B1 with special reference to microscopic effects.***Toxicology*. 2005; 215:37-47.

40. Dwivedi P, Burns RB and Maxwell MH. **Ultrastructural study of the liver and kidney in ochratoxicosis A in young broiler chicks**. *Res Vet Sci.* 1984; 36:104-16.

41. Hack R, Ebert E and Leist KH. **Chronic toxicity and carcinogenicity studies with the insecticide endosulfan in rats and mice**. *Food Chem Toxicol.* 1995; 33:941-50.

42. S. N. Kumar, A. G. Telang, K. P. Singh, B. Bastia and A. K. Jain. Toxic Manifestation of Endosulfan and Ochratoxin- A in Adult Male Rats. *MOJ Toxicol.* 2015; 1:00012.

8

CHAPTER

HISTOCHEMICAL AND HISTOMORPHOMETRICAL STUDIES ON THE EFFECT OF AQUEOUS STEM BARK EXTRACT OFANOGEISSUS LEIOCARPUS ON ADULT WISTAR RAT OVERIES

Murtala M. Jibril, Ojo S. Adeniyi, Bawa E. Kambai and Zubairu S. Rayyan

Keywords: Anogeissus leiocarpus, ovaries, histochemistry, histomorphometry

INTRODUCTION

Anogeissus leiocarpus (DC) Guill. & Perr. is a common plant distributed across the African savanna region, mostly across the West and Central Africa [3]. It has many local names in different languages across Africa. It is referred to as «*Orin-odan*" in Yoruba, and "*Marke*" in Hausa. *A. leiocarpus* is still locally used for problems associated with reproduction in many parts of Northern Nigeria.

The effect of *A. leiocarpus* extract on reproduction and fertility has not been investigated. Many of the plant materials used in traditional medicine are readily available in rural areas and this has made traditional medicine relatively cheaper than modern medicine [4]. Over Sixty percent of Nigeria rural populations depend on traditional medicine for their healthcare need [4].

Phytochemical studies conducted on *A. leiocarpus* revealed that the stem bark extracts has various chemical constitutions such as alkaloids, glycosides, steroid, anthraquinone, phenol, tannins, saponins, calcium and fluorides [1].

Citation: Jibril MM, Adeniyi OS, Kambai BE and Rayyan ZS. Histochemical and histomorphometrical studies on the effect of aqueous stem bark extract of Anogeissus leiocarpus on adult wistar rat overies. J Histol Histopathol. 2015; 2:20. http://dx.doi.org/10.7243/2055-091X-2-20.

MATERIALS AND METHODS

Experimental animals

Twenty-four young adult Wistar rats weighing between 135-150g per group were obtained from the department of pharmacology of Ahmadu Bello University Zaria, Kaduna state, Nigeria. They were kept in plastic cages and maintained under laboratory condition at room temperature and humidity. Water and standard pellet diet were provided to the rats ad libitum. All animals received care in compliance with the guidelines of the ethical committee of medical research, ABU Zaria. There after, the animals were divided into four groups of six animals each.

Plant Material

The fresh stem bark of *A. leiocarpus*, readily available within the Ahmadu Bello University Zaria, were collected and authenticated in the herbarium of Biological Sciences Department of ABU Zaria by a taxonomist U. S. Gallah with a voucher specimen number 1738 for future reference. Two kilogram of *A. leiocarpus* stem bark was air dried, minced and powdered using a clean, sterile laboratory mortar. 50g of the resulting powder was dissolved in 0.5 liters of distilled water using a soxhlet extractor. The solution was allowed to settle for twenty-four hours and filtered with Whartmann's filter paper. The resultant solute was allowed to settle for one hour, and placed in water bath under reduced pressure at 35°C for evaporation.The extract was weighed and dissolved in distilled water to prepare the stock solution.

Experimental Procedure

Twenty-four (n=24) adult female wistar rats were used for the study. The animals were randomly assigned into four groups I, II, III and IV, each group consisting of six animals selected at random. Each group was placed in a separate cage. The experimental groups were given rat pellets and various concentrations of aqueous extract of *A. leiocarpus* of varying concentrations of the extract gavage, corresponding to 600mg/kg (½LD_{50}) for group VI, 400mg/kg (⅓LD_{50}) for group III, and 200mg/kg (¼LD_{50}) for group II, the control group I, were given food and distilled water for the period of six weeks.

Histological Studies

The reproductive organs; Ovaries, uterus and the uterine horns, were harvested immediately after the rats were sacrificed. They were weighed in analytical balance, and fixed in 10% Bouin's fixative solution. Tissue sections were prepared and stained using Hematoxylin & Eosin stain for light microscopy. Photomicrographs were obtained using a microscope eyepiece attached to a computer.

Histometrical Studies

Histometrical study was conducted using the method of [2]. Paraffin sections of 3μm thickness were cut on a microtome and stained with Hematoxylin and eosin (H&E)

for morphometry and enumeration of ovarian follicles. Homologous cross sections of the entire ovary showing a better area of vision were chosen. The ovarian section was traced around the tissue boundaries with the computerized software and a sampling grid was superimposed over the section. Each square of the sampling grid represent a sampled area measuring 6400μm. A counting frame was then used to sample a pre-determined area within each square of the sampling grid. Section area was calculated by integrating the area inside the traced perimeter and volume calculated by multiplying the section thickness.

Statistical Analysis

The results obtained were analyzed using Statistics 5.0 software and Microsoft Excel 2007. All results were expressed a mean value±SEM. The variance of the data and the confidence interval were determined using the analysis of variance (ANOVA) and a value of $P<0.05$ was considered as statistically significant. Dunnet's post hoc tests were used to determine where the level of significance lies.

RESULTS

Effect of *anogeissus leiocarpus* extract on body weight of the animals

The effects of the extract on body weight showed a slight increase in weight of the animals across the experimental groups (Table 1). It is more visible in experimental groups II and III compared to the control. However, the mean weight taken at the end of the experiment showed that the increase in weight is not statistically significant ($P\leq0.05$).

Table 1: Effect of extract administration of Anogeissus leiocarpus on body weight of rats after 6 week

Group	n	Mean weight (g)±SEM	Mean weight (g)±SEM	Mean weight(g) ±SEM	Mean weight (g)±SEM	Mean weight(g) ±SEM	Mean weight(g) ±SEM	Mean weight(g) ±SEM	P-value
		0week	1st	2nd	3rd	4th	5th	6th	
I-Control	6	146±5.1	145±5.0	146±5.1	146±5.1	147±5.3	146±5.1	147±4.0	0.47
II-200mg/kg	6	142±4.2	142±4.2	143±4.3	145±4.8	144±4.5	146±4.7	146±4.9	0.46
III-400mg/kg	6	137±4.1	137±4.1	138±4.2	139±4.3	140±5.3	141±3.9	141±5.1	0.46
IV-600mg/kg	6	135±4.5	134±4.7	135±4.5	137±4.1	137±3.9	138±4.0	141±5.3	0.49

Effect of Different Doses of Extract on the Weight of the Reproductive tract of the Animals

The reproductive tract (fallopian tubes, ovaries, and the uterus) of the experimental rats, showed no significant difference in weight ($P\leq0.05$) at the end of the extract administration in groups II and III when compared with the control group (Table 2). There is a statistically significant increase however in the high dose group (IV) ($P\leq0.05$) compared to the control.

Table 2: Weight of the uterus, fallopian tubes, and ovaries across the experimental groups

Group	Weight of Uterus, fallopian tubes, and Ovaries Mean weight (g)±SEM	Body weight/ Organ ratio Mean weight (g)±SEM	P- value
I-Control	0.54±0.04	242±5.3	0.043
II-200mg/kg	0.56±0.04	260±5.1	0.047
III-400mg/kg	0.56±0.04	251±4.9	0.046
IV–600mg/kg	0.57±0.06	272±4.0	0.057*

P<0.05; SEM=Standard Error in Mean; *=Statistically significant

Effect of Different Doses of Extract on the Number of Ovarian Follicles

There was an increased folliculogenesis, which shows an increase in the number of tertiary follicles in the treatment group that received 200mg/kg (group II) compared with the control (Table 3). An increase in primary and secondary follicles was also observed in the group that received extract concentration of 400mg/kg (group III) was also observed ($P \leq 0.05$) compared to the control group.

Table 3: Number of follicles across each experimental group

Group	Follicles		
	Primary follicles Mean±SEM	Secondary follicles Mean±SEM	Tertiary follicles Mean±SEM
I-Control	96.3±3.70*	39.8±2.90	13.6±1.47
II-200mg/kg	94.2±3.70	37.1±2.90	14.2±1.47*
III-400mg/kg	98.7±3.70	47.1±2.90*	12.5±1.47
IV-600mg/kg	87.1±3.70	34.1±2.90	2.8±1.47

P<0.05; SEM=Standard error in mean; *=Statistically Significant

Histological Slides

The histological features of the ovaries in the experimental group (II) showed normal features of the ovary as evidence by the presence of follicles in different stages of development, as in the control group (Figure 1). There is normal histological architecture of the ovary with the cortex and the medulla clearly visible, and the presence of oocytes at different stages of development. There was an increase in the number of secondary follicles in the treatment group that received extract concentration of 400mg/kg (group III), a distinct follicles can be seen in the ovarian surface (Figure 2), with the outer surface epithelium, and the tunica albuginea, as seen in the control group.

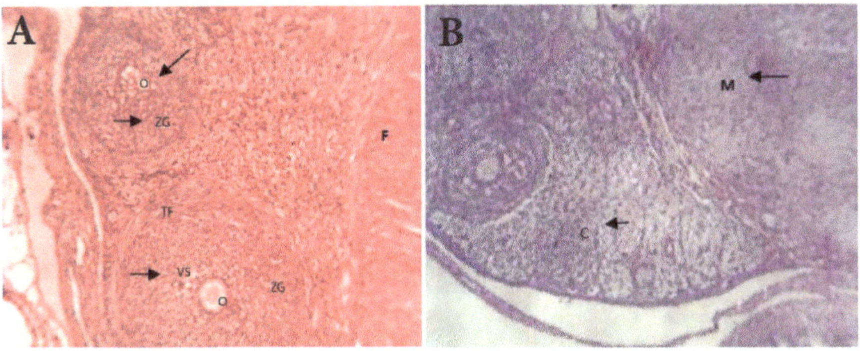

Figure 1: Photomicrograph showing a cross section of the ovary of (A) Group that received 200mg/kg body weight, (B) Control group, showing normal architecture of the ovary with primary Oocyte (O); Theca Folliculi (TF); Vesicular Spaces (VS); Zona Granulosa (ZG); Ovarian Cortex (C); Ovarian Medulla (M). (H&Ex100).

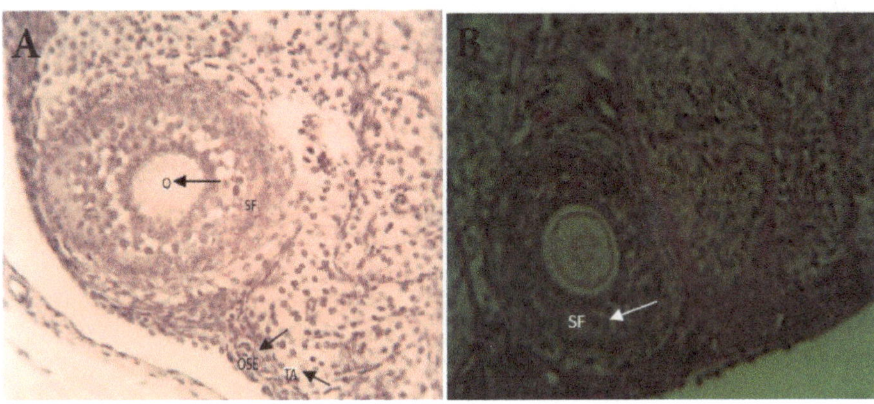

Figure 2: Photomicrograph showing a cross section of the ovary of (A) Group III received 400mg/kg body weight, and (B) Control group, both showing normal architecture of the ovary with primary Oocyte (O); Outer Surface Epithelium (OSE); TunicaAlbuginea (TA). (Pasx250).

The presence of more primary follicle (PF) was observed in the group that received extract concentration of 200mg/kg (group II), as compared with the control. The presence of outer surface epithelium (OSE) and the tunica albuginea can also be seen (Figure 3).

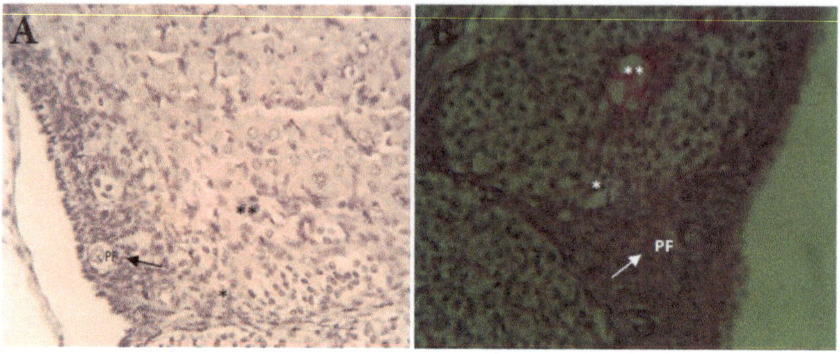

Figure 3: Photomicrograph showing the cross section of the ovary with a primary follicle from (A) Group II that received 200mg/kg, and (B) Control group; (*) positive PAS reaction. (PASx250).

DISCUSSION

Changes in body weight were observed across all the experimental groups. This increase was more pronounced in the treatment groups (I, II and III). The increase in the weight of the control group was non-significant. This suggests that the extract did have an effect on the rate of food intake and utilization, thus confirming the studies conducted by [6], on the hypoglycemic effect of the leaf extract of *A. leiocarpus* on blood glucose utilization in wistar rats, which has more effect at a dose of 400mg/kg.

The histological slides of the ovaries showed no gross or histological changes as a result of the extract administration. There was simple cuboidal epithelium with typical features throughout its extent. The medulla was well formed and contains blood vessels and abundant amount of fibroconnective tissue. The medulla was well formed and shows normal histological structure of the wistar rat ovary.

A precise border between the cortex and the medulla cannot be distinguished, characteristics of the normal structure of the mouse ovary. There was a significant decrease in the number of primary and tertiary follicles (2.8±1.47; 87.1±3.70), compared with the control group (96.8±3.70). Also, a significant increase in the number of primary follicle in group II (400mg/kg), compared with the control group was observed, (98.7±3.70), and (96.8±3.70). This finding is the first reported on the effect of the stem bark extract of Anogeissus leiocarpus on follicular dynamics.

AUTHORS' CONTRIBUTIONS

Authors' contributions	MMJ	OSA	BEK	**ZSR**
Research concept and design	√	√	--	--
Collection and/or assembly of data	√	√	√	√
Data analysis and interpretation	√	√	√	--
Writing the article	√	--	--	--

Critical revision of the article	√	√	√	√
Final approval of article	√	√	√	√
Statistical analysis	√	--	√	--

ACKNOWLEDGEMENT

We wish to acknowledge the contribution of Umar Ahmad of the Universiti Putra Malaysia (UPM) for his contribution to data analysis, and Mr. Mairiga of the department of histopathology ABUTH Shika, Zaria for helping during my slide preparation.

REFERENCES

1. Mann A, Y. Yahaya, A. Banso and G. O. Ajayi. Phytochemical andantibacterialscreening of Anogeissus leiocarpus against some microorganisms associated withinfectious wounds. *Academic Journals*. 2010.
2. Plowchalk D.R, B.J. Smith and D.R. Mattison. Methods in toxicology. *Academic Press Inc*. 1993; 57-66.
3. Takahashi T and Ohnishi J. **Molecular mechanism of follicle rupture during ovulation**. *Zoolog Sci*. 1995;12:359-65.
4. Apulu N, Dada J. O, Odama L. E. and Galadima M. Antibacterial activity of aqueousextract of some Nigerian medicinal plants. *Nigerian Journal of Botany*. 1994; 7:45-48.
5. Smith BJ, Plowchalk DR, Sipes IG and Mattison DR. **Comparison of random and serial sections in assessment of ovarian toxicity**. *Reprod Toxicol*. 1991; 5:379-83.
6. Chen TH, Chen SC, Chan P, Chu YL, Yang HY and Cheng JT. **Mechanism of the hypoglycemic effect of stevioside, a glycoside of Stevia rebaudiana**. *Planta Med*. 2005; 71:108-13.

9
CHAPTER

EVALUATION OF HISTOPATHOLOGICAL AND ULTRASTRUCTURAL CHANGES IN THE TESTIS OF TADALAFIL TREATED ADULT MALE ALBINO RATS

Hagar A. Hashish

Keywords: Tadalafil, testis, sertoli cells, seminefrous tubules, leydig cells

INTRODUCTION

Male infertility is a private problem. However the assisted reproductive technology (ART) is a line of management for infertility due to male etiology, significant percent of infertile males still infertile after intrauterine insemination or *in vitro*fertilization (IVF) techniques. There was no ideal medication for treatment of the infertile males. So, it appears that modern medication with a positive effect on male infertility is essential. PDE5 (PhosphoDiestrase Enzyme) inhibitors are line of management for male infertility [1].

It is known that inhibition of the enzyme phosphodiesterase (PDE) type 5 can maintain nitric oxide induced smooth muscle relaxation in the corpus cavernosum of penis and socause penile erection [2,3]. PDE5 is well expressed in the smooth muscle cells of the penile corpus cavernosum and the smooth muscle cells in blood vesselsin the lung, so PDE5 inhibitors can manage erectile dysfunction (ED) [4] and pulmonary hypertension [5].

Although the most of the data about PDE5 inhibitors and ED comes from studies on sildenafil [6], two new PDE5 inhibitors; tadalafil [7] and vardenafil [8] are recently available for the treatment of ED.

Citation: Hagar A. Hashish, Evaluation of histopathological and ultrastructural changes in the testis of tadalafil treated adult male albino rats, DOI : http://dx.doi.org/10.7243/2055-091X-2-18.

The three PDE-5 inhibitors have same mode of action, but their selectivity differs for PDE-5. Sildenafil and vardenafilless selective for PDE5 than tadalafil [9].

Tadalafil is efficient, reversible and selective PDE5 Inhibitor. It is used as an oral therapy in ED casused by psychological, organic or mixed factor [7]. It is a long-acting therapy [10]. Its half-life is about 17.5 hour, high-fat foods do not interfere with tadalafil's absorption rate in contrast with Sildenafil and vardenafil [11]. Tadalafil is also known to cause less visual manifistations like abnormal color vision in contrast to the other two drugs [9].

This study was designed to evaluate the effect of tadalafil on the histologicsl structure and ultrastructure ofadult male albino rats testis.

MATERIALS AND METHODS

Experimental animals

Twenty-four adult male albino rats (4-6 months old, 200-350gm weight) were used. The use of the animals was prospectively approved by the Committee at Mansoura University, Faculty of Medicine. The rats were housed in the Animal Care Centre of Mansoura faculty of Pharmacy. The rats were provided with fresh food and water daily and inspected for any possible signs of infection (e.g., redness or ulceration of skin).

Experimental design

Animals were divided into four groups (6 rats each). The first group used as a control group. The other three groups were used as treated groups.

Tadalafil administration

Group 1 (Control group): received oral saline solution via orogastric feeding tube for 4 weeks.

Group 2 (treated): 9mg/kg tadalafil dissolved in distilled water daily for 30 days, through orogastric feeding tube (equivalent to 10 mg adult human dose).

Group 3 (treated): received 1.8mg/kg tadalafil dissolved in distilled water daily for 30 days, through orogastric feeding tube(equivalent to 20 mg adult human dose) [12].

Group 4 (treated): received 2.6mg/kg body weight of tadalafil dissolved in distilled water daily for 30 days, through orogastric feeding tube. The giving doses were similar to the recommended human oral doses 40 mg. Tadalafil was supplied from Pfizer Inc. (Pfizer, Egypt), stored at 2-4°C and protected from sunlight.

Histological analysis

At the end of treatment, rats of each group were anaesthetized with with Ketamine (60 mg/kg i.p.) and perfused intracardially with 0.9% NaCl, followed by 4% paraformaldehyde in 0.1 M phosphate buffer (PB) pH 7.2. The testis was carefully dissected and removed. Both testiswere taken and weighted. one of them was immersed in 0% paraformaldehyde solution for 24 hours. The specimens were processed for paraffin sections of 5 µm-thickness and stained with H&E for histological examination.

Tissue preparation for ultrastructural study

The other testis was cut into small pieces 1mm^3 each. Specimens were immediately fixed in cold 3.5% glutaraldehyde and washed in 0.1 M phosphate buffer (PH 7.2). Then, postfixed with 1% osmium tetraoxide (OsO4), dehydrated and embedded in epoxy resin. Semithin sections (1µm thick) were cut on an LKB ultratome and stained with toluidine blue stain and examined by light microscope. Ultrathin sections (50-70nm thick) were cut, mounted on copper grids, stained with uranyl acetate and lead citrate [13]. Sections were examined by JEOL-100SX transmission electron microscope provided with a digital camerain the Electron Microscopic Unit of Tanta Faculty of Medicine.\

Quantitative analysis

The transverse and longitudinal diameters of the seminiferous tubules were measured. The number of cells in tests were measured in a fixed field in serial sections by LeicaQuin 500" image analyzer computer system (England). The cells were counted in five fixed non-overlapping microscopic fields using a 100×objective lens.

Statistical analysis

Statistical analysis was done using computer software SPSS program (statistical package for social science) version 10. All data were expressed as the mean±SD. The significance level considered was $P \leq 0.05$.

RESULTS

Light microscopic examination

Group 1 (control group)

Histological examination of H&E and toluidine blue stained sections in the testis of the control group showed multiple rounded seminiferous tubules with regular outlines. They were lined by 4-6 layers of germinal epithelium at different stages of spermatogenesis. The flagella of mature sperms were seen in the lumen of the tubules. The lining epithelium consisted of Sertoli cells and other germinal cells. Sertoli cells appeared pyramidal in shape and resting on the basement membrane. The germinal epithelium consisted of spermatogonia, 1ry spermatocytes, rounded spermatids and elongated spermatids. The interstitial spaces in-between the tubules contained Leydig cells and some blood vessels (Figure 1).

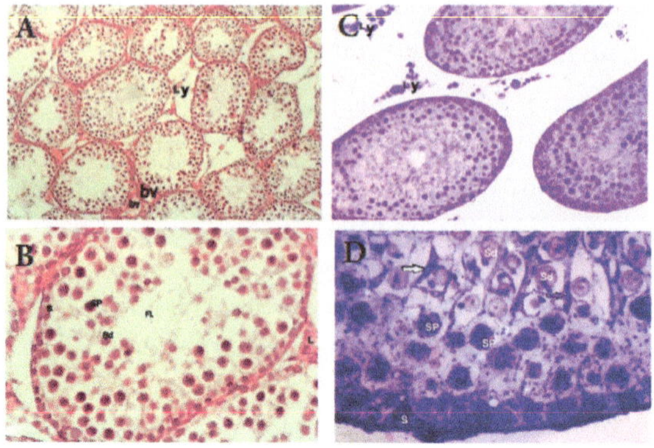

Figure 1: Photomicrograph of sections in control tests; A. Multiple rounded seminiferous tubules with regular outlines, lined by layers of germinal epithelium. The interstitial spaces in-between the tubules contain Leydig cells (Ly) and some blood vessels (bv) (H&E x100). B. The flagella of mature sperms are seen in the lumen of the tubules (FL), Sertoli cells (S), 1ry spermatocyte (Sp), rounded spermatids (Sd) (H&E x400). C. Seminefrous tubules with interstial cells of leydig (Ly) (Touldine blue x100). D. Higher magnification of C, showing Sertoli cells (S), 1ry spermatocyte (Sp), rounded spermatids (Sd), elongated spermatid (arrows) (Touldine blue x400).

Group 2 (treated-T1)

L/M examination of testicular sections of this group showed seminiferous tubules with germinal epithelium. The flagella of sperms were obvious in the lumen. Sertoli cells were seen resting on the basement membrane. The spermatogenic cells were noticed; 1ry spermatocyte, round spermatid and elongated sperms. Areas of intercellular vacuoles were detected. The interstitial space showed some Leydig cells seperated bycongested blood vessels (Figure 2).

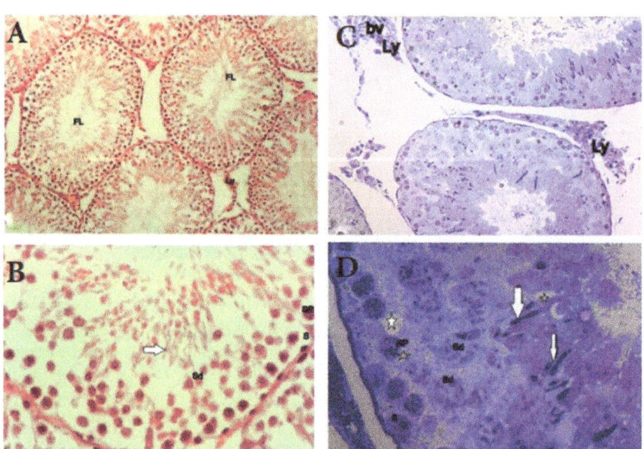

Figure 2: Photomicrograph of sections in treated tests (T1); A. Seminiferous tubules with germinal epithelium. The flagella of mature sperms are seen in the lumen of the tubules (FL). The

interstitial spaces in-between the tubules contain Leydig cells (Ly) (H&E x100). B. Sertoli cells are resting on the basement membrane (S). The spermatogenic cells are noticed; 1ry spermatocyte (Sp), round spermatid (Sd) elongated sperms (arrow) (H&E x400). C. Seminefrous tubules with interstial cells of leydig (Ly) and congested blood vessels (bv) (Touldine blue x100). D. Higher magnification of C, showing Sertoli cells (S), 1ry spermatocyte (Sp), rounded spermatids (Sd), elongated spermatid (arrows) Areas of intercellular vacuoles are detected (*) (Touldine blue x400).

Group 3 (treated-T2)

L/M examination of testicular sections of this group showed some seminiferous tubules with irregular outline. The flagella of sperms were obvious in the lumen. Sertoli cells were seen resting on the thin, irregular basement membrane. The spermatogenic cells were noticed; 1ry spermatocyte, round spermatid and elongated sperms. More areas of intercellular vacuoles were detected. The interstitial space showed some Leydig cells seperated by congested blood vessels (Figure 3).

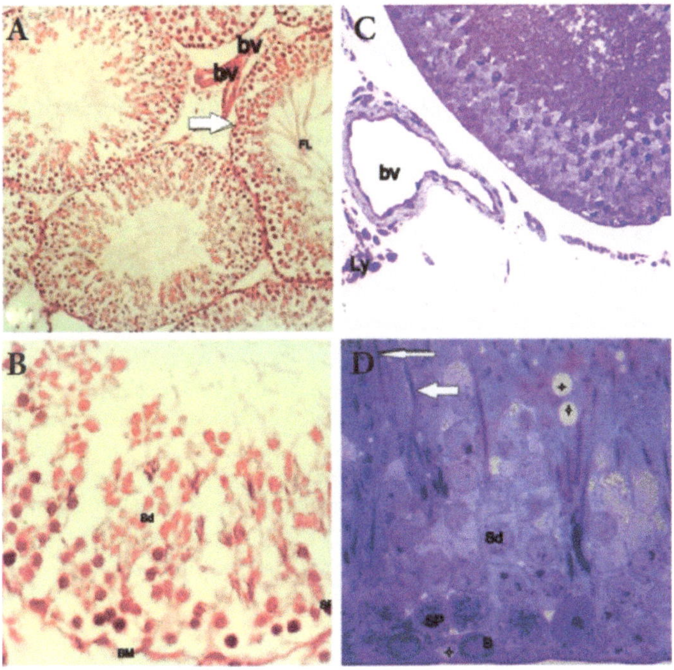

Figure 3 : Photomicrograph of sections in treated tests (T2); A. Some seminiferous tubules with irregular outline (arrow). The flagella of mature sperms are seen in the lumen of the tubules (FL). The interstitial spaces in-between the tubules contain Leydig cells (Ly), congested blood vessels (bv) (H&E x100). B. 1ry spermatocyte (Sp), round spermatid (Sd) resting on thin, irregular basement membrane (BM) (H&E x400). C. Seminefrous tubules with interstial cells of leydig(Ly) and blood vessel (bv) (Touldine blue x100). D. Higher magnification of C, showing Sertoli cells (S), 1ry spermatocyte (Sp), rounded spermatids (Sd), elongated spermatid (arrows) Areas of intercellular vacuoles are detected (*) (Touldine blue x400).

Group 4 (treated-T3)

L/M examination of testicular sections of this group showed seminiferous tubules with irregular outline with acidophilic exudate in their lumen. Some spermatogenic cells showed signs of degeneration, vacuolated cytoplasm and pyknotic nuclei. Increased areas of cellular loss and vaculation. Congested blood vessels between tubules (Figure 4).

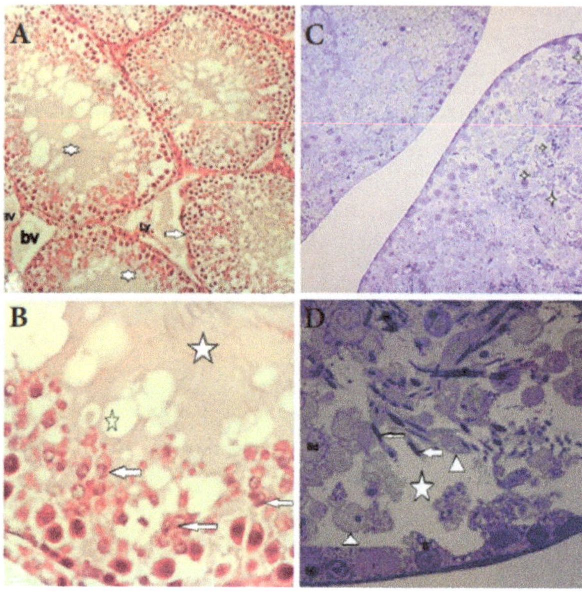

Figure 4: Photomicrograph of sections in treated tests (T3); A. Some seminiferous tubules with irregular outline (arrow), and acidophilic exudate in their lumen and interestial space (*). Interstial cells of leydig (Ly) and congested blood vessel (bv) are noticed (H&E x100). B. Some spermatogenic cells showed signs of degeneration, vacuolated cytoplasm and pyknotic nuclei (arrows). Incresed areas of cellular loss and vaculation. And acidophilic exudate in the lumen (*) (H&E x400). C. Seminefrous tubules with intercellular vaculation(*) (Touldine blue x100). D. Higher magnification of C, showing Sertoli cells (S), rounded spermatids (Sd), elongated spermatid (arrows) Areas of intercellular vacuoles are detected (*). Degnerated cells with pyknotic nuclei (arrow heads) (Touldine blue x400).

Transmission electron microscopic results (TEM)

Group 1 (control group)

The ultrastructure of the control testis showed Sertoli cell, were resting on the basement membrane with adjacent myoid cell. The nucleus appeared triangular and euchromatic with welldeveloped nucleolus. The cytoplasm showed some organelles like mitochondria, and ribosomes. The inter-Sertoli junctional specialization with adjacent cells was apparent (Figure 5A). The germinal epithelium showed different stages of maturation. The primary spermatocytes appeared as large rounded cells, with rounded nucleus and dispersed granular chromatin. The cytoplasm showed mitochondria, ribosomes, and lysosmoes (Figure 5B). The rounded spermatids showed rounded nucleus with fine granular chromatin. Acrosomal vesicle was apparent over the anterior part of the nucleus to form acrosomal cap. The cytoplasm contained mitochondria and ribosomes (Figure 5C). The fusiform spermatids showed elongated pyriform nuclei. Acrosomal cap could be noticed on the anterior part of the nucleus (Figures 5D and 5E). The interstitial cells of Leydig showed nuclei with thin peripheral rim of chromatin. The cytoplasm showed organelles like mitochondria, lysosomes and smooth endoplasmic reticulum (Figure 5F).

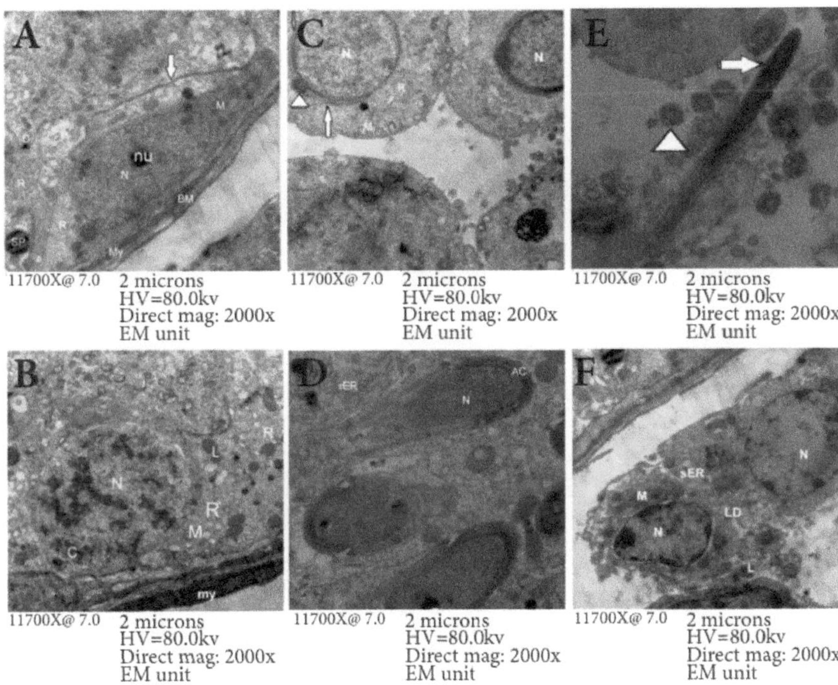

Figure 5: Photomicrogragh of ultrastructure of the control testis A. Sertoli cell, resting on the basement membrane(BM) with adjacent myoid cell (My). The nucleus appears triangular and euchromatic (N) with well developed nucleolus (nu). The cytoplasm shows some organelles, mitochondria (M), and ribosomes (R). The inter-Sertolijunctional specialization with adjacent cells is apparent (arrow). B. The primary spermatocytes appear as large rounded cells, with rounded nucleus (N) and dispersed granular chromatin (C).The cytoplasm shows mitochondria(M), ribosomes(R)lysosmoes (L). C. The rounded spermatids with rounded nucleus with fine granular chromatin (N). Acrosomal vesicle is apparent (arrow head) to form acrosomal cap (arrows). The cytoplasm contains mitochondria (M) and ribosomes(R). D. The fusiform spermatids with elongated pyriform nuclei (N). Acrosomal cap is noticed (Ac). (E) Mature sperm (arrow), multiple cross sections of sperm middle piece (arrow head). (F) The interstitial cells of Leydig, nucleus with thin peripheral rim of chromatin (N). The cytoplasm organelles like mitochondria (M), lysosomes(L), lipid droplet (LD) and smooth endoplasmic reticulum (sER).

Group 2 (treated-T1)

The ultrastructure of the treated testis revealed normal Sertoli cells, which showed triangular nucleus with prominent nucleolus and fine granular chromatin. The cytoplasm contained some normal and some dilated mitochondria (Figure 6A). The spermatogonia appeared large rounded cell, with irregular nuclear membrane, the cytoplasm contained ballooned mitochondria, lysosmomes, vacuoles, ribosomes and smooth endoplasmic reticulum. 1ry spermatocyte appear with large rounded nucleus (Figures 6B and 6C). Rounded spermatids appeared with spherical nuclei and incomplete acrosomal caps. Cross sections of the middle pieces of numerous spermatozoa could be also seen (Figure 6D). The elongated spermatids showed pyriform shaped nuclei with acrosomal cap (Figure 6E). The interstitial cells of Leydig appeared with slight indentation in the nuclear membrane. The cytoplasm contained mitochondria, lysosomes and vacuoles (Figure 6F).

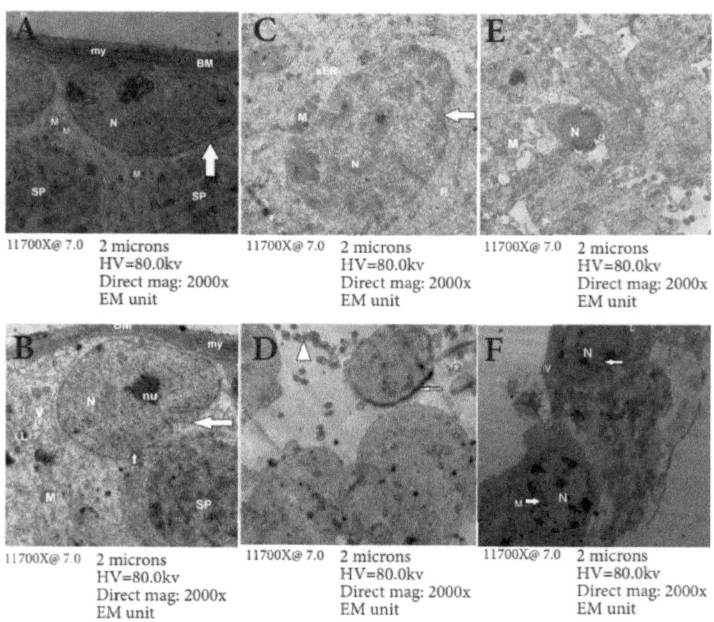

Figure 6: Photomicrogragh of ultrastructure of the treated testis (T1) A. Sertoli cells, with triangular nucleus with prominent nucleolus (nu) and fine granular chromatin (N). The cytoplasm contains some normal and some dilated mitochondria (M). B&C. The spermatogonia appear large rounded cell, with irregular nuclear membrane (arrows). The cytoplasm with ballooned mitochondria (M), lysosmomes (L), vacuoles (V), ribosomes (R), smooth endoplasmic reticulum (sER). 1ry spermatocyte appear with large rounded nucleus (sp) D. Rounded spermatids with spherical nuclei and incomplete acrosomal caps (arrow). Cross sections of the middle pieces of spermatozoa could be also seen (arrow head). E. The elongated spermatids show pyriform shaped nucleus (N) with acrosomal cap (AC). F. The interstitial cells of Leydig appeared with slight indentation in the nuclear membrane (arrows). The cytoplasm contained mitochondria (M), lysosomes (L) and vacuoles (V).

Group 3 (treated-T2)

The examination of the treated testis in this group showed abnormal structure of Sertoli cells, its nucleus appeared with irregular nuclear membrane, the cytoplasm contained ballooned mitochondria. The inter-Sertolijunctional specialization with adjacent cells was interrupted (Figure 7A). The spermatogonia showed nucleus with irregular nuclear membrane, the cytoplasm contained ballooned mitochondria, ribosomes, dilated smooth cytoplasmic reticulum and some vaculated areas (Figure 7B). Round spermatid showed rounded nucleus with incomplete acrosomal caps. The cytoplasm contained rounded mitochondriaand ribosomes (Figure 7C). The elongated spermatids showed pyriform shaped nuclei. Ectoplasmic specialization could be observed between the Sertoli cell and the spermatids. The ectoplasmic specialization composed of three layers; Sertoli cell plasma membrane, surface cistern of smooth endoplasmic reticulum that lies parallel to the plasma membrane, and layer of actin filaments located between the plasma membrane and surface cistern (Figure 7D). Some abnormal forms of sperms could be seen (Figures 7D and 7E). The interstitial cells of Leydig appeared with indented nuclei. The cytoplasm contained lysosomes, mitochondria, and vacuoles (Figure 7F).

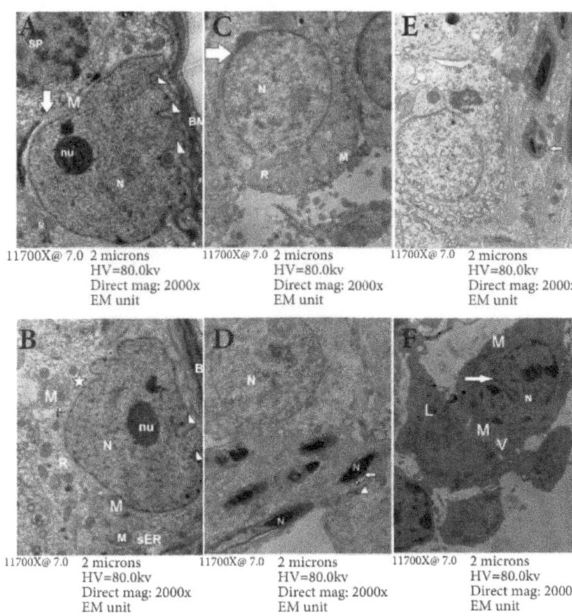

Figure 7: Photomicrogragh of ultrastructure of the treated testis (T2) A. Sertoli cell nucleus with irregular nuclear membrane (arrow heads) and fine granular chromatin. The cytoplasm contains ballooned mitochondria (M). The inter-Sertoli junctional specialization with adjacent cells is interrupted (arrow). B. The spermatogonia showed nucleus with irregular nuclear membrane (arrow heads). The cytoplasm shows ballooned mitochondria (M), ribosomes (R), dilated smooth cytoplasmic reticulum (sER) and some vaculated areas (*). C. Round spermatid with rounded nucleus and incomplete acrosomal caps (arrow). The cytoplasm contains rounded mitochondria (M) and ribosomes(R). D. The elongated spermatids with pyriform shaped nuclei (N). Ectoplasmic specialization can be observed between the Sertoli cell and the spermatids. It is made of three

layers; Sertoli cell plasma membrane (arrow head), surface cistern of smooth endoplasmic reticulum that lies parallel to the plasma membrane (*), and layer of actin filaments located between the plasma membrane and surface cistern (arrow). E. Some abnormal forms of sperms can be seen (arrow). F. The interstitial cells of Leydig appear with indented nuclei (arrow). The cytoplasm contains lysosomes (L), rounded mitochondria (M), and vacuoles (V).

Group 4 (treated-T3)

The examination of the treated testis in this group showed abnormal structure of Sertoli cells. It showed triangular nucleus with irregular membrane, prominent nucleolus, the cytoplasm contained large cytoplasmic clear vacuole, dilated smooth endoplasmic reticulum and lysosome. The inter-Sertolijunctional specialization with adjacent cells was disturbed (Figure 8A). The adjoining primary spermatocytes cells exhibited large nucleus with irregular membrane and clumped chromatin (Figure 8B). Round spermatid showed indented nucleus with dense clumped chromatin. There was complete loss of acrosomal caps. The cytoplasm showed vacuoles and ballooned mitochondria. Some abnormal forms of elongated spermatids were also noticed (Figure 8C). The interstitial cells of Leydig appeared with indented nuclei and clumped chromatin. The cytoplasm contained lysosomes, mitochondria, lipid droplets and vacuoles (Figure 8D).

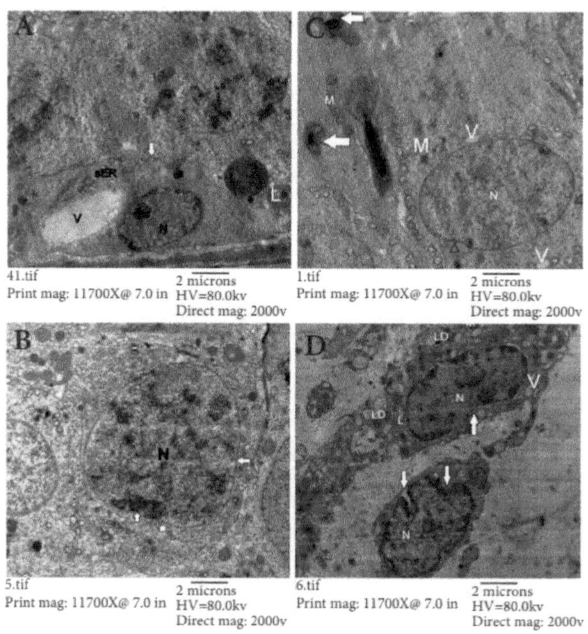

Figure 8: Photomicrogragh of ultrastructure of the treated testis (T3) A. Sertoli cells with triangular nucleus with irregular membrane (N), prominent nucleolus (nu). The cytoplasm contains large cytoplasmic clear vacuole (V), dilated smooth endoplasmic reticulum (sER) and lysosome (L). The interSertoli junctional specialization with adjacent cells is disturbed (arrow). B. The adjoining Primary spermatocytes cells shows large nucleus with irregular membrane and clumped chromatin (arrows). C. Round spermatid shows indented nucleus with dense clumped chromatin

(arrow head). There is complete loss of acrosomal caps. The cytoplasm contains vacuoles (V) and ballooned mitochondria (M). Some abnormal forms of elongated spermatids are noticed (arrows). D. The interstitial cells of Leydig with indented nuclei and (arrows) and clumped chromatin. The cytoplasm shows lysosomes (L), mitochondria (M), lipid droplets (LD) and vacuoles (V).

Morphometric results and statistical analysis

Weight of testis

There was no significant change in testicular weight between control and treated groups (Graph 1).

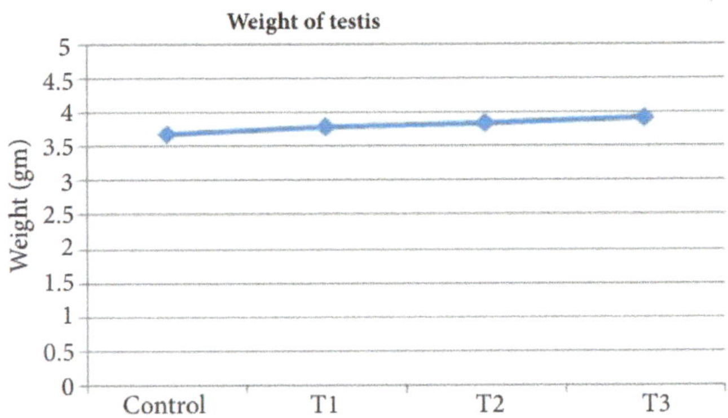

Graph 1: Changes in the weight of tests in all groups.

The mean diameter of seminefrous tubules

In comparison with thecontrol group, the mean diameter of seminiferous tubules showed a significant increase in the treated groups (Graph 2).

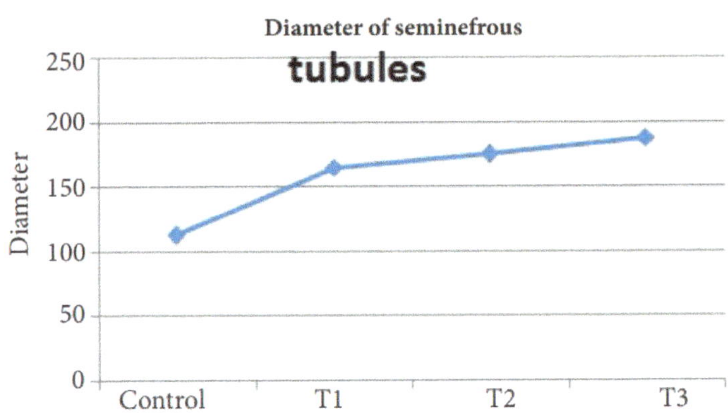

Graph 2: Changes in the diameter in seminefroustubules in all groups.

The number of germ cells

In comparison with the control group, the mean number of germ cells showed a significant decrease in the treated groups (Graph 3).

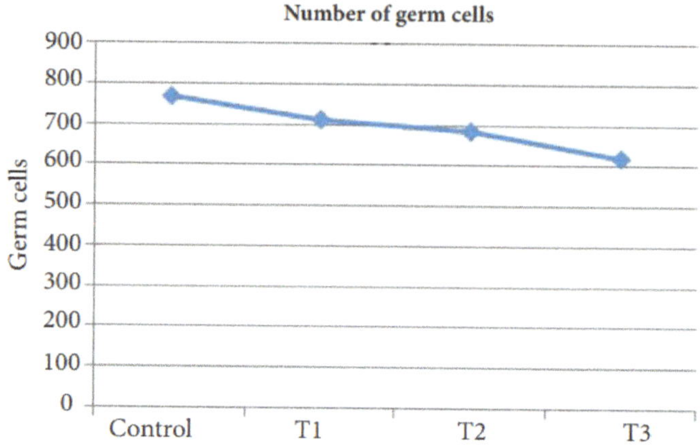

Graph 3: Changes in the number of germ cells in all groups.

DISCUSSION

The PDE-5 inhibitors; sildnafile, tadalafil and vardenafil helped to treat the erectile dysfunction. All three drugs are safe and tolerable. Tadalafil improved erectile dyfunction even in males with type 1 or type 2 diabetes [14].

In this study, the control rat testis showed multiple rounded seminiferous tubules with regular outlines. The lining epithelium consisted of Sertoli cells and other germinal cells. Sertoli cells appeared pyramidal in shape and resting on the basement membrane. The germinal epithelium consisted of spermatogonia, 1ry spermatocytes, rounded spermatids and elongated spermatids. The interstitial spaces in-between the tubules contained Leydig cells and some blood vessels.

The ultrastructure of the Sertoli cell showed that the nucleus appeared triangular and euchromatic with well developed nucleolus. The inter-Sertoli junctional specialization with adjacent cells was apparent. The primary spermatocytes appeared as large rounded cells, with rounded nucleus and dispersed granular chromatin. The rounded spermatids showed rounded nucleus with fine granular chromatin. Acrosomal vesicle was apparent over the anterior part of the nucleus. The fusiform spermatids showed elongated pyriform nuclei. Acrosomal cap could be noticed on the anterior part of the nucleus. The interstitial cells of Leydig showed nuclei with thin peripheral rim of chromatin. This comes in agreement with the histological and ultrasructure of the controladult rat testis [15].

The treated group testicular sections which received the least dose of tadalafil, 0.9 mg/kg orally, showed seminiferous tubules with germinal epithelium. The flagella of sperms were obvious in the lumen. Areas of intercellular vacuoles were detected.

The interstitial space showed some Leydig cells separated by congested blood vessels. The ultrastructure of the treated testis revealed normal Sertoli cells, which showed triangular nucleus with prominent nucleolus and fine granular chromatin. The cytoplasm contained some normal and some dilated mitochondria. The spermatogonia appeared as rounded cell, with irregular nuclear memmbrane. Rounded spermatids appeared with spherical nuclei and incomplete acrosomal caps. Cross sections of the middle pieces of numerous spermatozoa could be also seen. The elongated spermatids showed pyriform shaped nuclei with acrosomal cap. The interstitial cells of Leydig appeared with slight indentation in the nuclear membrane. The cytoplasm contained mitochondria, lysosomes and vacuoles. The diameter of seminefrous tubule increased in this group when compared with control group. The number of germ cells showed significant decrease in this group when compared with the control group.

In contrast to this study, It was reported that single dose of sildenafil increased the total sperm count and the percente of motile sperms in semen samples after sildenafil intake compared with semen samples before use of sildenafil. However, long time use of sildenafil treatment is associated with a significant decrease in total sperm count. In another study, vardenafil administration (10 mg) showed a significantly increase in the number of spermatozoa and percentage of morphologically normal spermatozoa [16].

In this research, L/M examination of testicular sections of treated group received 1.8 mg/kg, showed some seminiferous tubules with irregular outline. The basement appeared thin,more areas of intercellular vacuoles were detected. The interstitial space showed some Leydig cells seperated by congested blood vessels. The ultrastructure examination, showed abnormal structure of Sertoli cells, the nucleus with irregular nuclear membrane, the cytoplasm contained ballooned mitochondria. The inter-Sertoli junctional specialization with adjacent cells was interrupted. The spermatogonia showed nucleus with irregular nuclear membrane, the cytoplasm contained ballooned mitochondria, ribosomes, dilated smooth cytoplasmic reticulum and some vaculated areas. Round spermatid showed rounded nucleus with incomplete acrosomal caps. The elongated spermatids showed pyriform shaped nuclei. The interstitial cells of Leydig appeared with indented nuclei, the cytoplasm contained lysosomes, mitochondria, and vacuoles. The diameter of seminefrous tubule increased in this group when compared with control group. The number of germ cells showed significant decrease in this group when compared with the control group.

In agreement with this result, it was concluded that tadalafil caused a significant decrease in sperm count and motility with increased incidence of abnormal forms. Histological examination showed loosely packed stroma around seminiferous tubules with reduction in number of spermatogenic cells [12]. Also, it was documented that administration of 50 mg sildenafil caused degeneration of somniferous tubules and the spermatogenic cells. The interstitial tissue showed congested blood vessels, degenerated leydig cells. The basement membrane was thin [17]. It was concluded that of sildenafil citrate (50 mg) administration caused significant reduction in the number of sperms [18].

In contrast, it was reported that administration of 10-mg and 20-mg tadalafil in human every day for six months, showed insignificant change in the sperm morphology

[19]. Also, it was found that administration of single dose of sildenafil (50 mg) in young infertile males resulted in significant increase in sperm motility, while, tadalafil single dose (20 mg) caused reduction in the motility of the sperms. It was found that impact of sildenafil on the motility of sperms mightbe due tochanges in mitochondria and calcium channels [20].

The Sertoli cell tight junctions is a vital component of the blood-testis barrier which is essential for normal spermatogenesis. The interrupted inter-Sertoli junctional specialization in case of tadalafil administration may be explained by the fact defective testicular blood barrier could cause opening of the testicular blood barrier gate. This disturb the protective and nutritional function of the barrier and impair spermatogenesis [21]. L/M examination of testicular sections of the group received 2.6 mg/kg showed seminiferous tubules with irregular outline with acidophilic exudate in their lumen and congested blood vessels in between. Some spermatogenic cells showed signs of degeneration; vacuolated cytoplasm and pyknotic nuclei. Increased areas of cellular loss and vaculation in the tubules. The ultrastructure of treated testis in this group showed abnormal structure of Sertoli cells. It showed triangular nuclei with irregular membrane, the cytoplasm contained large cytoplasmic clear vacuoles, dilated smooth endoplasmic reticulum and lysosome. The inter-Sertoli functional specialization with adjacent cells was disturbed. Round spermatid showed indented nucleus with dense clumped chromatin. There was complete loss of acrosomal cap. The cytoplasm showed vacuoles and ballooned mitochondria. Some abnormal forms of elongated spermatids were also noticed with defected ectoplamic specialization. The interstitial cells of Leydig appeared with indented nuclei, the cytoplasm contained lysosomes, mitochondria, lipid droplets and vacuoles. The diameter of seminefrous tubule increased in this group when compared with control group. The number of germ cells showed significant decrease in this group when compared with the control group.

In agreement with this result, it was documented that administration of 100 mg sildenafil caused degeneration of somniferous tubules with thin basement membrane and the spermatogenic cells, the interstitial tissue showed congested blood vessels, degenerated leydig cells [17]. However, it was noticed that 100-mg sildenafil citrate in diabetic patients increased sperm motility and semen volume [22].

In the same time, it was documented that administration of 100-mg singledose of sildenafil had no significant effect on sperm motility, sperm count or morphology in human [23]. Also, single dose of vardenafil (20 mg) had no significant effects on sperm motility, sperm viability, and sperm morphology in males [24].

In this study, round spermatid in treated rats showed incomplete or absent acrosomal cap. Some elongated spermatids showed abnormal nuclei, shape and defective ectoplasmic specialization. According to some authors, the ectoplasmic specialization, which is unique to the testis, have an essential role in spermatid nuclear shaping. F-actin filaments from normal Sertoli cells enhance spermatid head elongation [25]. So, abnormal Sertoli cell may affect spermatid nuclear shaping.

On the other hand, it was reported that PDE5 inhibitors may enhance the capacitation of spermatids [18,26,27]. cGMPcan opencyclic nucleotide-gated channels for calcium entry inside he spermatozoa to initiate the acrosome reaction. However, PDE5 cause hydrolysis of cGMP, so, inhibition of PDE5 by sildenafil citrate can trigger the effect of cGMP on sperm acrosomal reaction [28].

In this investigation, the diameter of seminefrous tubules increased in treated rats when compared with control rats. Similar result was reported in case of sildenafil and explained by the vasoactive of the drug, which may occur in other PDE5 inhibitors [29].

CONCLUSION

It can be concluded that, long-term daily use of tadalafil can lead to noticeable pathological effect in the testis which may be implicated in male fertility and this effect is dose dependent, so the effect of tadalafil necessitates further investigations.

ACKNOWLEDGEMENT

The author thanks Prof. Dr. Amany M Shams professor of Anatomy and all the staff members of Anatomy and Embryology Department in Faculty of Medicine, Mansoura University, Egypt, for their cooperation and helpful comments during this work.

REFERENCES

1. Dimitriadis F, Tsampalas S, Tsounapi P, Giannakis D, Chaliasos N, Baltogiannis D, Miyagawa I, Saito M, Takenaka A and Sofikitis N. Effects of phosphodiesterase-5 inhibitor vardenafil on testicular androgen-binding protein secretion, the maintenance of foci of advanced spermatogenesis and the sperm fertilising capacity in azoospermic men. *Andrologia*. 2012; 44 Suppl 1:144-53.
2. Boolell M, Allen MJ, Ballard SA, Gepi-Attee S, Muirhead GJ, Naylor AM, Osterloh IH and Gingell C. Sildenafil: an orally active type 5 cyclic GMP-specific phosphodiesterase inhibitor for the treatment of penile erectile dysfunction. *Int J Impot Res*. 1996; 8:47-52.
3. Rosen RC and Kostis JB. Overview of phosphodiesterase 5 inhibition in erectile dysfunction. *Am J Cardiol*. 2003; 92:9M-18M.
4. Lue TF. Erectile dysfunction. *N Engl J Med*. 2000; 342:1802-1813.
5. Galie N, Ghofrani HA, Torbicki A, Barst RJ, Rubin LJ, Badesch D, Fleming T, Parpia T, Burgess G, Branzi A, Grimminger F, Kurzyna M and Simonneau G. Sildenafil citrate therapy for pulmonary arterial hypertension.*N Engl J Med*. 2005; 353:2148-57.
6. Burls A, Gold L and Clark W. Systematic review of randomised controlled trials of sildenafil (Viagra) in the treatment of male erectile dysfunction. *Br J Gen Pract*. 2001; 51:1004-12.
7. Padma-Nathan H and Giuliano F. Oral drug therapy for erectile dysfunction. *Urol Clin North Am*. 2001;28:321-34.
8. Porst H, Rosen R, Padma-Nathan H, Goldstein I, Giuliano F, Ulbrich E and Bandel T. The efficacy and tolerability of vardenafil, a new, oral, selective

phosphodiesterase type 5 inhibitor, in patients with erectile dysfunction: the first at-home clinical trial. *Int J Impot Res*. 2001; 13:192-9.

9. Gresser U and Gleiter CH. Erectile dysfunction: comparison of efficacy and side effects of the PDE-5 inhibitors sildenafil, vardenafil and tadalafil--review of the literature. *Eur J Med Res*. 2002; 7:435-46. | Pdf |PubMed
10. Kulkarni SK and Patil CS. Phosphodiesterase 5 enzyme and its inhibitors: update on pharmacological and therapeutical aspects. *Methods Find Exp Clin Pharmacol*. 2004; 26:789-99.
11. Arlond LM. Vardenafil and tadalafil Options for erectile dysfunction, Two new PDE-5 inhibitors have demonstrated efficacy and tolerability in clinical trials. *Current Pyscatry*. 2004; 3:51-52.
12. Khalaf MA, Abbas MF and El-Fakahany HM. Effects of chronic tadalafil use on the testes and sperm parameters of old albino rats. *Andrologia*. 2012; 44 Suppl 1:370-5.
13. Hayat M. Principles and techniques of electron microscopy, biological applications. 3rd ed. *CRC press*. 1989; 24-74.
14. Saenz de Tejada I, Anglin G, Knight JR and Emmick JT. Effects of tadalafil on erectile dysfunction in men with diabetes. *Diabetes Care*. 2002; 25:2159-64.
15. Halawa AM. Effect of Sildenafil Adminstration on Ischemia/Reperfusion of the Testis in Adult Albino Rat Light and Electron Microscopic Study. Egypt. *J. Histol*. 2010; 33:380–395.
16. Dimitriadis F, Giannakis D, Pardalidis N, Zikopoulos K, Paraskevaidis E, Giotitsas N, Kalaboki V, Tsounapi P, Baltogiannis D, Georgiou I, Saito M, Watanabe T, Miyagawa I and Sofikitis N. Effects of phosphodiesterase-5 inhibitors on sperm parameters and fertilizing capacity. *Asian J Androl*. 2008; 10:115-33.
17. Al-Fartosi KG. Effect of Long Term Adminstration of Sildenafil Citrate (Viagra) on Some Sperm Characteristic and Tests Architecture of Male Rats. *Bas. J. Vet. Res*. 2009; 8:91-103. | Pdf
18. Glenn DR, McVicar CM, McClure N and Lewis SE. Sildenafil citrate improves sperm motility but causes a premature acrosome reaction in vitro. *Fertil Steril*. 2007; 87:1064-70.
19. Hellstrom WJ, Gittelman M, Jarow J, Steidle C, McMurray J, Talley D, Watts S, Mitchell CL and McGill JM. An evaluation of semen characteristics in men 45 years of age or older after daily dosing with tadalafil 20mg: results of a multicenter, randomized, double-blind, placebo-controlled, 9-month study. *Eur Urol*. 2008; 53:1058-65.
20. Pomara G, Morelli G, Canale D, Turchi P, Caglieresi C, Moschini C, Liguori G, Selli C, Macchia E, Martino E and Francesca F. Alterations in sperm motility after acute oral administration of sildenafil or tadalafil in young, infertile men. *Fertil Steril*. 2007; 88:860-5.

21. McCabe MJ, Tarulli GA, Meachem SJ, Robertson DM, Smooker PM and Stanton PG. Gonadotropins regulate rat testicular tight junctions in vivo. *Endocrinology*. 2010; 151:2911-22.

22. Ali ST and Rakkah NI. Neurophysiological role of sildenafil citrate (Viagra) on seminal parameters in diabetic males with and without neuropathy. *Pak J Pharm Sci*. 2007; 20:36-42.

23. Purvis K, Muirhead GJ and Harness JA. The effects of sildenafil on human sperm function in healthy volunteers. *Br J Clin Pharmacol*. 2002; 53 Suppl 1:53S-60S.

24. Bauer R. J and Rohde G. A single oral dose of vardenafil had no acute effect on sperm motility in healthy males. 27th Annual Meeting of the American Society of Andrology. April 24-27, 2002. Seattle, Washington, USA. J Androl. 2002; 26.

25. Kierszenbaum AL and Tres LL. The acrosome-acroplaxome-manchette complex and the shaping of the spermatid head. *Arch Histol Cytol*. 2004; 67:271-84.

26. Lefievre L, De Lamirande E and Gagnon C. The cyclic GMP-specific phosphodiesterase inhibitor, sildenafil, stimulates human sperm motility and capacitation but not acrosome reaction. *J Androl*. 2000;21:929-37.

27. Cuadra DL, Chan PJ, Patton WC, Stewart SC and King A. Type 5 phosphodiesterase regulation of human sperm motility. *Am J Obstet Gynecol*. 2000; 182:1013-5.

28. Biel M, Sautter A, Ludwig A, Hofmann F and Zong X. Cyclic nucleotide-gated channels--mediators of NO:cGMP-regulated processes. *Naunyn Schmiedebergs Arch Pharmacol*. 1998; 358:140-4.

29. Erol B, Tokgoz H, Hanci V, Bektas S, Akduman B, Yencilek F, Mungan G and Mungan A. Vardenafil reduces testicular damage following ischemia/reperfusion injury in rats. *Kaohsiung J Med Sci*. 2009; 25:374-80.

10

CHAPTER

THE POTENTIAL PROTECTIVE EFFECT OF PROPOLIS ON EXPERIMENTALLY INDUCED HEPATITIS IN ADULT MALE ALBINO RATS. HISTOLOGICAL AND IMMUNOHISTOCHEMICAL STUDY

Abeer M. El-Mahalaway, Amal A. Selim and Faiza Abdul Razzak Mahboub

Keywords: Acute hepatitis, D–galactosamine, lipopolysaccharide, immunohistochemistery, propolis

INTRODUCTION

The liver is a vital organ that plays a key role in the detoxification of exogenous and endogenous substances. It also performs a wide range of metabolic activities required for homeostasis, nutrition and immune defense. A variety of pathological factors including viral hepatitis (especially hepatitis B and C), alcohol and drug abuse, metabolic diseases, autoimmune diseases and congenital abnormalities can cause hepatic injury. Liver fibrosis is the final stage of all chronic hepatic disease. Hepatic stellate cells (HSCs) play a principal role in liver fibrosis. It is a well-known fact that fibrosis has lots of important complications such as portal hypertension, hepatocellular carcinoma, hepatic encephalopathy, spontaneous bacterial peritonitis and hepatorenal syndrome [1,2].

Hepatitis is a major public health problem worldwide, responsible for considerable morbidity and mortality from liver disease. Common causes of hepatitis include viral infection, side effects of certain prescription drugs and overdoses of the over-counter drugs [3].

Among the numerous models of experimental hepatitis, Lipopolysaccharide (LPS)/D-galactosamine (D-GalN) are a well-established hepatotoxicant, inducing liver

Citation: El-Mahalaway AM, Selim AA and Mahboub FAR. The potential protective effect of propolis on experimentally induced hepatitis in adult male albino rats. Histological and immunohistochemical study. J Histol Histopathol. 2015; 2:14. http://dx.doi.org/10.7243/2055-091X-2-14.

damage which closely resembling to human viral hepatitis in its morphological and functional features [4].

LPS is a toxic component of the cell walls of gram-negative bacteria and is widely present in the digestive tracts of humans and animals [5]. D-GalN is an amino sugar selectively metabolized by hepatocytes [6]. The toxicity of D- Gal N is mainly related to depletion of uridine pools that are associated with limited ribonucleic acid (RNA), glycogen and protein synthesis, thus altering hepatocellular function [4].

Currently, hepatoprotective drugs are inadequate, so far no therapy has successfully prevented the progression of hepatic disease; even though newly developed drugs have been used to treat chronic liver disorders, these drugs have often have side effects. Therefore, a special interest has been directed to the use of dietary antioxidants of natural products in the treatment of such disorders and may have a significant role in maintaining health [7,8].

Propolis is considered as one of the most promising natural products has therapeutic and preventive actions. It contains more than 300 compounds from different groups. It contains mostly a mixture of polyphenols, flavonoids (major ingredients). Propolis can be used for treatment of cardiovascular, blood system, respiratory disorders, cancer, digestive tract disorders and dermatological disorders [9-11].

Propolis exhibits a wide spectrum of pharmacological properties such as antioxidant, anti-inflammatory, antibacterial, antiviral, anti-ulcerous, anticarcinogenic properties and immune system support [10,12].

The aim of this study was to evaluate the possible protective effect of propolis on experimental induced hepatitis in adult male albino rats.

MATERIALS AND METHODS

In this study, 40 adult male rats of average weight 150-250 g were used The animals obtained from the animal house, Moshtohor faculty of Veterinary Medicine, Benha University, Moshtohor city, Egypt. Animals were housed in the animal laboratory at the medical research center of Benha faculty of medicine. Strict care and cleaning measures were utilized to keep the animal in a normal healthy state, the animals were kept in animal cages under the prevailing atmospheric conditions and also were fed to standard basal diet and liberal supply of tap water. All ethical protocols for animal treatment were followed and were supervised by the animal facilities. The experimental protocol was approved by the Ethical Committee of Benha faculty of medicine.

Used Drugs

LPS (lipopolysaccharide from Escherichia coli, O55:B5), and N-acetyl D-GalN, were purchased from Sigma-Aldrich Company- Saint Louis, Missouri, USA. Propolis was purchased from a beekeeper. It was dissolved in 1% gum acacia, forming an aqueous solution.

Diagnostic kits

1 For the determination of alanine aminotransferase (ALT), aspartate aminotransferase (AST), and bilirubin using kits were purchased from Bio diagnostic Co, Cairo, Egypt.
2 For the determination of Tumour necrosis factor α (TNF-α): using the a commercially available enzyme-linked immunosorbent assay (ELISA) Ray Bio Rat TNF-α kit (Catalogue number ELR-TNF-α 001, Ray Biotech Inc., 3607 Parkway Lane, Suite 100, Norcross GA 30092, USA).

Experimental procedure

Rats were divided into 4 groups, included 10 rats for each as follows

Group I (Control group)

The 5 rats received intraperitoneally injection of phosphatebuffered saline as vehicle for D-GalN and LPS. They were sacrificed at the same time as the corresponding experimental groups. The other 5 rats received 0.5 ml gum acacia dissolved in distilled water as vehicle for propolis. They were sacrificed at the same time as the corresponding experimental groups.

Group II (Propolis group)

Rats received an aqueous suspension of propolis 200 mg/kg orally by gastric tube daily for 2 weeks [7].

Group III (Hepatitis model group)

Rats received single intraperitoneally injection of D-GalN and LPS (300 mg/kg body weight and 30 μg/kg body weight) dissolved in phosphate-buffered saline 18 hrs before the end of experiment [8].

Group IV (Propolis and hepatitis model group)

Rats received an aqueous suspension of propolis 200 mg/kg orally by gastric tube daily for 2 weeks and received single intraperitoneally injection of D-GalN and LPS (300 mg/kg body weight and 30 μg/kg body weight) dissolved in phosphatebuffered saline 18 hrs before the end of experiment.

The blood was drained from the tail vein by using capillary tubes immediately before the end of the experiment into Eppendorf tubes containing heparin (20 ml, 200 IU/ml). The plasma was separated by centrifugation (5000 rpm for 5 min) and used for biochemical analysis.

Biochemical measurements

Liver function tests

Plasma alanine aminotransferase (ALT), aspartate aminotransferase (AST) [13], total bilirubin [14], albumin [15] were measured.

Tumor necrosis factor α (TNF-α)

Quantitive determination of serum(TNF-α) a hepatic proin flammatory cytokine was carried by using the a commercially available enzyme-linked immunosorbent assay [16].

At the end of the experiment, the rats were scarified by cervical decapitation. Specimens of liver were taken. Paraffin sections of about 5-6 μm were prepared and stained with hematoxylin and eosin(H&E) to verify the histological details & Masson's trichrome to demonstrate the collagen fibers [17].

Imunohistochemistery study

1. Imunohistochemical staining for detection of antiproliferating cell nuclear antigen (PCNA); the primary monoclonal antibody used was anti–PCNA IgG antibody (Santa Cruz Biotechnology Inc., Santa Cruz, CA, USA). The cellular site of the reaction was nuclear and brown color.
2. Imunohistochemical staining for detection of antiTransforming growth factor (TGF β1); the primary monoclonal antibody used was TGF-β1 IgG antibody (Biogen Inc. ,Cambridge, Massachusetts, USA). The cellular site of the reaction was cytoplasmic and brown color.

Imunohistochemical study was conducted using the avidin– biotin peroxidase method. Briefly, sections of about 5 μm were deparaffinized, rehydrated, rinsed in tap water, and embedded in 3% H2O2 for 10 min to block endogenous peroxidase. The sections were treated initially with 2% trypsin at 37°C for 10 min in order to increase the sensitivity of the immunoperoxidase staining method. Sections were immersed in an antigen retrieval solution (10mmol/l sodium citrate buffer, pH 6) and subjected to heat-induced antigen retrieval for 20 min in a microwave. Nonspecific protein binding was blocked by a blocking solution (phosphate buffer solution (PBS) and 10%normal goat serum). The slides were incubated for 30 min with the diluted primary antibody using PBS. Drops of streptavidin peroxidase were added to the slide, left for 20 min and then washed with PBS for 5 min. Diaminobenzidine (Dakopatts, Glostrup, Denmark) was added to slides as a chromogen, after which the slides were washed with distilled water. Finally, the sections were counterstained with hematoxylin, dehydrated, rendered transparent with xylene, mounted and observed under a light microscope. For the negative control the specific primary antibody was replaced by phosphate-buffered saline.

Morphometric study

The mean area percentage (%) of PCNA and TGF-β1 reaction were quantified in 10 images for each group using Image-Pro Plus program version 6.0 (Media Cybernetics Inc., Bethesda, Maryland, USA). Mean area percentage of PCNA reaction and TGF-β1 in group IV (Propolis and hepatitis model group) compared with group III (Hepatitis model group) using the t-test, with $P<0.05$ as the level of statistical significance.

Statistical analysis

Statistical analyses were carried out using IBM SPSS statistics software for Windows, Version 20 (IBM Corp., Armonk, NY, USA). All data were expressed as mean±SD. The significance of dif ferences between mean values was analyzed by using the t-test, with $P<0.05$ as the level of statistical significance.

RESULT

Biochemical results

As shown in Table 1. In group III compared to control group, the liver injury markers of ALT, AST, total Bilirubin and TNF-α were very highly significant increase ($p<0.001$), but albumin was very highly significant decrease ($p<0.001$). In group IV compared to group III, ALT was significant decrease ($p<0.05$), AST was very highly significant decrease ($p<0.001$), total Bilirubin was highly significant decrease ($p<0.01$) and TNF-α was very highly significant decrease ($p<0.001$), but albumin was highly significant increase ($p<0.01$).

Table 1: Showing changes in liver function tests and TNF-α in all experimental groups

	Group I	Group II	Group III	Group IV
Serum AlT (U/L)	31.36±2.6	33.40±8.2	98.27±5.4*	61.74±4.8[a]
Serum AST (U/L)	80.18±4.5	85.50±18.9	250.50±18.9*	180.90±9.5[c]
Albumin (g/dl)	4.52±0.25	4.25±0.15	1.99±0.14*	2.62±0.26[b]
Total bilirubin (mg/dl)	0.70±0.03	0.75±0.02	1.55±0.14*	0.92±0.04[b]
TNF-α (Pg/ml)	21.5±2.55	22.6±2.61	130.7±0.96*	45.14±4.81[c]

Values are presented as mean±SD. P values:*<0.001 (Group III compared with control group I). P values: a<0.05, b<0.01, c<0.001 (Group IV compared with group III).

Histological results

Haematoxylin and eosin

Group I (Control group)

The liver sections of the group I showed cords of normal hepatocytes radiating from central vein. Hepatocytes are polyhedral in shape with central vesicular nuclei with prominent nucleoli and acidophilic cytoplasm. Some hepatocytes may be binucleated. Slit like spaces lined by endothelial cells and kupffer cells representing blood sinusoid were seen between the cords of hepatocytes (Figure 1A). The portal tract contained a branch of portal vein, a branch of hepatic artery and a branch of bile duct (Figure 1B).

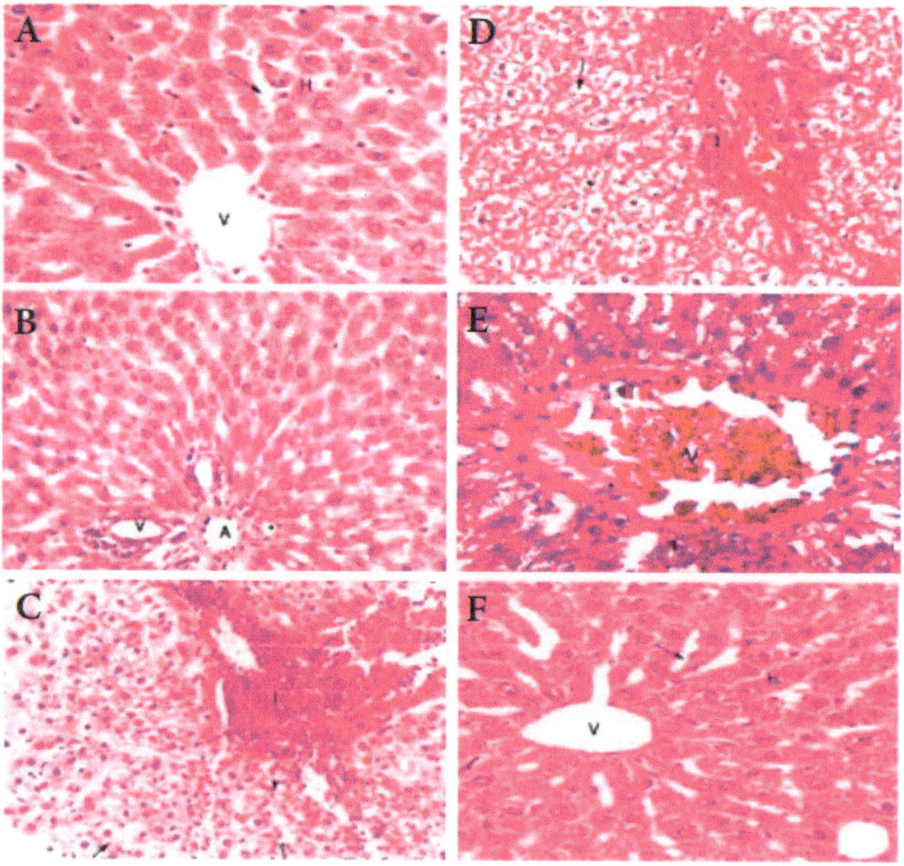

Figure 1: Photomicrograph of liver sections stained with hematoxylin and eosin. (A) Liver section from group I showing cords of normal hepatocytes (H) radiating from central vein (V). Hepatocytes are polyhedral in shape with central vesicular nuclei and acidophilic cytoplasm. Slit like spaces lined by endothelial cells representing blood sinusoid are seen between the cords of hepatocytes (↑) [H&E X400]. (B) Liver section from group I showing portal tract with portal vein

(V), hepatic artery (A) and bile duct (*) [H&E X400]. (C) Liver section from group III showing monocellular infiltration (I). Some swollen hepatocytes show finely granular cytoplasm (↑). The hepatocytes show small hyperchromatic nuclei (arrow head ^). Notice collapse of sinusoids between hepatocytes. [H&E X400]. (D) Liver section from group III showing empty hepatocytes that contain wisp of cytoplasmic remnants (*). The nuclei of some hepatocytes show karyolytic changes (↑) and the wall of blood vessel is thickened by inflammatory cells (I). [H&E X400]. (E) Liver section from group III showing dilated congested central vein (V). Notice swelling and proliferation of endothelial cells of central vein (*) and its wall show inflammatory cells (I). [H&E X630]. (F) Liver section from group IV showing more or less normal hepatocytes (H), central vein (V) and blood sinusoids (↑). [H&E X400].

Group II (Propolis group)

No histological changes were observed in the group II as compared to that of the control group.

Group III (Hepatitis model group)

Showed signs of degeneration and necrosis as some swollen hepatocytes had finely granular cytoplasm , other hepatocytes had small hyperchromatic nuclei. Monocellular infiltration and collapse of sinusoids between hepatocytes were seen (Figure 1C). Empty hepatocytes that contained wisp of cytoplasmic remnants were seen. The nuclei of some hepatocytes showed karyolytic changes and the wall of blood vessel was thickened by inflammatory cells (Figure 1D). Dilated congested central vein, swelling and proliferation of endothelial cells of central vein(central phlebitis) were seen and its wall showed inflammatory cells (Figure 1E).

Group IV (Propolis and hepatitis model group)

Showed preserved hepatic architecture as more or less normal hepatocytes, central vein and blood sinusoids were seen (Figure 1F).

Masson's trichrome stain

Group I (Control group)

The liver sections of the group I showed little amount of collagen fibers around central vein and portal tract (Figure 2A and 2B).

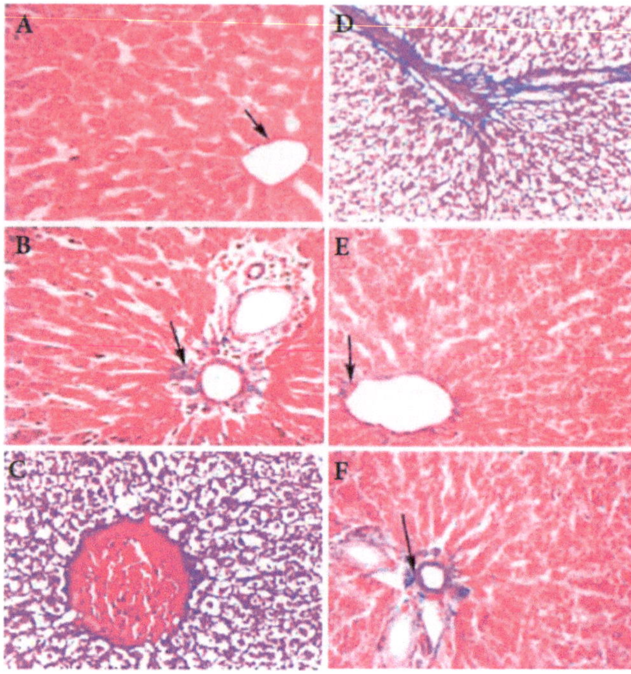

Figure 2: Photomicrograph of liver sections stained with masson trichrome. (A) Liver section from group I showing few collagen fibers around central vein (↑). [Masson's Trichrome X400]. (B) Liver section from group I showing few collagen fibers around portal tract (↑). [Masson's Trichrome X400]. (C) Liver section from group III showing an apparent increase of collagen fibers around dilated congested central vein and blood sinusoids. [Masson's Trichrome X400]. (D) Liver section from group III showing an apparent increase of collagen fibers around portal area and blood sinusoids. [Masson's Trichrome X400]. (E) Liver section from group IV showing apparent scanty collagen fibers around central vein (↑). [Masson's Trichrome X400]. (F) Liver section from group IV showing apparent scanty collagen fibers in the portal area (↑). [Masson's Trichrome X400].

Group II (Propolis group)

No detectable changes were observed in the distribution of collagen fibers in the liver of the group II as compared to that of the control group.

Group III (Hepatitis model group)

Showed apparent increase of collagen fibers around the central vein and portal tract and between cords of hepatocytes and blood sinusoids (Figures 2C and 2D).

Group IV (Propolis and hepatitis model group)

Showed apparent scanty collagen fibers around the central vein and portal tract (Figures 2E and 2F).

Immunohisochemistery results

PCNA immunohistochemical stain

Group I (Control group)

The liver sections of the control group showed few brown PCNA positive nuclei among few hepatocytes (Figure 3A).

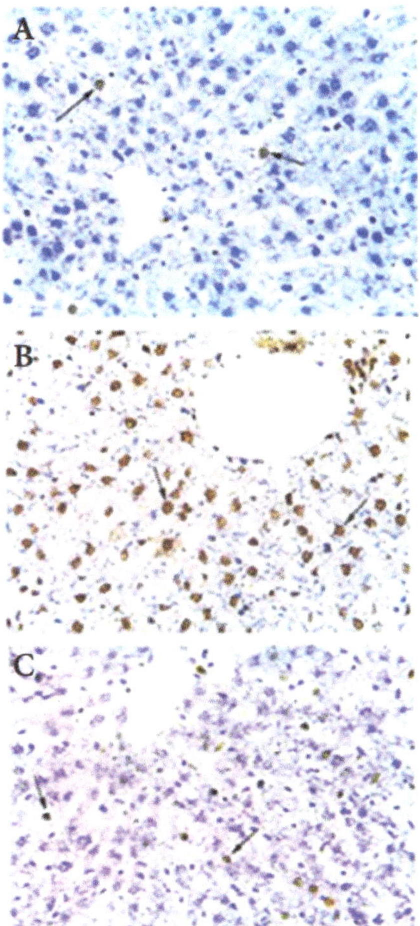

Figure 3: Photomicrograph of liver sections stained with anti-proliferating cell nuclear antigen (PCNA). (A) Liver section from group I showing few brown PCNA positive nuclei among few hepatocytes (↑) [Immunostaining for PCNA X400]. (B) Liver section from group III showing increase the number of brown PCNA positive nuclei among hepatocytes (↑) [Immunostaining for PCNA X400]. (C) Liver section from group IV showing decrease the number of brown PCNA positive nuclei among hepatocytes (↑). [Immunostaining for PCNA X400].

Group II (Propolis group)

No detectable changes were observed to PCNA expression in the group II as compared to that of the control group.

Group III (Hepatitis model group)

Showed increase the number of brown PCNA positive nuclei among hepatocytes (Figure 3B).

Group IV (Propolis and hepatitis model group)

Showed decrease the number of brown PCNA positive nuclei among hepatocytes (Figure 3C).

TGF-β1 immunohistochemical stain

Group I (Control group)

The liver sections of the control group showed weak positive immunoreaction for TGFβ1 in the wall of central vein and blood sinusoids (Figure 4A).

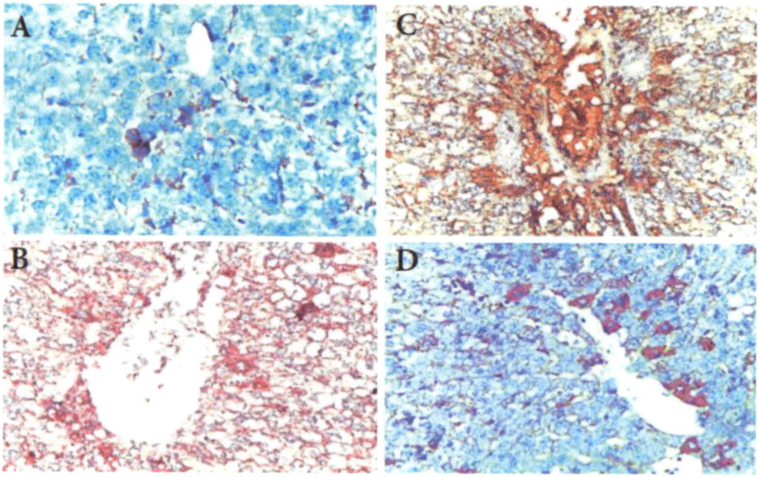

Figure 4: Photomicrograph of liver sections stained with transforming growth factor-β1 (TGF-β1). (A) Liver section from group I showing weak positive immunoreaction for TGF-β1 in the wall of central vein and blood sinusoids [Immunostaining for TGF-β1 X400]. (B) Liver section from group III showing strong positive immunoreaction for TGF-β1 in the wall of central vein and blood sinusoids [Immunostaining for TGF-β1 X400]. (C) Liver section from group III strong positive immunoreaction for TGF-β1 in the wall of portal vein and blood sinusoids. [Immunostaining for TGF-β1 X400]. (D) Liver section from group IV showing moderate positive immunoreaction for TGF-β1 in the wall of central vein and blood sinusoids. [Immunostaining for TGF-β1 X400].

Group II (Propolis group)

No detectable changes were observed to TGFβ1 expression in the group II as compared to that of the control group.

Group III (Hepatitis model group)

Showed strong positive immunoreaction for TGF-β1 in the wall of central vein, portal vein and blood sinusoids (Figures 4B and 4C).

Group IV (Propolis and hepatitis model group)

Showed moderate positive immunoreaction for TGF-β1 in the A B C A B D wall of central vein and blood sinusoids (Figure 4D).

Morphometric results

The mean area % of PCNA and TGF-β1 reaction for studied experimental groups was represented in (Tables 2 and3) and Histograms 1 and 2). There were significantly decreased ($P<0.05$) in PCNA and TGF-β1 reaction in group IV compared with group III.

Table 2: Showing the mean area % and ±SD of PCNA reaction in all experimental groups

	Group I	Group II	Group III	Group V
Mean area %	0.06	0.07	3.63	0.18
±SD	0.027	0.03	0.484	0.096
P value	--	--	--	0.000
Significance	--	--	--	S

SD: Standard deviation; S: Significant at $P<0.05$
Group IV compared with group III.

Table 3: Showing the mean area % and ±SD of TGF-β1 reaction in all experimental groups

	Group I	Group II	Group III	Group V
Mean area %	2.16	2.02	21.90	3.14
±SD	0.161	0.141	0.650	0.765
P value	--	--	--	0.000
Significance	--	--	--	S

SD: Standard deviation; S: Significant at $P<0.05$
Group IV compared with group III.

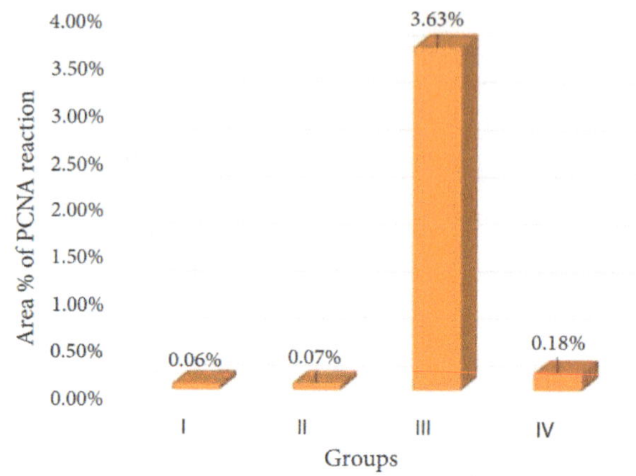

Histogram 1: Showing the mean area % of PCNA reaction in all experimental groups.

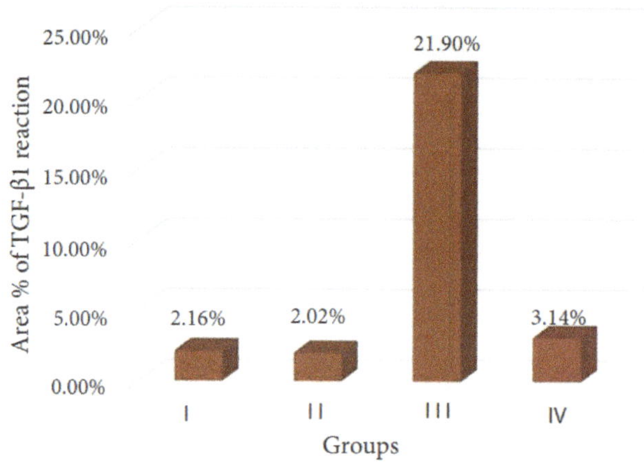

Histogram 2: Showing the mean area % of TGF-β1 reaction in all experimental groups.

DISCUSSION

Hepatitis remains as a clinical challenge and a problem of great importance in the worldwide today and affect a great number of population especially in Egypt [18].

In the present study our group III revealed a very highly significant increase of AST, ALT, total bilirubin and TNF-α but there was a very highly significant decrease of albumin as compared to control group.

Serum ALT and AST a cytoplasmic enzymes were released into circulation after cellular damage in acute hepatoxicity and were considered the most sensitive markers used in the diagnosis of hepatic damage [19].

Our results were in agreement with the findings of some investigators who reported that a liver damage induced by D-GalN/LPS reflected the disturbances of liver cell metabolism which leads to characteristic changes in the liver serum enzymes and albumin [3,4,18,20].

Serum bilirubin was considered as an index for the assessment of hepatic function and any abnormal increase indicates hepatobiliary disease [21].

D-galactosamine (D-GaIN) together with lipopolysaccharide (LPS) can lead to pronounced secretion of pro-inflammatory cytokine such as TNF-α by Kupffer, stellate and sinusoidal endothelial cells which had been shown to be early and important mediators of liver injury and hepatic necrosis [3,22]. Some authors clarified that the D-GaIN/LPS induced hepatocyte apoptotic changes and enhance the expression of cytokines TNF-α [6,18].

The histological examination of liver sections of group III of the present study revealed signs of degeneration and necrosis such as some swollen hepatocytes had finely granular cytoplasm, other hepatocytes had small hyperchromatic nuclei or karyolytic changes. Monocellular infiltration and collapse of sinusoids between hepatocytes were seen. Empty hepatocytes that contained wisp of cytoplasmic remnants were seen. The wall of blood vessel was thickened by inflammatory cells. Central vein was dilated and congested and its wall infiltrated by inflammatory cells. Swelling and proliferation of endothelial cells of central vein(central phlebitis) were seen.

These result were in agreement with previous studies indicated that during D-GalN/LPS induced hepatitis, there were severe hepatocellular degeneration , necrosis and mononuclear cellular infiltration [20,23,24].

Some authors clarified that the D-GalN/LPS induced marked cellular infiltration, is due to ROS production that indirectly regulate chemokine receptor expression and promote cytokine IL-6, IL-8 and TNF-α which are key modulators of inflammatory response [4].

Some investigators reported that central phlebitis characterized by swelling and proliferation of endothelial cells of central vein [25].

The release of aminotransferases by the damaged hepatocytes was strongly support the previous histological observations.

An apparent increase in collagen fibers around the central vein and the portal areas was seen in the present study. This was supported with strong positive immunoreaction for TGF-β1 in the wall of central vein, portal vein and blood sinusoids. Our results were in accordance with other researchers who stated the expression of TGF-β1 could be correlated with the degree of liver damage to cirrhosis in chronic viral hepatitis [26]. Liver fibrosis, an early stage of cirrhosis, was a common consequence of chronic injury from many causes as infection and toxic drugs and characterized by the accumulation of extracellular matrix (ECM) proteins which; due to imbalance in their production, deposition, and breakdown. Prolonged liver injury result in hepatocytes damage, which triggers activation of hepatic stellate cells(HSCs). TGF-β1 was produced by HSCs and Kupffer cells and was believed to be involved in the synthesis and deposition of extracellular matrix components like fibronectin, collagens type I, III, and IV. TGF-β1 had a dual impact on the progression of liver disease by promoting fibrogenesis and inducing hepatocytes apoptosis [27-29].

Liver fibrosis was caused by a combination of multiple mechanisms, such as acute and chronic hepatocyte damage, recruitment and activation of inflammatory cells as macrophages, eosinophil and neutrophils, release of inflammatory and fibrogenic cytokines, production of reactive oxygen species; activation of hepatic stellate cells (HSCs) , periportal or perivenular fibroblasts, circulating fibrocytes, and bone marrow cells that transdifferentiate into collagen producing myofibroblats [29-31].

Portal hypertension was a major complication of advanced liver cirrhosis. The main reason of portal hypertension was pathologically elevated intrahepatic resistance to portal blood flow due to fibrosis or cirrhosis caused by different chronic mainly inflammatory stimuli. The site of the increased resistance may be prehepatic (portal vein obstruction) or posthepatic (hepatic vein obstruction) [32].

An increase in the number of brown PCNA positive nuclei among hepatocytes were seen in group III of the present study. Proliferating cell nuclear antigen (PCNA) was a marker of cell proliferation.

PCNA found in cell nucleus and was directly involved in DNA replication. Its expression was increased at late G1 stage and early S stage. Previous studies had demonstrated that PCNA labeling index increased sequentially from normal tissue through premalignant stage to carcinoma of various tumors [33,34].

Some investigators reported PCNA had been also found to induce apoptosis in cells subjected to oxidative stress [35].

Our findings were in accordance with those of previous studies who suggested that the ability of cell proliferation become stronger and this was closely related to malignant cell proliferation and carcinogenesis in livers of D-GalN/LPS treated rats [36-38].

In many liver disorders, inflammation , fibrosis and apoptosis are important pathogenic components, finally leading to acute liver failure [39].

Some researchers demonstrated that the mechanism of action of D-GalN/LPS induced hepatitis mediated through release of the oxidized products of oxidative stress such as reactive oxygen species (ROS) and different cytokines released by Kupffer cells (KC) of the liver such as tumor necrosis factor (TNF-α) , Interleukin-1 (IL-1) and Interleukin-6 (IL-6). These ROS of oxidative stress were altering and damaging the cell compounds as protein and lipid as well as membranes and leading to increase lipid peroxidation and hepatic damage characterized by hepatocellular necrosis, inflammation and apoptosis [4,5,22,40].

In the present study group IV revealed a marked improvement of biochemical parameter, histological changes of liver. Moreover, a decrease in the number of brown PCNA positive nuclei among hepatocytes and moderate positive immunoreaction for TGF-β1 in the wall of portal vein and blood sinusoids.

These results are in agreement and confirming the findings of some researchers who reported the protective effect of propolis against hepatotoxicity as it contains higher content of total phenolic compounds [7,9,41].

Some researchers reported that the protective effect of propolis was due to its antioxidant properties, as it acts as a free-radical scavenger and lipid peroxidation inhibitor. Further it was increasing the intracellular concentration of glutathione and superoxide anions and antioxidant enzymes [42]. Moreover propolis was improving the activity of hepatic microsomal drug metabolizing enzymes [10].

Propolis had potent anti-inflammatory and immunomodulatory agents which acted through inhibiting neutrophil infiltration, suppression of proinflammatory cytokines or mediators as tumor necrosis factor-α and interleukins and stimulation of macrophages and thus influencing specific and nonspecific immune defense mechanisms [11,43]. Some researcher reported that propoils had been shown to ameliorate fibrosis due to its antioxidant properties [12]. Other investigators had reported that propolis might exert a modulatory effect on cytokine TGF-β1 induced fibrosis [44]. Some investigators reported that the propolis had antiproliferative and anticarcinogenic activity [34,45].

CONCLUSION

Acute D-GAlN/ LPS induced hepatitis model caused an increase of oxidative stress and degenerative changes of liver. Propolis had a potential protective effect and preventing degenerative changes of liver caused by D-GAlN/LPS as it had antioxidant, anti-inflammatory enzyme and antiapoptotic activities. These results should provide a new insight in treating patients with acute hepatitis and thus the intake of propolis as supplement should be advised and might serve as clinically useful hepatoprotective natural product in future.

AUTHORS' CONTRIBUTION

Authors' contributions	**AMEM**	**AAS**	**FARM**
Research concept and design	√	--	--
Collection and/or assembly of data	√	√	√
Data analysis and interpretation	√	√	√
Writing the article	√	--	--
Critical revision of the article	√	√	√
Final approval of article	√	√	√
Statistical analysis	--	√	--

ACKNOWLEDGEMENT

The authors thank all the staff members of Histology and Cell Biology Department in Benha Faculty of Medicine, Benha University, Egypt and professor Amany Elshawarby, head of Histology and Cell Biology Department, Ain Shams Faculty of Medicine, Cairo, Egypt for their cooperation and helpful comments during this work.

REFERENCES

1. Abdel-Mohsen AF, Salama NM, Elgendy MS and Elsayed AM. Histological study on the effect of stem cells and hepatocyte growth factor on induced liver fibrosis in male albino rats. *The Egyptian Journal of Histology*. 2014; 37:615-628.
2. Ahmed SK, Mohammed SA, Khalaf G and Fikry H. Role of Bone Marrow Mesenchymal Stem Cells in the Treatment of CCL4 Induced Liver Fibrosis in Albino Rats: A Histological and Immunohistochemical Study. *Int J Stem Cells*. 2014; 7:87-97.
3. Jihan H, Eman R, Safaa M, Dalia M and Fatma O. Green tea attenuates experimental hepatitis in context of oxidative stress. *Journal of Applied Pharmaceutical Science*. 2013; 3:124-128.
4. Padmanabhan P and Jangle SN. Hepatoprotective activity of herbal preparation (HP-4) against D-Galactosamine induced hepatotoxicity in mice. *International Journal of Pharmaceutical Sciences and Drug Research*. 2014; 6:31-37.
5. Wang X, Zhang L, Wei Z, Zhang X, Gao Q, Ma Y, Liu X,Jiang Y and Guo C. The inhibitory action of PDCD4 in lipopolysaccharide/D-galactosamine-induced acute liver injury. *Lab Invest*. 2013; 93:291-302.
6. Wu YH, Hu SQ, Liu J, Cao HC, Xu W, Li YJ and Li LJ. Nature and mechanisms of hepatocyte apoptosis induced by D-galactosamine/lipopolysaccharide challenge in mice. *Int J Mol Med*. 2014; 33:1498-506.
7. Bhadauria M. Propolis prevents hepatorenal injury induced by chronic exposure to carbon tetrachloride.*Evid Based Complement Alternat Med*. 2012; 2012:235358.
8. El-Meligy RM, Zain ME and Ahmed FA. Protective role of Cynanchum acutum L. extracts on carbon tetrachloride-induced hepatotoxicity in rat. *Int. J. Chem. Appl. Biol. Sci*. 2014; 1:8-13.
9. Saleh EM. Antioxidant effect of aqueous extract of propolis on hepatotoxicity induced by octylphenol in male rats. *Acta Toxicol. Argent*. 2012; 20:68-81.
10. Mahmoud EF and Mahmoud MF. Evaluation of The effect of Propolis extract on the Tongue mucosa of an Induced toxic rabbit by Fenitrothion. *Life Science Journal*. 2013; 10:767-775.
11. Nakamura T, Ohta Y, Ohashi K, Ikeno K, Watanabe R, Tokunaga K and Harada N. Protective Effect of Brazilian Propolis against Liver Damage with Cholestasis in Rats Treated with alpha-Naphthylisothiocyanate. *Evid Based Complement Alternat Med*. 2013; 2013:302720.
12. Araujo MAR, Libério SA, Guerra RNM, Ribeiro MNS and Nascimento FRF. Mechanisms of action underlying the anti-inflammatory and immunomodulatory effects of propolis: a brief review. *Braz. J. Pharmacognosy*. 2012; 22:208-219.
13. Reitman S and Frankel S. A colorimetric method for the determination of serum glutamic oxalacetic and glutamic pyruvic transaminases. *Am J Clin Pathol*. 1957; 28:56-63.

14. Walter M and Gerade RW. Bilirubin direct/total. *Microchem. J.* 1970; 15:231-233.

15. Doumas BT, Watson WA and Biggs HG. Albumin standards and the measurement of serum albumin with bromcresol green. *Clin Chim Acta.* 1971; 31:87-96.

16. Corti A, Fassina G, Marcucci F, Barbanti E and Cassani G. Oligomeric tumour necrosis factor alpha slowly converts into inactive forms at bioactive levels. *Biochem J.* 1992; 284:905-10.

17. Bancroft JD and Layton C. The hematoxylin and eosin, connective and mesenchymal tissues with their stains In. S. Kim suvarna, Christopher Layton and John D. Bancroft editors. Bancroft s Theory and practice of histological techniques. 7th ed. Churchill Livingstone: Philadelphia. 2013; 173-212.

18. Mahmoud M and Hamdan D. Naringin and rutin prevent D-galactosamine-induced hepatic injury in rats via attenuation of the inflammatory cascade and oxidative stress. *European Scientific Journal.* 2013;9:141-155.

19. Heikal TM, Mossa AH, Abdel Rasoul MA and Marei GH. The ameliorating effects of green tea extract against cyromazine and chlorpyrifos induced liver toxicity in male rats. *Asian. J. Pharm .Clin. Res.* 2013;6:48-55.

20. Fyiad AA, Abd El-Kader MA and Abd El-Haleem AH. Modulatory effects of pomegranate juice on nucleic acids alterations and oxidative Stress in experimentaly hepatitis rats. *Life Science Journal.* 2012; 9:676-682.

21. El-Alfy NZ, Ahmed HH, Mahmoud MF and Yahya SM. Regression of liver fibrosis by punica granatum peel extract in the experimental model. *World Journal of Pharmacy and Pharmaceutical Sciences.* 2014; 3:22-44.

22. Kim SJ, Kim JK, Lee DU, Kwak JH and Lee SM. Genipin protects lipopolysaccharide-induced apoptotic liver damage in D-galactosamine-sensitized mice. *Eur J Pharmacol.* 2010; 635:188-93.

23. Taye A, El-Moselhy MA, Hassan MK, Ibrahim HM and Mohammed AF. Hepatoprotective effect of pentoxifylline against D-galactosamine-induced hepatotoxicity in rats. *Ann Hepatol.* 2009; 8:364-70.

24. Sheriff SA and Devaki T. Lycopene stabilizes lipoprotein levels during D-galactosamine/lipopolysaccharide induced hepatitis in experimental rats. *Asian Pac J Trop Biomed.* 2012; 2:975-80.

25. Rubin R and Strayer DS. Rubin pathology. 5th ed. Lippincott Williams and Wilkins. 2008; 642-643.

26. Tache DE, Stanciulescu CE, Banita IM, Purcaru SO, Andrei AM, Comanescu V and Pisoschi CG. Inducible nitric oxide synthase expression (iNOS) in chronic viral hepatitis and its correlation with liver fibrosis.*Rom J Morphol Embryol.* 2014; 55:539-43.

27. Bai T, Lian LH, Wu YL, Wan Y and Nan JX. Thymoquinone attenuates liver fibrosis via PI3K and TLR4 signaling pathways in activated hepatic stellate cells. *Int Immunopharmacol.* 2013; 15:275-81.

28. Noh DH, Lee EJ, Kim AY, Lee EM, Min CW, Kang KK, Lee MM, Kim SH,

Sung SE, Hwang M, Yu DY and Jeong KS. Alcohol induced hepatic degeneration in a hepatitis C virus core protein transgenic mouse model. *Int J Mol Sci.* 2014; 15:4126-41.

29. Zhong L, Wang X, Wang S, Yang L, Gao H and. Yang C. The anti-fibrotic effect of bone morphogenic protein-7(BMP-7) on liver fibrosis. *Int J Med Sci.* 2013; 10:441-50.

30. Friedman SL. Evolving challenges in hepatic fibrosis. *Nat Rev Gastroenterol Hepatol.* 2010; 7:425-36.

31. Yao QY, Xu BL, Wang JY, Liu HC, Zhang SC and Tu CT. Inhibition by curcumin of multiple sites of the transforming growth factor-beta1 signalling pathway ameliorates the progression of liver fibrosis induced by carbon tetrachloride in rats. *BMC Complement Altern Med.* 2012; 12:156.

32. Liedtke C, Luedde T, Sauerbruch T, Scholten D, Streetz K, Tacke F, Tolba R, Trautwein C, Trebicka J and Weiskirchen R. Experimental liver fibrosis research: update on animal models, legal issues and translational aspects. *Fibrogenesis Tissue Repair.* 2013; 6:19.

33. Ismail MF, Ali DA, Fernando A, Abdraboh ME, Gaur RL, Ibrahim WM, Raj MH and Ouhtit A. Chemoprevention of rat liver toxicity and carcinogenesis by Spirulina. *Int J Biol Sci.* 2009; 5:377-87.

34. El-kott AF, Kandeel AA, Abed El-Aziz SF and Ribea HM. Effects of bee honey on PCNA and P53 expression in the rat hepatocarcinogenesis. *International Journal of Cancer Research.* 2012; 8:130-139.

35. Hidaka M, Takagi Y, Takano TY and Sekiguchi M. PCNA-MutSalpha-mediated binding of MutLalpha to replicative DNA with mismatched bases to induce apoptosis in human cells. *Nucleic Acids Res.* 2005;33:5703-12.

36. Nafees S, Ali N, Rashid S, Hasan SK and Sultana S. Chemopreventive Effect of Bauhinia Purpurea Against Chemically Induced Hepatocarcinogenesis via Amelioration of Oxidative Damage, Cell Proliferation and Induction of Apoptosis in Wistar Rats. *Toxicol Int.* 2013; 20:117-25.

37. Nitha A, Prabha SP, Ansil PN and Larha MS. Curative effect of woodfordia fruticosa kurz flowes on N- nitrosodiethylamine induced hepatocellular carcinoma in rats. *Int. J. Pharm. Pharm. Sci.* 2014; 6:150-155.

38. Shen T, Khor SC, Zhou F, Duan T, Xu YY, Zheng YF, Hsu S, J DES, Yang J, Xu LH and Zhu XQ.Chemoprevention by lipid-soluble tea polyphenols in diethylnitrosamine/phenobarbital-induced hepatic pre-cancerous lesions. *Anticancer Res.* 2014; 34:683-93.

39. Aigner T. Apoptosis, necrosis, or whatever: how to find out what really happens? *J Pathol.* 2002; 198:1-4.

40. Lekic N, Cerny D, Horinek A, Provaznik Z, Martinek J and Farghali H. Differential oxidative stress responses to D-galactosamine-lipopolysaccharide hepatotoxicity based on real time PCR analysis of selected oxidant/antioxidant and apoptotic gene expressions in rat. *Physiol Res.* 2011; 60:549-58.

41. Banskota AH, Tezuka Y, Adnyana IK, Midorikawa K, Matsushige K, Message D, Huertas AA and Kadota S.Cytotoxic, hepatoprotective and free radical scavenging effects of propolis from Brazil, Peru, the Netherlands and China. *J Ethnopharmacol.* 2000; 72:239-46.

42. Newairy AA and Abdou HM. Effect of propolis consumption on hepatotoxicity and brain damage in male rats exposed to chlorpyrifos. *African Journal of Biotechnology*. 2013; 12:5232-5243.

43. Korish AA and Arafa MM. Propolis derivatives inhibit the systemic inflammatory response and protect hepatic and neuronal cells in acute septic shock. *Braz J Infect Dis*. 2011; 15:332-8.

44. de Moura SA, Ferreira MA, Andrade SP, Reis ML, Noviello Mde L and Cara DC. Brazilian green propolis inhibits inflammatory angiogenesis in a murine sponge model. *Evid Based Complement Alternat Med*. 2011; 2011:182703.

45. El-Kott AF and Owayss AA. Protective Effects of Propolis Against the Amitraz Hepatotoxicity in Mice.*Journal of Pharmacology and Toxicology*. 2008; 3:402-408.

11
CHAPTER

THERAPEUTIC INNOVATIONS: TYROSINE KINASE INHIBITORS IN CANCER

Nikolaos Dervisis and Shawna Klahn

Keywords: Tyrosine kinase inhibitors, comparative, cancer, chemotherapy, dog, cat, human

INTRODUCTION

Kinases are among the first oncogenes identified. Initial understanding of oncogene function originates from experiments utilizing retroviruses expressing oncogenic kinases. Murine, feline, and avian retroviruses were the first to demonstrate integration into the host genome, thereby transducing genes harbored at the insertion site. Src kinase is transduced within the avian genome by the Rous sarcoma virus and is the driving force behind Rous sarcoma. Similarly, Raf kinase is transduced by the same retrovirus. Activation of genes encoding kinases contribute to oncogenic transformation of the infected cell. An array of over 500 kinases have since been identified using animal tissue culture models and genetic methodologies [1,2]. Their role in tumorigenesis, tumor progression, and metastasis has been expanding, along with pharmacological attempts to therapeutically intervene the aberrant functions.

DIGITAL AGE IN CELLULAR BIOLOGY

Kinases catalyze the transfer of the gamma-phosphate group of ATP onto a substrate. Kinases mediate nearly all signal transductions, thereby regulating multiple cellular

Citation: Nikolaos Dervisis and Shawna Klahn, Therapeutic Innovations: Tyrosine Kinase Inhibitors in Cancer, doi:10.3390/vetsci3010004.

activities such as proliferation, survival, apoptosis, metabolism, transcription, differentiation [3,4]. Accumulating pharmacological and pathological evidence demonstrate that kinases are promising drug targets for the treatment of numerous diseases, such as cancer, inflammatory diseases, central nervous system disorders, cardiovascular diseases, and diabetes [5]. The catalytic activity depends on the phosphorylation status of specific amino-acid residues. Conformational and other changes induced by phosphorylation events result in dramatic shifts in the kinase catalytic activity, manifesting as a binary switch in functional behavior of the enzyme [6,7,8].

Kinases are located at key positions within the cell. Intercellular communication and the extracellular environment are monitored through signal receptors, while intracellular communication is conducted through secondary signaling molecules and at specific functional checkpoints. Individual subcircuits representing relative simplified functions, such as cellular growth and energy metabolism, have multiple interconnections and crosstalk, forming a functional signaling network that is characterized by higher-level complexity [9]. Kinases have an important role in the amplification and termination of signals, facilitating communication between integral parts of the cell, and between cells. Thus, kinases can be thought as the molecular receptors, amplifiers and transducers of extra and intracellular signals, facilitating the cell's response to the challenges of life.

A consequence of this complex and intricate signaling network is that kinases exhibit pleiotropy and locus heterogeneity. Mutations within the same gene may result in several phenotypes, while the same disease phenotype can sometimes result from mutations in different kinase genes. For example, gain-of-function mutations in the region of the immunoglobulin domain of fibroblast growth factor receptor 1 (FGFR1) result in Pfeiffer syndrome and osteoglophonic dysplasia, whereas loss-of-function mutations throughout the protein cause hypogonadotrophic hypogonadism [10,11].

DISEASE AS A KINASE DYSFUNCTION

Despite the enormous amount of research and rapid developments during the past decades, cancer continues to be a worldwide killer. In the USA, cancer accounts for 23% of the total deaths, and is the second most common cause of death after heart disease. It is expected to surpass heart disease as the leading cause of death in the next few years [12,13]. The intense research in the molecular biology of cancer resulted in an explosion of candidate genes that drive oncogenesis. Nearly simultaneous with the discovery of cancer-associated genes, strategies to repair them were explored. Early attempts focusing on gene replacement therapies were not translated into clinical use due to technological, ethical, and biological barriers. Efforts were soon turned towards pharmacologic methods of blocking specific aberrant oncogenic signaling.

Mutations in protein kinases are overrepresented approximately four-fold compared with a random selection of genes, and reportedly the most frequently mutated family of genes contributing to neoplastic diseases [14,15]. Protein kinases may act as tumor suppressors or proto-oncogenes in normal, healthy cells. Aberrations in protein kinase function can lead to tumorigenesis through numerous mechanisms, including the activation of proliferative pathways, genomic instability, reduction of the DNA damage response, deactivation of apoptotic pathways and/or the promotion of angiogenesis and cellular motility [15]. Gain-of-function mutations typically increase constitutive kinase activity, leading to unrestrained cellular signaling, while loss of-function mutations can lead to a loss in cell signaling. The combined signal aberrations can have a profound effect on the cell, leading to oncogenesis, tumor growth and metastasis.

KINASES AS AN ATTRACTIVE DRUG TARGET

Protein kinases are considered to be the second most important group of drug targets after G-protein-coupled receptors [16,17]. Aberrant kinase activity is implicated in a large variety of diseases, particularly those involving inflammatory or proliferative responses, such as cancer, rheumatoid arthritis, cardiovascular and neurological disorders, asthma and psoriasis. Directly or indirectly, hundreds of human diseases have been connected to protein kinase dysfunction. The ability to modulate kinase activity therefore represents an attractive therapeutic strategy for the treatment of human illnesses [18].

Kinase activity is typically regulated by interconverting between two structural conformations via phosphorylation of key amino acid residues, shifting the balance between active and inactive. These two states are characterized by movements in conformationally mobile loops that border or block the ATP binding site of the kinase. For this reason, the dissociation constant for ATP may be significantly higher for the inactive conformation than for the active conformation. This kinase activation model provides the framework for drugs designed to interact with specific kinase domains. A large number of kinase inhibitors selectively target the inactive conformation, whereas other compounds bind to both conformations with similar affinity [19,20,21]. Inhibitors that bind to the inactive conformation likely face weaker competition with cellular ATP. The potential result is enhanced activity *in vivo*, acting primarily to shift equilibria between conformational states to prevent kinase activation, indirectly inhibiting activity [22].

The modulation of kinase activity can be achieved through either direct or indirect strategies (Figure 1). Imatinib (Gleevec; Novartis) is the prototype of direct protein-tyrosine kinase inhibitors that inhibits the BCR-ABL phosphorylation activity through blocking ATP binding. Imatinib has been approved for the treatment of patients with BCR-ABL positive chronic myeloid leukemia (CML) and patients with Kit (CD117)-positive gastrointestinal stromal tumors. BCR-ABL is the constitutively active tyrosine kinase in CML and in certain forms of acute lymphoblastic leukemia. Imatinib also inhibits the kinase activity of platelet derived growth factor receptor, stem-cell factor receptor and c-kit. Indirect kinase inhibition involves disruption of protein-protein interactions. Cetuximab (Erbitux; ImClone/Bristol-Myers Squibb) is a monoclonal antibody that selectively binds to the extracellular domain of human epidermal growth factor receptor (EGFR), and competitively inhibits binding of epidermal growth factor (EGF) to its receptor tyrosine kinase. Bevacizumab (Avastin; Genentech) is the first anti-angiogenesis cancer drug approved by the FDA. Bevacizumab binds to human vascular endothelial growth factor A (VEGF-A), and prevents it from binding to its receptor tyrosine kinases, Flt-1/VEGFR1 and KDR/VEGRF2. Inhibition of VEGF signaling interferes with tumor blood vessel development, a process that is crucial for tumor growth and metastasis [23].

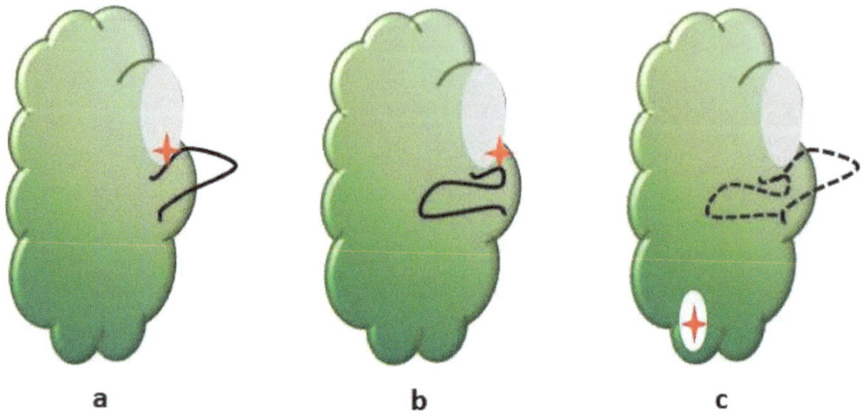

Figure 1: The activation loop of the protein kinase domain regulates access to the ATP binding site. The conformation of a conserved Asp-Phe-Gly (DFG) motif within the activation loop is used to categorize the binding mode of inhibitors. The common types of kinase—kinase inhibitor interactions include: (a) Type I inhibitors (red star) bind the ATP binding site (grey) of the protein kinase domain (green). The aspartate side chain in the conserved DFG motif at the beginning of the activation loop (black) faces into the active site; (b) Type II inhibitors bind a flipped conformation of the DFG motif in which the aspartate side chain faces outwards; (c) Allosteric ligands bind to binding pockets (white) that do not overlap with the active site of the kinase. The DFG motif conformation is not important. These binding pockets can be adjacent to the active site or distant from the active site.

Compounds that bind to protein kinases outside of the ATP-binding pocket may possess advantages over ATP-competitive counterparts. Drugs can be administered at concentrations closer to their biochemical inhibition constant, as inhibition is not affected by fluctuations in the cellular concentration of ATP. There is a potential for greater selectivity as residues outside the ATP binding pocket tend to be less conserved. In certain cases, noncompetitive inhibitors can be substrate selective, inhibiting the activity of a kinase against only a subset of its targets. Rapamycin, the first noncompetitive kinase inhibitor to be identified, is a cyclic macrolide that inhibits the protein kinase mammalian target of rapamycin (mTOR) [24]. MEK1 inhibitor PD098059, the first synthetic noncompetitive kinase inhibitor to be described, acts by binding to inactive MEK1 and preventing its phosphorylation by the upstream kinase Raf [25,26]. Several such inhibitors, termed allosteric, have been described, targeting kinases such as Akt, and inhibitor of nuclear factor kappa-B kinase (IKK-2) [27,28].

The target regions for most kinase inhibitors are intracellular. As small molecules, kinase inhibitors enter the cell by diffusion down the concentration gradient that exists across the membrane. The rate at which this process occurs, and the rate of active efflux, are important determinantsof the intracellular bioavailability of a kinase. How quickly the intracellular inhibitor concentration reaches a steady state and the relative concentrations of inhibitor inside and outside the cell at steady state rely on the relative lipophilicity *vs.* hydrophilicity characteristics of the drug. The rate that it permeates the cellular membrane and non-specific binding to proteins and may affect the route of administration and dosing schedule [29,30]. Expression of drug efflux pump transporters has been shown to reduce the steady-state intracellular drug concentration, although most mammalian cells in culture appear to have less efflux activity for kinase inhibitors compared to chemotherapeutics such as doxorubicin.

HITTING THE TARGET

The transition from cytotoxic chemotherapy to molecularly targeted cancer drug discovery and development has resulted in an increasing number of successful therapies that have impacted the lives of a large number of cancer patients. The BCR-ABL inhibitor imatinib is generally regarded as a trailblazer drug that most impressively validated the concept of designing a small molecule therapeutic. Imatinib is designed to treat a defined patient population with chronic myeloid leukemia in which the malignancy is driven by the BCR-ABL translocation. The improvement in survival has been dramatic [31]. These successes were followed by a number of other small molecule drugs inhibiting critical cancer targets, essentially changing the anti-neoplastic armamentarium of modern Oncology. There has been an explosion of approved kinase inhibitors, with nearly 20 drugs approved by the FDA in a four-year period (Table 1).Veterinary Oncology has been slowly following the fast pace of human Oncology, and there are currently three kinase inhibitors approved by FDA, and a number of small molecular inhibitors under various stages of development (Table 2).

The clinical success of such targeted therapeutics depends to a large degree to the availability of predictive markers. The specific histopathologic diagnosis may not be of such importance, as the presence of markers associated with specific genetic aberrations (mutations, internal tandem duplications, gene amplifications) [32,33,34,35]. For example, the anaplastic lymphoma kinase (ALK) was first implicated in the pathogenesis of an aggressive type of non-Hodgkin's lymphoma [36]. Rearrangements of the ALK gene were subsequently discovered to be are present in 3% to 5% of non-small-cell lung cancers (NSCLC) [37]. These genetic lesions define a distinct subgroup of NSCLC that typically occurs in younger patients who have never smoked or have a history of light smoking [38]. Knowing the presence of these rearrangements can guide the treatment protocol selection, alter the prognosis, and essentially result in a truly personalized approach in cancer therapy [29,35].

Table 1: Approved tyrosine kinase inhibitors in human medicine, 2011–2015 [a]

Drug	Target	Year Approved	Indication
Vandetanib (Caprelsa®)	Flt1, Flt4, KDR, EGFR, Ret	2011	MTC
Crizotinib (Xalkori®)	ALK, MET, EML4-ALK fusion protein	2011	NSCLC
Ruxolitinib (Jakafi®/Jakavi®)	JAK1, JAK2	2011	Myelofibrosis
Vemurafenib (Zelboraf®)	BRAF	2011	Melanoma
Bosutinib (Bosulif®)	BCR/ABL1	2012	CML
Axitinib (Inlyta®)	Flt1, Flt4, KDR, Kit, PDGF-Rα/β	2012	RCC
Cabozantinib (Cometriq®)	KDR, Mek	2012	MTC
Regorafinib (Stivarga®)	KDR, TEK	2012	CC, GIST
Ponatinib (Iclusig®)	BCR/ABL1	2012	CML, ALL
Dabrafenib (Tafinlar®)	BRAF	2013	Melanoma
Trametinib (Mekinist®)	MEK1, MEK2	2013	Melanoma
Afatinib (Gilotrif®)	ERBB2, EGFR	2013	NSCLC
Ibrutinib (Imbruvica®)	BTK	2013	MCL, CLL
Tofacitinib (Xeljanz®)	JAK3	2013	Rheumatoid arthritis
Idelalisib (Zydelig®)	PI3-K	2014	CLL Follicular B-cell NHL
Ceritinib (Zykadia®)	ALK	2014	ALK⁺ NSCLC
Lenvatinib (Lenvima®)	VEGFR2 and VEGFR3	2015	Radioactive iodine-refractory DTC
Palbociclib (Ibrance®)	CDK4 and CDK6	2015	Breast carcinoma

[a] Abbreviations: ALL, acute lymphoblastic leukemia; CC, colorectal cancer; CML, chronic myelogenous leukemia; DTC, differentiated thyroid cancer; GIST, gastrointestinal stromal tumor; MCL, mantle cell lymphoma; MTC, medullary thyroid carcinoma; NHL, Non-Hodgkin's lymphoma; NSCLC, non-small-cell lung carcinoma; RCC, renal cell carcinoma.

Table 2: Approved tyrosine kinase inhibitors in veterinary medicine, all drugs

Drug	Targets	Year Approved	Indication
Toceranib (Palladia®)	VEGF-R2 PDGF-Rα Kit Flt-3 *RET* *JAK family*	2009	Patnaik grade 2 or 3, recurrent, cutaneous mast cell tumors with or without regional lymph node involvement in dogs
Masitinib (Kinavet-CA1®)	Kit PDGF-Rα/β Lyn FGF-R3	2010 [a]	Nonresectable grade 2 and 3 cutaneous mast cell tumors in dogs that have not previously received radiotherapy and/or chemotherapy except corticosteroids
Oclacitinib (Apoquel®)	JAK1 JAK 2	2013	Control of pruritus associated with allergic dermatitis and control of atopic dermatitis in dogs at least 12 mos of age

[a] Conditional approval by the FDA expired in December 2015 and the drug is not commercially available in the US. The drug can only be obtained through the FDA's personal import mechanism.

MISSING THE POINT

The high specificity of the kinase inhibitors appears to be their Achilles heel. As many of the kinase inhibitors exert their tumoricidal effects primarily by inhibiting a specific kinase, there is a strong selective pressure for cells to acquire resistance through mutations in the kinase gene that abrogate drug binding. Additional non-mutation kinase inhibitor resistance mechanisms have been documented, including target amplification and upregulation of alternative kinase pathways such as hepatocyte growth factor receptor in the acquisition of resistance to EGFR kinase inhibitors in lung cancer [30,39,40]. The rapid proliferation of cancer cells and the acquisition of mutations conferring drug resistance has become a recurring theme in the clinic. To date the most extensive clinical and laboratory characterization of resistance-causing mutations has been performed for BCR–ABL in the context of imatinib and second-generation inhibitors. Furthermore, it has been shown in specific hematological tumors that quiescent stem cells are refractory to tyrosine kinase inhibitors, and these cell populations may be instrumentally involved in resistance mechanisms [41].

Inhibitor resistance conferred by mutations at the gatekeeper residue appears to be the common theme for a variety of kinases. The gatekeeper residue term refers to the amino acid side chain at the position that determines the relative accessibility of the hydrophobic pocket located near the ATP/drug binding site. Access to this pocket is important to many kinase inhibitors because hydrophobic interactions in this site are crucial for the binding affinity of the drug. Several strategies are being investigated to overcome kinase inhibitor resistance mutants. A first approach was to develop inhibitors that can tolerate diverse amino acids at the gatekeeper position [42,43]. A second approach is to target the kinase with inhibitors that bind at alternative binding sites [44]. A third approach involves targeting other molecules that may be required for signal transduction in the specific kinase pathway [45]. These approaches have been demonstrated to work in cell culture, and rodent models and clinical trials are currently underway.

UNANSWERED QUESTIONS

Considerable progress made with the new molecularly targeted therapies. Significant advances have occurred in the treatment of diseases in which few treatment options are available, such NSCLC and melanoma. However, for many patients the therapeutic options are still limited, and the process of bringing a new drug to patients is frustratingly slow with very high failure rates [46,47]. The point of failure between basic research and new drug approval has often referred to as the "Valley of Death" [48,49].

The current model of targeted drug development is severely flawed. The inefficiency of translating seemingly important discoveries from the lab to the clinic can be demonstrated by a simple comparison between the research publications on kinase function and the drug approvals. Multiple obstacles within the current framework severely restrict the timely exploration of combinatorial kinase inhibitor therapies. Regulatory, patent secrets, and risk-averse corporate cultures need to be quickly remedied in order to be prepared, as cancer is becoming the leading cause of death in both humans and veterinary patients.

Scientific questions potentially affecting patient clinical management and treatment options include:

- When to treat with kinase inhibitors?

- What is the biologically sound way to combine kinase inhibitors with cytotoxic chemotherapy?
- How to combine multiple kinase inhibitors in a treatment protocol
- How to determine efficacy when tumor size is not an appropriate measure
- How to manage treatment failure? Switch to different kinase inhibitors, or add different kinase inhibitors to the current therapy?

The canine cancer patient can help in answering some of these questions. Spontaneous cancers in pet dogs offer a unique and largely unexploited translational research opportunity for cancer imaging, device and drug development. Dogs suffer from spontaneous malignancies at similar rates and types as humans. Limitations with rodent models stem from development from inbred strains of mice kept in controlled environments. Companion animals, like humans, are genetically diverse and are exposed to many of the same environmental influences. Furthermore, purebred dogs represent unique gene pools, with genetic predisposition to cancers segregating within specific breeds. This provides the opportunity to study complex phenotypes in a relatively simplified genetic background, allowing the identification of critical genetic events that drive malignant behavior.

Dogs suffering from cancer have been successfully used in elegantly designed studies, providing useful and translatable pharmacokinetic/pharmacodynamic data [50,51,52,53,54,55]. Data from canine clinical trials have informed on the scheduling and dosing of small molecular inhibitors in human cancer patients [56]. The availability of the canine genome and growth of high throughput genomic technologies and informatics has enabled comparative oncology to describe canine cancer biology and define potential therapeutic targets in many of the same ways as human cancers [57,58]. Canine cancer patients offer an unparalleled resource for targeting the tumor stroma and tumor/host immune interactions, due to the presence of syngeneic host-tumor relationship and a competent immune function [50].

Using spontaneous pet dog oncology modeling does not require up-front treatment with specific cancer treatment regimens. Thus, novel therapeutic agents can be offered through clinical trials at any stage in cancer presentation. The disease progression times in pet dogs is compressed, allowing for evaluation of a variety of pharmacodynamics intervention outcomes and providing longitudinal endpoints of cancer response through serial sampling. Randomized controlled trials can be conducted in the newly-diagnosed, adjuvant, or metastatic settings, evaluating the utility of drug combinations and drug selection algorithms across a range of tumor and genetic background scenarios [51].

Finally, the infrastructure and resources to realize the potential of the canine cancer patient as an additional tool in conquering cancer exists. The National Cancer Institute's Comparative Oncology Trials Consortium (NCI-COTC;http://ccr.cancer.gov/resources/cop/COTC.asp) brings together study sponsors with academic veterinary oncology centers in North America to support multicenter clinical trials of investigational therapeutics [59]. High-quality biologic samples (tumor, normal, biologic fluids) from dogs with various malignancies are available via the Pfizer-Canine Comparative Oncology and Genomics Consortium (CCOGC) biospecimen repository (www.ccogc.

net) [60]. As a direct result of such mechanisms drugable target identification and signaling pathway similarities have been identified between canine and human cancer patients [61,62,63,64,65].

FUTURE DIRECTIONS

The use of pet dogs in translational medicine may be the "bridge" to the Death Valley [66]. Translational medicine is the process of applying knowledge gained from basic biomedical research to clinical practice. It involves bridging new research findings, scientific discoveries and new techniques to approaches in the prevention, diagnosis or treatment of diseases. The ultimate outcome is the patient's health. The paradigm shift is that scientific discoveries should not only be celebrated in basic laboratories and research institutes, or published (and archived) in prestigious medical journals—they need to make their way to hospitals, clinics, and into patients' lives to be real successes. Translational medicine involves a longer-term strategy for research that is beyond the immediate outcomes of a research project [67].

A major hurdle in therapeutic development is the translation of efficacy determined during the drug discovery phase into efficacy in the clinic. There are often discrepancies between drug efficacy, demonstrated in the current preclinical experimental models, and final efficacy, or lack thereof, in patients. Tissue culture and various rodent models have been and are used as potential predictive models for response in human cancers. It remains to be decided which model is most predictive, however, it is clear that none can reliably predict significant clinical efficacy.

CONCLUDING REMARKS

Veterinary cancer patients can provide the solution for some of the current limitations faced in targeted therapies. Several of the features that define human cancer, including long periods of latency, the complex biology of cancer recurrence and metastasis, the stromal interactions, and outcomes to novel therapies are frequently not adequately represented in murine cancer [68]. Dogs develop cancer and are diagnosed, staged, and treated in an almost identical manner to human cancer patients. Canine tumors develop in a complex genetic background, in the backdrop of intact immune system, and are exposed to the same environmental carcinogens as their human counterparts. Many dogs are essentially family members. Their owners are motivated to treat their pets, and as advocates for their pet, they actively seek participation in Clinical Trials. With the continuous improvement of the canine genomic annotation, dogs with cancer may represent an excellent opportunity for bridging the Valley of Death. One of the payoffs for human cancer patients is reduced exposure to ineffective clinical trials. The partnership under One Medicine of basic science researchers, veterinary and human oncologists, and pharmaceutical industry, has significant potential to advance drug discovery and approval. Ultimately, this ideal could result in improved cancer management, regardless of species.

AUTHOR CONTRIBUTIONS

Nikolaos Dervisis and Shawna Klahn equally contributed to the writing, revisions and editing of the paper. They are both veterinary oncologists with extensive experience in cancer chemotherapy.

REFERENCES

1. Zhang, J.; Yang, P.L.; Gray, N.S. Targeting cancer with small molecule kinase inhibitors. *Nat. Rev. Cancer* 2009, *9*, 28–39.
2. Tsatsanis, C.; Spandidos, D.A. Oncogenic kinase signaling in human neoplasms. *Ann. N. Y. Acad. Sci.* 2004, *1028*, 168–175.
3. Johnson, L.N.; Lewis, R.J. Structural basis for control by phosphorylation. *Chem. Rev.* 2001, *101*, 2209–2242.
4. Adams, J.A. Kinetic and catalytic mechanisms of protein kinases. *Chem. Rev.* 2001, *101*, 2271–2290.
5. Rask-Andersen, M.; Zhang, J.; Fabbro, D.; Schioth, H.B. Advances in kinase targeting: Current clinical use and clinical trials. *Trends Pharmacol. Sci.* 2014, *35*, 604–620.
6. Burnett, G.; Kennedy, E.P. The enzymatic phosphorylation of proteins. *J. Biol. Chem.* 1954, *211*, 969–980.
7. Cohen, P. The origins of protein phosphorylation. *Nat. Cell Biol.* 2002, *4*, 127–130.
8. UniProt, C. Uniprot: A hub for protein information. *Nucleic Acids Res.* 2015, *43*, 204–212. [Google Scholar]
9. Hanahan, D.; Weinberg, R.A. Hallmarks of cancer: The next generation. *Cell* 2011, *144*, 646–674.
10. Muenke, M.; Schell, U.; Hehr, A.; Robin, N.H.; Losken, H.W.; Schinzel, A.; Pulleyn, L.J.; Rutland, P.; Reardon, W.; Malcolm, S.; *et al.* A common mutation in the fibroblast growth factor receptor 1 gene in Pfeiffer syndrome. *Nat. Genet.*1994, *8*, 269–274.
11. Pitteloud, N.; Acierno, J.S., Jr.; Meysing, A.; Eliseenkova, A.V.; Ma, J.; Ibrahimi, O.A.; Metzger, D.L.; Hayes, F.J.; Dwyer, A.A.; Hughes, V.A.; *et al.* Mutations in fibroblast growth factor receptor 1 cause both kallmann syndrome and normosmic idiopathic hypogonadotropic hypogonadism. *Proc. Natl. Acad. Sci. USA* 2006, *103*, 6281–6286.
12. CDC. Leading Causes of Death. Available online: http://www.cdc.gov/nchs/fastats/leading-causes-of-death.htm(accessed on 19 January 2016).
13. Siegel, R.L.; Miller, K.D.; Jemal, A. Cancer statistics, 2015. *CA Cancer J. Clin.* 2015, *65*, 5–29.
14. Futreal, P.A.; Coin, L.; Marshall, M.; Down, T.; Hubbard, T.; Wooster, R.; Rahman, N.; Stratton, M.R. A census of human cancer genes. *Nat. Rev. Cancer* 2004, *4*, 177–183.

15. Lahiry, P.; Torkamani, A.; Schork, N.J.; Hegele, R.A. Kinase mutations in human disease: Interpreting genotype-phenotype relationships. *Nat. Rev. Genet.* 2010, *11*, 60–74.

16. Vlahovic, G.; Crawford, J. Activation of tyrosine kinases in cancer. *Oncologist* 2003, *8*, 531–538.

17. Cohen, P. Protein kinases—The major drug targets of the twenty-first century? *Nat. Rev. Drug Discov.* 2002, *1*, 309–315.

18. Melnikova, I.; Golden, J. Targeting protein kinases. *Nat. Rev. Drug Discov.* 2004, *3*, 993–994.

19. Schindler, T.; Bornmann, W.; Pellicena, P.; Miller, W.T.; Clarkson, B.; Kuriyan, J. Structural mechanism for STI-571 inhibition of abelson tyrosine kinase. *Science* 2000, *289*, 1938–1942.

20. Wan, P.T.; Garnett, M.J.; Roe, S.M.; Lee, S.; Niculescu-Duvaz, D.; Good, V.M.; Jones, C.M.; Marshall, C.J.; Springer, C.J.; Barford, D.; *et al.* Mechanism of activation of the RAF-ERK signaling pathway by oncogenic mutations of β-RAF. *Cell* 2004, *116*, 855–867.

21. Frantz, B.; Klatt, T.; Pang, M.; Parsons, J.; Rolando, A.; Williams, H.; Tocci, M.J.; O'Keefe, S.J.; O'Neill, E.A. The activation state of p38 mitogen-activated protein kinase determines the efficiency of ATP competition for pyridinylimidazole inhibitor binding. *Biochemistry* 1998, *37*, 13846–13853.

22. Knight, Z.A.; Shokat, K.M. Features of selective kinase inhibitors. *Chem. Biol.* 2005, *12*, 621–637.

23. Ferrara, N.; Hillan, K.J.; Novotny, W. Bevacizumab (avastin), a humanized anti-VEGF monoclonal antibody for cancer therapy. *Biochem. Biophys. Res. Commun.* 2005, *333*, 328–335.

24. Benjamin, D.; Colombi, M.; Moroni, C.; Hall, M.N. Rapamycin passes the torch: A new generation of mTOR inhibitors.*Nat. Rev. Drug Discov.* 2011, *10*, 868–880.

25. Alessi, D.R.; Cuenda, A.; Cohen, P.; Dudley, D.T.; Saltiel, A.R. PD 098059 is a specific inhibitor of the activation of mitogen-activated protein kinase kinase *in vitro* and *in vivo*. *J. Biol. Chem.* 1995, *270*, 27489–27494.

26. Dudley, D.T.; Pang, L.; Decker, S.J.; Bridges, A.J.; Saltiel, A.R. A synthetic inhibitor of the mitogen-activated protein kinase cascade. *Proc. Natl. Acad. Sci. USA* 1995, *92*, 7686–7689.

27. Lindsley, C.W.; Zhao, Z.; Leister, W.H.; Robinson, R.G.; Barnett, S.F.; Defeo-Jones, D.; Jones, R.E.; Hartman, G.D.; Huff, J.R.; Huber, H.E.; *et al.* Allosteric AKT (PKB) inhibitors: Discovery and SAR of isozyme selective inhibitors. *Bioorg. Med. Chem. Lett.* 2005, *15*, 761–764.

28. Yang, J.; Amiri, K.I.; Burke, J.R.; Schmid, J.A.; Richmond, A. Bms-345541 targets inhibitor of κβ kinase and induces apoptosis in melanoma: Involvement of nuclear factor κβ and mitochondria pathways. *Clin. Cancer Res.* 2006, *12*, 950–960.

29. Shaw, A.T.; Kim, D.W.; Nakagawa, K.; Seto, T.; Crino, L.; Ahn, M.J.; de Pas, T.;

Besse, B.; Solomon, B.J.; Blackhall, F.; *et al.* Crizotinib versus chemotherapy in advanced alk-positive lung cancer. *N. Engl. J. Med.* 2013, *368*, 2385–2394.

30. le Coutre, P.; Tassi, E.; Varella-Garcia, M.; Barni, R.; Mologni, L.; Cabrita, G.; Marchesi, E.; Supino, R.; Gambacorti-Passerini, C. Induction of resistance to the abelson inhibitor sti571 in human leukemic cells through gene amplification. *Blood* 2000, *95*, 1758–1766.
31. Druker, B.J.; Guilhot, F.; O'Brien, S.G.; Gathmann, I.; Kantarjian, H.; Gattermann, N.; Deininger, M.W.; Silver, R.T.; Goldman, J.M.; Stone, R.M.; *et al.* Five-year follow-up of patients receiving imatinib for chronic myeloid leukemia. *N. Engl. J. Med.* 2006, *355*, 2408–2417.
32. Yang, J.C.; Sequist, L.V.; Geater, S.L.; Tsai, C.M.; Mok, T.S.; Schuler, M.; Yamamoto, N.; Yu, C.J.; Ou, S.H.; Zhou, C.; *et al.* Clinical activity of afatinib in patients with advanced non-small-cell lung cancer harbouring uncommon EGFR mutations: A combined post-hoc analysis of LUX-Lung 2, LUX-Lung 3, And LUX-Lung 6. *Lancet Oncol.* 2015, *16*, 830–838.
33. Lorenzen, S.; Riera Knorrenschild, J.; Haag, G.M.; Pohl, M.; Thuss-Patience, P.; Bassermann, F.; Helbig, U.; Weissinger, F.; Schnoy, E.; Becker, K.; *et al.* Lapatinib *versus* lapatinib plus capecitabine as second-line treatment in human epidermal growth factor receptor 2-amplified metastatic gastro-oesophageal cancer: A randomised phase II trial of the arbeitsgemeinschaft internistische onkologie. *Eur. J. Cancer* 2015, *51*, 569–576.
34. London, C.A.; Malpas, P.B.; Wood-Follis, S.L.; Boucher, J.F.; Rusk, A.W.; Rosenberg, M.P.; Henry, C.J.; Mitchener, K.L.; Klein, M.K.; Hintermeister, J.G.; *et al.* Multi-center, placebo-controlled, double-blind, randomized study of oral toceranib phosphate (SU11654), a receptor tyrosine kinase inhibitor, for the treatment of dogs with recurrent (either local or distant) mast cell tumor following surgical excision. *Clin. Cancer Res.* 2009, *15*, 3856–3865.
35. Solomon, B.J.; Mok, T.; Kim, D.W.; Wu, Y.L.; Nakagawa, K.; Mekhail, T.; Felip, E.; Cappuzzo, F.; Paolini, J.; Usari, T.; *et al.* First-line crizotinib *versus* chemotherapy in ALK-positive lung cancer. *N. Engl. J. Med.* 2014, *371*, 2167–2177.
36. Duyster, J.; Bai, R.Y.; Morris, S.W. Translocations involving anaplastic lymphoma kinase (ALK). *Oncogene* 2001, *20*, 5623–5637.
37. Rikova, K.; Guo, A.; Zeng, Q.; Possemato, A.; Yu, J.; Haack, H.; Nardone, J.; Lee, K.; Reeves, C.; Li, Y.; *et al.* Global survey of phosphotyrosine signaling identifies oncogenic kinases in lung cancer. *Cell* 2007, *131*, 1190–1203.
38. Blackhall, F.H.; Peters, S.; Bubendorf, L.; Dafni, U.; Kerr, K.M.; Hager, H.; Soltermann, A.; O'Byrne, K.J.; Dooms, C.; Sejda, A.; *et al.* Prevalence and clinical outcomes for patients with ALK-positive resected stage I to III adenocarcinoma: Results from the european thoracic oncology platform lungscape project. *J. Clin. Oncol.* 2014, *32*, 2780–2787.
39. Engelman, J.A.; Zejnullahu, K.; Mitsudomi, T.; Song, Y.; Hyland, C.; Park, J.O.; Lindeman, N.; Gale, C.M.; Zhao, X.; Christensen, J.; *et al.* Met amplification

leads to gefitinib resistance in lung cancer by activating ERBB3 signaling. *Science* 2007, *316*, 1039–1043.

40. Cui, J.J. Targeting receptor tyrosine kinase met in cancer: Small molecule inhibitors and clinical progress. *J. Med. Chem.* 2014, *57*, 4427–4453.
41. Copland, M.; Hamilton, A.; Elrick, L.J.; Baird, J.W.; Allan, E.K.; Jordanides, N.; Barow, M.; Mountford, J.C.; Holyoake, T.L. Dasatinib (BMS-354825) targets an earlier progenitor population than imatinib in primary cml but does not eliminate the quiescent fraction. *Blood* 2006, *107*, 4532–4539.
42. Weisberg, E.; Manley, P.W.; Breitenstein, W.; Bruggen, J.; Cowan-Jacob, S.W.; Ray, A.; Huntly, B.; Fabbro, D.; Fendrich, G.; Hall-Meyers, E.; *et al.* Characterization of AMN107, a selective inhibitor of native and mutant BCR-ABL.*Cancer Cell* 2005, *7*, 129–141.
43. Shah, N.P.; Lee, F.Y.; Luo, R.; Jiang, Y.; Donker, M.; Akin, C. Dasatinib (BMS-354825) inhibits kitd816v, an imatinib-resistant activating mutation that triggers neoplastic growth in most patients with systemic mastocytosis. *Blood* 2006,*108*, 286–291.
44. Gumireddy, K.; Reddy, M.V.; Cosenza, S.C.; Boominathan, R.; Baker, S.J.; Papathi, N.; Jiang, J.; Holland, J.; Reddy, E.P. ON01910, a non-ATP-competitive small molecule inhibitor of Plk1, is a potent anticancer agent. *Cancer Cell* 2005, *7*, 275–286.
45. Copland, M.; Pellicano, F.; Richmond, L.; Allan, E.K.; Hamilton, A.; Lee, F.Y.; Weinmann, R.; Holyoake, T.L. BMS-214662 potently induces apoptosis of chronic myeloid leukemia stem and progenitor cells and synergizes with tyrosine kinase inhibitors. *Blood* 2008, *111*, 2843–2853.
46. Yap, T.A.; Workman, P. Exploiting the cancer genome: Strategies for the discovery and clinical development of targeted molecular therapeutics. *Annu. Rev. Pharmacol. Toxicol.* 2012, *52*, 549–573.
47. DiMasi, J.A.; Grabowski, H.G. Economics of new oncology drug development. *J. Clin. Oncol.* 2007, *25*, 209–216.
48. Adams, D.J. The valley of death in anticancer drug development: A reassessment. *Trends Pharmacol. Sci.* 2012, *33*, 173–180.
49. Wong, T.Y. How to bridge the "valley of death" between a research discovery and clinical application? *Ann. Acad. Med. Singap.* 2014, *43*, 422–424.
50. Paoloni, M.; Mazcko, C.; Selting, K.; Lana, S.; Barber, L.; Phillips, J.; Skorupski, K.; Vail, D.; Wilson, H.; Biller, B.; *et al.* Defining the pharmacodynamic profile and therapeutic index of NHS-IL12 immunocytokine in dogs with malignant melanoma. *PLoS ONE* 2015.
51. Paoloni, M.; Webb, C.; Mazcko, C.; Cherba, D.; Hendricks, W.; Lana, S.; Ehrhart, E.J.; Charles, B.; Fehling, H.; Kumar, L.; *et al.* Prospective molecular profiling of canine cancers provides a clinically relevant comparative model for evaluating personalized medicine (PMed) trials. *PLoS ONE* 2014.
52. Paoloni, M.; Lana, S.; Thamm, D.; Mazcko, C.; Withrow, S. The creation of the

comparative oncology trials consortium pharmacodynamic core: Infrastructure for a virtual laboratory. *Vet. J.* 2010, *185*, 88–89.

53. Paoloni, M.C.; Mazcko, C.; Fox, E.; Fan, T.; Lana, S.; Kisseberth, W.; Vail, D.M.; Nuckolls, K.; Osborne, T.; Yalkowsy, S.;*et al.* Rapamycin pharmacokinetic and pharmacodynamic relationships in osteosarcoma: A comparative oncology study in dogs. *PLoS ONE* 2010.
54. Gordon, I.; Paoloni, M.; Mazcko, C.; Khanna, C. The comparative oncology trials consortium: Using spontaneously occurring cancers in dogs to inform the cancer drug development pathway. *PLoS Med.* 2009.
55. Paoloni, M.C.; Tandle, A.; Mazcko, C.; Hanna, E.; Kachala, S.; Leblanc, A.; Newman, S.; Vail, D.; Henry, C.; Thamm, D.; *et al.* Launching a novel preclinical infrastructure: Comparative oncology trials consortium directed therapeutic targeting of TNFα to cancer vasculature. *PLoS ONE* 2009, *4*, e4972.
56. London, C.A.; Bernabe, L.F.; Barnard, S.; Kisseberth, W.C.; Borgatti, A.; Henson, M.; Wilson, H.; Jensen, K.; Ito, D.; Modiano, J.F.; *et al.* Preclinical evaluation of the novel, orally bioavailable selective inhibitor of nuclear export (SINE) KPT-335 in spontaneous canine cancer: Results of a phase I study. *PLoS ONE* 2014.
57. Lindblad-Toh, K.; Wade, C.M.; Mikkelsen, T.S.; Karlsson, E.K.; Jaffe, D.B.; Kamal, M.; Clamp, M.; Chang, J.L.; Kulbokas, E.J., 3rd; Zody, M.C.; *et al.* Genome sequence, comparative analysis and haplotype structure of the domestic dog. *Nature* 2005, *438*, 803–819.
58. Hoeppner, M.P.; Lundquist, A.; Pirun, M.; Meadows, J.R.; Zamani, N.; Johnson, J.; Sundstrom, G.; Cook, A.; FitzGerald, M.G.; Swofford, R.; *et al.* An improved canine genome and a comprehensive catalogue of coding genes and non-coding transcripts. *PLoS ONE* 2014.
59. LeBlanc, A.K.; Mazcko, C.N.; Khanna, C. Defining the value of a comparative approach to cancer drug development.*Clin. Cancer Res.* 2015.
60. Webster, J.D.; Simpson, E.R.; Michalowski, A.M.; Hoover, S.B.; Simpson, R.M. Quantifying histological features of cancer biospecimens for biobanking quality assurance using automated morphometric pattern recognition image analysis algorithms. *J. Biomol. Tech.* 2011, *22*, 108–118.
61. Simpson, R.M.; Bastian, B.C.; Michael, H.T.; Webster, J.D.; Prasad, M.L.; Conway, C.M.; Prieto, V.M.; Gary, J.M.; Goldschmidt, M.H.; Esplin, D.G.; *et al.* Sporadic naturally occurring melanoma in dogs as a preclinical model for human melanoma. *Pigment Cell Melanoma Res.* 2014, *27*, 37–47.
62. Bushell, K.R.; Kim, Y.; Chan, F.C.; Ben-Neriah, S.; Jenks, A.; Alcaide, M.; Fornika, D.; Grande, B.M.; Arthur, S.; Gascoyne, R.D.; *et al.* Genetic inactivation of TRAF3 in canine and human B-cell lymphoma. *Blood* 2015, *125*, 999–1005.
63. Elvers, I.; Turner-Maier, J.; Swofford, R.; Koltookian, M.; Johnson, J.; Stewart, C.; Zhang, C.Z.; Schumacher, S.E.; Beroukhim, R.; Rosenberg, M.; *et al.* Exome sequencing of lymphomas from three dog breeds reveals somatic mutation patterns reflecting genetic background. *Genome Res.* 2015, *25*, 1634–1645.

64. Mochizuki, H.; Kennedy, K.; Shapiro, S.G.; Breen, M. BRAF mutations in canine cancers. *PLoS ONE* 2015.

65. Decker, B.; Parker, H.G.; Dhawan, D.; Kwon, E.M.; Karlins, E.; Davis, B.W.; Ramos-Vara, J.A.; Bonney, P.L.; McNiel, E.A.; Knapp, D.W.; *et al.* Homologous mutation to human BRAF V600E is common in naturally occurring canine bladder cancer—Evidence for a relevant model system and urine-based diagnostic test. *Mol. Cancer Res.* 2015, *13*, 993–1002.

66. Butler, D. Translational research: Crossing the valley of death. *Nature* 2008, *453*, 840–842.

67. Jiang, F.; Zhang, J.; Wang, X.; Shen, X. Important steps to improve translation from medical research to health policy.*J. Transl. Med.* 2013.

68. Ranieri, G.; Gadaleta, C.D.; Patruno, R.; Zizzo, N.; Daidone, M.G.; Hansson, M.G.; Paradiso, A.; Ribatti, D. A model of study for human cancer: Spontaneous occurring tumors in dogs. Biological features and translation for new anticancer therapies. *Crit. Rev. Oncol. Hematol.* 2013, *88*, 187–197.

12

CHAPTER

MAST CELL ACTIVATION DISEASE: A CONCISE PRACTICAL GUIDE FOR DIAGNOSTIC WORKUP AND THERAPEUTIC OPTIONS

Gerhard J Molderings, Stefan Brettner, Jürgen Homann and Lawrence B Afrin

INTRODUCTION

The term *mast cell activation disease* (MCAD) denotes a collection of disorders characterized by (1) accumulation of pathological mast cells in potentially any or all organs and tissues and/or (2) aberrant release of variable subsets of mast cell mediators. A classification has been proposed which differentiates several types and subclasses of MCAD (Table 1). The traditionally recognized subclass termed *systemic mastocytosis*(SM) includes disorders characterized by certain pathological immunohistochemical and mutational findings (the WHO criteria; Table 2; [1, 2]) which are divided into several subtypes (Table 1). On the other hand, *mast cell activation syndrome* (MCAS) presents a complex clinical picture of multiple mast cell mediator-induced symptoms, failure to meet the WHO criteria for diagnosis of SM, and exclusion of relevant differential diagnoses [1, 3, 4, 5]. Symptoms observed in patients with MCAS are little, if any, different from those seen in patients with SM [6, 7, 8]. Patients present variable and often fluctuating patterns of symptoms (Table 3; [9,10, 11, 12, 13, 14, 15]) which depend on the tissue responses to mast cell mediators released both spontaneously and in response to trigger stimuli.

Citation: Gerhard J Molderings, Stefan Brettner, Jürgen Homann3 , Lawrence B Afrin, Mast cell activation disease: a concise practical guide for diagnostic workup and therapeutic options, DOI: 10.1186/1756-8722-4-10.

Table 1: Classification of mast cell activation disease (modified from [2, 3, 4])

Mast cell activation disease (MCAD)	
Mast cell activation syndrome (MCAS)	
Systemic mastocytosis (SM) defined by the WHO criteria	• Indolent systemic mastocytosis • Isolated bone marrow mastocytosis • Smoldering systemic mastocytosis • Systemic mastocytosis with an associated clonal hematologic non-mast cell lineage disease • Aggressive systemic mastocytosis
Mast cell leukemia (MCL)	

Table 2: Criteria proposed to define mast cell activation disease (for references, see text).

Criteria to define *mast cell activation syndrome*	**WHO criteria to define *systemic mastocytosis***
Major criteria	**Major criterion**
1. Multifocal or disseminated dense infiltrates of mast cells in bone marrow biopsies and/or in sections of other extracutaneous organ(s) (e.g., gastrointestinal tract biopsies; CD117-, tryptase- and CD25-stained)	Multifocal dense infiltrates of mast cells (>15 mast cells in aggregates) in bone marrow biopsies and/or in sections of other extracutaneous organ(s) (CD117-, tryptase- and CD25-stained)
2. Unique constellation of clinical complaints as a result of a pathologically increased mast cell activity (mast cell mediator release syndrome)	
Minor criteria	**Minor criteria**
1. Mast cells in bone marrow or other extracutaneous organ(s) show an abnormal morphology (>25%) in bone marrow smears or in histologies	1. Mast cells in bone marrow or other extracutaneous organ(s) show an abnormal morphology (>25%) in bone marrow smears or in histologies

2. Mast cells in bone marrow express CD2 and/or CD25	2. Mast cells in bone marrow express CD2 and/or CD25
3. Detection of genetic changes in mast cells from blood, bone marrow or extracutaneous organs for which an impact on the state of activity of affected mast cells in terms of an increased activity has been proved.	3. c-kit mutation in tyrosine kinase at codon 816 in mast cells in extracutaneous organ(s)
4. Evidence of a pathologically increased release of mast cell mediators by determination of the content of	4. Serum total tryptase >20 ng/ml (does not apply in patients who have associated hematologic non-mast-cell lineage disease)
• tryptase in blood	
• N-methylhistamine in urine	
• heparin in blood	
• chromogranin A in blood	
• other mast cell-specific mediators (e.g., leukotrienes, prostaglandin D_2)	

The diagnosis *mast cell activation syndrome* is made if both major criteria or the second criterion and at least one minor criterion are fulfilled. According to the WHO criteria [1], the diagnosis *systemic mastocytosis* is established if the major criterion and at least one minor criterion or at least three minor criteria are fulfilled.

Table 3: Frequent signs and clinical symptoms ascribed to episodic unregulated release of mast cell mediators (modified from [12]; further references therein; an exhaustive survey is given in [50])

Signs and Symptoms	
Abdominal	abdominal pain, intestinal cramping and bloating, diarrhea and/or obstipation, nausea, non-cardiac chest pain, Helicobacter pylori-negative gastritis, malabsorption
Oropharyngeal	burning pain, aphthae
Respiratory	cough, asthma-like symptoms, dyspnea, rhinitis, sinusitis
Ophthalmologic	conjunctivitis, difficulty in focusing
Hepatic	splenomegaly, hyperbilirubinemia, elevation of liver transaminases, hypercholesterolemia
Splenomegaly	
Lymphadenopathy	

Cardiovascular	tachycardia, blood pressure irregularity (hypotension and/or hypertension), syncope, hot flush
Neuropsychiatric	headache, neuropathic pain, polyneuropathy, decreased attention span, difficulty in concentration, forgetfulness, anxiety, sleeplessness, organic brain syndrome, vertigo, lightheadedness, tinnitus
Cutaneous	urticaria pigmentosa, hives, efflorescences with/without pruritus, telangiectasia, flushing, angioedema
Abnormal bleeding	
Musculoskeletal	muscle pain, osteoporosis/osteopenia, bone pain, migratory arthritis
Interstitial cystitis	
Constitutional	fatigue, asthenia, fever, environmental sensitivities

A rare variant of MCAD is mast cell leukemia (MCL; Table 1). This aggressive mast cell neoplasm is defined by increased numbers of mast cells in bone marrow smears (≥20%) and by circulating mast cells (reviewed in [2]). Patients typically suffer from rapidly progressive organopathy involving the liver, bone marrow and other organs. The bone marrow typically shows a diffuse, dense infiltration with mast cells. In typical MCL, mast cells account for more than 10% of blood leukocytes. In a smaller group of patients, pancytopenia occurs and mast cells account for less than 10% (aleukemic variant of MCL). The prognosis in MCL is poor. Most patients survive less than 1 year and respond poorly to cytoreductive drugs or chemotherapy.

Mast cell activation disease in general has long been thought to be rare. However, although SM and MCL as defined by the WHO criteria are truly rare, recent findings suggest MCAS is a fairly common disorder. Evidence has been presented for a causal involvement of pathologically active mast cells not only in the pathogenesis of SM and MCAS but also in the etiology of idiopathic anaphylaxis [16, 17, 18], interstitial cystitis [19], some subsets of fibromyalgia [20, 21] and some subsets of irritable bowel syndrome [22, 23, 24].

Pathogenesis

Mutations in kinases (particularly in the tyrosine kinase Kit) and in enzymes and receptors (JAK2, PDGFRα, RASGRP4, Src-kinases, c-Cbl-encoded E3 ligase, histamine H4 receptor) which are crucially involved in the regulation of mast cell activity have been identified as necessary to establish a clonal mast cell population, but other abnormalities yet to be determined must be added for the development of a clinically symptomatic disease ([7, 8, 25, 26]; further references therein). The observations that the same KIT mutation (e.g. D816V) can be associated with both good prognosis as well as progression to advanced disease [27] and that the D816V mutation has also been detected in healthy subjects [28] highlight the potential role of other factors in determining the progression/outcome of the disease. Recent findings suggest that the immunohistochemical and morphological alterations which constitute the WHO criteria for SM (formation of mast cell clusters; spindle-shaped morphology of mast cells; expression of CD25 on mast cells; Table 2) are causally related to and specific for the occurrence of a mutation in codon 816 of tyrosine kinase Kit in the affected mast cells [6,29, 30, 31]. Another aspect that limits the diagnostic value of this mutation is that during progression of SM the Kit mutant D816V may disappear ([32]; own unpublished observation). Taken together, the recent genetic findings suggest that the clinically different subtypes of MCAD (encompassing SM, MCL, and MCAS) should be more accurately regarded as varying presentations of a common generic root process of mast cell dysfunction than as distinct diseases [4, 7, 8, 11].

Clinical Diagnostics

MCAD is first suspected on clinical grounds, based on recognition of compatible mast cell mediator-related symptoms and, in some, identification of typical skin lesions. The clinical presentation of MCAD is very diverse, since due to both the widespread distribution of mast cells and the great heterogeneity of aberrant mediator expression patterns, symptoms can occur in virtually all organs and tissues (Table 3). Moreover, symptoms often occur in a temporally staggered fashion, waxing and waning over years to decades. Symptoms often initially manifest during adolescence or even childhood or infancy but are recognized only in retrospect as MCAD-related. Clinical features and courses vary greatly and range from very indolent with normal life expectancy to highly aggressive with reduced survival times. Physical examination should include inspection for a large assortment of types of skin lesions, testing for dermatographism (Darier's sign), and palpating for hepatosplenomegaly and lymphadenopathy. A diagnostic algorithm is shown in Figure 1. Recognition of a mast cell mediator release syndrome, i.e. a pattern of symptoms caused by the unregulated increased release of mediators from mast cells, can be aided by use of a validated checklist [2, 11, 12, 33] which lists the complaint complexes to be considered. In addition to the detection of the characteristic clinical constellation of findings, it must be investigated whether levels of the mast cell-specific mediators tryptase, histamine, and heparin are elevated in the blood, whether the excretion of the histamine metabolite methylhistamine into the urine is increased, and whether mast cell activity-related eosinophilia, basophilia or monocytosis in the blood can be observed. Other useful markers fairly specific to mast cells include serum chromogranin A (in the absence of cardiac and renal failure, neuroendocrine cancer, and proton pump inhibitor use) and serum and urinary leukotriene and prostaglandin isoforms (e.g., leukotriene E_4, prostaglandin D_2, and prostaglandin $9\alpha,11\beta PGF_2$). Together with a characteristic clinical presentation, abnormal markers can be of diagnostic, therapeutic and prognostic relevance. However, it remains unsettled whether demonstration of an elevation of mast cell activity markers is absolutely necessary for diagnosis of MCAD because (1) many conditions (e.g., degrading enzymes, complexing molecules, tissue pH) may attenuate or impede spill-over of exocytosed mediators from tissues into the blood, (2) only a handful of the more than 60 releasable mast cell mediators can be detected by routine commercial techniques, and (3) mediator release syndrome may be due to an amplification cascade of basophil, eosinophil, and general leukocyte activation induced by liberation of only a few mast cell mediators [34] which, again, may not be detectable by present techniques.

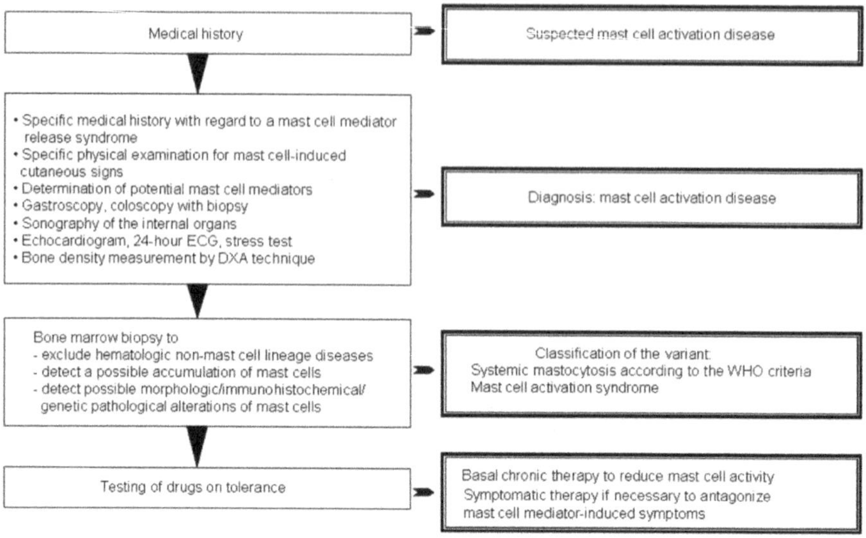

Figure 1: Diagnostic algorithm.

When relevant differential diagnoses of a mast cell activation disease (Table 4) which may present mast cell mediator-induced symptoms by activation of normal mast cells (e.g., allergy) or as result of non-mast-cell-specific expression of mediators (e.g., neuroendocrine cancer) are excluded, the cause of the mast cell mediator release syndrome must lie in the uncontrolled increase in activity of pathologically altered mast cells. Patients with most types of MCAD often initially enjoy symptom-free intervals interspersed amongst symptomatic periods. Over time, symptom-free intervals shorten, and finally symptoms become chronic with intensity which fluctuates but with an overall trend toward steadily increasing intensity. Following the proposed revised diagnostic criteria (Table 2; [3, 4, 5, 9, 35]), MCAD is diagnosed if either both major criteria or one major criterion and at least one minor criterion are met. After clinical diagnosis, a bone marrow biopsy is usually recommended because based on current information it cannot be predicted whether the genetic alterations inducing pathological mast cell activity in affected mast cells have not also induced disturbances in hematopoietic non-mast cell lineages. SM due to codon 816 mutations has been shown to be associated with myeloid neoplasms (and, less frequently, with B-cell neoplasms) frequently enough to warrant routine marrow biopsy when SM is suspected (e.g., serum tryptase elevation per the WHO criteria, frequent unprovoked anaphylactoid events). The frequency of discovery of associated hematologic neoplasms on marrow biopsy at the time of diagnosis of MCAS remains unclear but in our experience appears very low. However, a byproduct of marrow biopsy is that immunohistochemical analysis of the specimen may permit the classification of the mast cell activation disease as SM defined by the WHO criteria or as MCAS (Table 2). In this context, it has to be considered that due to the typically patchy distribution of mast cell infiltration in the bones a single marrow biopsy fails to find systemic mastocytosis in the marrow approximately one-sixth of the time [36].

Table 4: Diseases which should be considered as differential diagnoses of mast cell activation disease, since they may mimick or may be associated with mast cell activation (diagnostic procedure of choice in parentheses)

Endocrinologic disorders	Diabetes mellitus (laboratory determination)
	Pancreatic endocrine tumours (gastrinoma, insulinoma, glucagonoma, somatostatinoma, VIPoma; laboratory determination, medical history)
	Porphyria (laboratory determination)
	Disorders of the thyroid gland (laboratory determination)
	Morbus Fabry (clinical picture, molecular genetic investigation)
Gastrointestinal disorders	Helicobacter-positive gastritis (gastroscopy, biopsy)
	Infectious enteritis (stool examination)
	Eosinophilic gastroenteritis (endoscopy, biopsy)
	Parasitic infections (stool examination)
	Inflammatory bowel disease (endoscopy, biopsy)
	Celiac disease (endoscopy, biopsy, laboratory determination)
	Primary lactose intolerance (molecular genetic investigation)
	Microscopic colitis (endoscopy, biopsy)
	Amyloidosis (endoscopy, biopsy)
	Intestinal obstructions by adhesions, volvulus and other reasons (medical history, imaging methods, laparoscopy)
	Hepatitis (laboratory determination)
	Cholelithiasis (imaging methods)
	Hereditary hyperbilirubinemia (laboratory determination)
Immunological/ neoplastic diseases	Carcinoid tumour (medical history, laboratory determination)
	Pheochromocytoma (medical history, laboratory determination)
	Primary gastrointestinal allergy (medical history)
	Hypereosinophilic syndrome (laboratory determination)
	Hereditary angioedema (medical history, laboratory determination)
	Vasculitis (medical history, laboratory determination)
	Intestinal lymphoma (imaging methods)

An aggressive course of MCAD is characterized and defined by organopathy caused by pathologic infiltration of various organs by neoplastic mast cells inducing an impairment of organ function. Organopathy due to mast cell infiltration is indicated by findings termed *C-findings*: (1) significant cytopenia(s); (2) hepatomegaly with impairment of liver function due to mast cell infiltration, often with ascites; (3) splenomegaly with hypersplenism; (4) malabsorption with hypoalbuminemia and weight loss; (5) life-threatening impairment of organ function in other organ systems; (6) osteolyses and/or severe osteoporosis with pathologic fractures. Urticaria pigmentosa-like skin lesions are usually absent. In contrast to MCL, the bone marrow smear shows fewer than 20% mast cells (reviewed in [2]). Mast cell infiltration with organomegaly but without end organ dysfunction (hepatomegaly, splenomegaly, lymphadenopathy, bone marrow alterations) is a *B-finding* and may occur in a subvariant of SM (smoldering SM) with high mast cell burden.

Treatment of mast cell Activation Diseases

The cornerstone of therapy is avoidance of identifiable triggers for mast cell degranulation such as animal venoms, extremes of temperature, mechanical irritation, alcohol, or medications (e.g., aspirin, radiocontrast agents, certain anesthetic agents). Individual patients may have variable tolerance patterns and avoidance lists, but it also is not uncommon to have no identifiable, reliable triggers.

Drug treatment of MCAD patients is highly individualized. Curative therapies are not avail-able, and each MCAD patient should be treated in accordance with his symptoms and complications. Irrespective of the specific clinical presentation of MCAD, evidence-based therapy consists of trigger avoidance, antihistamines, and mast cell membrane-stabilising compounds (basic therapy, Table 5) supplemented as needed by medications targeting individual mast cell mediator-induced symptoms or complications (symptomatic therapy, Table 5). First hints of success with any given therapy are usually seen within 4 weeks once suitable dosing has been achieved Multiple simultaneous changes in the medication regimen are discouraged since such can confound identification of the specific therapy responsible for a given improvement (or deterioration). Ineffective or harmful agents should be stopped promptly. If symptoms are resistant to therapy, as a next therapeutic step toward reducing mast cell activity and thereby decreasing mediator release, treatment with prednisone, ciclosporine (cyclosporine A), low dose methotrexate or azathioprine can be considered. Recently, anti-IgE treatment with the humanized murine monoclonal antibody omalizumab has alleviated high intensity symptoms of MCAD [37]. Since treatment with omalizumab has an acceptable risk-benefit profile, it should be considered in cases of MCAD resistant to evidence-based therapy. Recently, molecularly targeted therapy by tyrosine kinase inhibitors such as imatinib mesylate, dasatinib and midostaurin has been investigated. As with all drugs used in therapy of MCAD, their therapeutic success seems to be strongly dependent on the individual patient. In formal studies in SM patients, although the kinase inhibitors reduced mast cell burden as reflected by histological normalization in bone marrow and improved laboratory surrogate markers, at best only partial improvement of mediator-related symptoms was achieved [38, 39, 40, 41]. However, in some case reports, imatinib and dasatinib have been significantly effective at relieving symptoms. In spite of potential significant adverse effects of these drugs, a therapeutic trial may be justified in individual cases at an early stage. Given that PI3K/AKT/mTOR is one of the downstream signalling pathways upregulated by activated Kit, in theory mTOR inhibitors (e.g., sirolimus, temsirolimus, everolimus) may have utility in MCAD, but to date the one trial of this notion (everolimus in SM) showed no significant clinical activity [42].

Table 5: Treatment options for mast cell activation disease

Basic therapy (continuous oral combination therapy to reduce mast cell activity)	• H_1-histamine receptor antagonist (to block activating H_1-histamine receptors on mast cells; to antagonize H_1-histamine receptor-mediated symptoms) • H_2- histamine receptor antagonist (to block activating H_2-histamine receptors on mast cells; to antagonize H_2-histamine receptor-mediated symptoms) • Cromolyn sodium (stabilising mast cells) • Slow-release Vitamin C (increased degradation of histamine; inhibition of mast cell degranulation; not more than 750 mg/day) • If necessary, ketotifen to stabilise mast cells and to block activating H_1-histamine receptors on mast cells
Symptomatic treatment options(orally as needed)	• ***Headache***⇒ paracetamol; metamizole; flupirtine • ***Diarrhea***⇒ colestyramine; nystatin; montelukast; 5-HT_3 receptor inhibitors (eg. ondansetron); incremental doses (50-350 mg/day; extreme caution because of the possibility to induce mast cell degranulation) of acetylsalicylic acid; (in steps test each drug for 5 days until improvement of diarrhea) • ***Colicky abdominal pain*** due to distinct meteorism ⇒ metamizole; butylscopolamine • ***Nausea***⇒ metoclopramide; dimenhydrinate; 5-HT_3 receptor inhibitors; icatibant • ***Respiratory symptoms***(mainly increased production of viscous mucus and obstruction with compulsive throat clearing) ⇒ montelukast; urgent: short-acting ß-sympathomimetic • ***Gastric complaints***⇒ proton pump inhibitors (de-escalating dose finding) • ***Osteoporosis, osteolysis, bone pain***⇒ biphosphonates ([51]; vitamin D plus calcium application is second-line treatment in MCAD patients because of limited reported success and an increased risk for developing kidney and ureter stones; [52]) • ***Non-cardiac chest pain***⇒ when needed, additional dose of a H_2-histamine receptor antagonist; also, proton pump inhibitors for proven gastroesophageal reflux • ***Tachycardia***⇒ verapamil; AT1-receptor antagonists; ivabradin • ***Neuropathic pain and paresthesia***⇒ α-lipoic acid • ***Interstitial cystitis***⇒ pentosan, amphetamines • ***Sleep-onset insomnia/sleep-maintenance insomnia***⇒ triazolam/oxazepam • ***Conjunctivitis***⇒ exclusion of a secondary disease; otherwise preservative-free eye drops with glucocorticoids for brief courses • ***Hypercholesterolemia***⇒ (does not depend on the composition of the diet) therapeutic trial with HMG-CoA reductase inhibitors (frequently ineffective) • ***Elevated prostaglandin levels, persistant flushing***⇒ incremental doses of acetylsalicylic acid (50-350 mg/day; extreme caution because of the possibility to induce mast cell degranulation)

All drugs should be tested for tolerance in a low single dose before therapeutic use, if their tolerance in the patient is not known from an earlier application.

A difficult situation is the occurrence of life-threatening anaphylaxis in patients with MCAD. If anaphylaxis is provoked by a known allergen, especially hymenoptera venom, immunotherapy should be considered with recognition of potential risks [43, 44, 45]. In case of repeated life-threatening anaphylactoid episodes, the self-administration of epinephrine on demand has been recommended as an appropriate approach.

In patients with high-grade variants of MCAD (presence of C-findings) and a progressive clini-cal course, cytoreductive drugs are recommended and are prescribed together with anti-mediator-type drugs [46, 47]. Potential therapeutic options are interferon-α and 2-chlorodeoxyadenosine (2-CdA, cladribine). Interferon-α is frequently combined with prednisone and is commonly used as first-line cytoreductive therapy for aggressive SM. It ameliorates SM-related organopathy in a proportion of cases but is associated with considerable adverse effects (e.g., flu-like symptoms, myelosuppression, depression, hypothyroidism), which may limit its use in MCAD [48, 49]. PEGylated interferon-α has been shown to be as efficacious as, and less toxic than the non-PEGylated form in some chronic myeloproliferative diseases, but it has not been specifically studied in MCAD. 2-Chlorodeoxyadenosine (2-CdA) is generally reserved for last choice treatment of patients with aggressive SM who are either refractory or intolerant to interferon-α. Potential toxicities of 2-CdA include significant and potentially prolonged myelosuppression and lymphopenia with increased risk of opportunistic infections. Patients who fail interferon-α and 2-CdA therapy are candidates for experimental drugs. However, such therapeutic maneuvers and their potential beneficial effects have to be balanced against the long-term risk and serious side effects of these therapies (often immunosuppressive or/and mutagenic). Polychemotherapy including intensive induction regimens of the kind used in treating acute myeloid leukemia, as well as high-dose therapy with stem cell rescue, represent investigational approaches restricted to rare, selected patients. A variety of other agents have been reported to have in-vitro activity against at least some MCAD-associated mutations [3] and may have a future role in the treatment of this disease.

No tools yet exist to predict which specific therapeutic regimen will be optimal for the individual MCAD patient. However, especially in non-aggressive disease (comprising the great majority of patients), at least partial improvement is usually attainable with one regimen or another, and thus the practitioner is obligated to persist with therapeutic trials until no options remain. Finally, although clinical trials in MCAD are rare, enrolment in such must be a priority.

CONCLUSIONS

MCAD comprises disorders affecting functions in potentially every organ system by abnormal release of mediators from and/or accumulation of genetically altered mast cells. There is evidence that MCAD is a disorder with considerable prevalence and thus should be considered routinely in the differential diagnosis of patients with chronic multisystem polymorbidity of unknown cause. In most cases of MCAD, diagnosis is possible by relatively non-invasive investigation. Effective therapy often consists simply of antihistamines and mast cell membrane-stabilising compounds supplemented with medications targeted at specific symptoms and complications.

ACKNOWLEDGEMENTS

Publication of this article was supported by the *B.Braun-Stiftung* (Germany) and the *Förderclub Mastzellforschung e.V.* (Germany).

REFERENCES

1. Valent P, Horny HP, Escribano L, Longley BJ, Li CY, Schwartz LB, Marone G, Nuñez R, Akin C, Sotlar K, Sperr WR, Wolff K, Brunning RD, Parwaresch RM, Austen KF, Lennert K, Metcalfe DD, Vardiman JW, Bennett JM: Diagnostic criteria and classification of mastocytosis: a consensus proposal. Leuk Res. 2001, 25: 603-625. 10.1016/S0145-2126(01)00038-8.
2. Valent P, Akin C, Escribano L, Födinger M, Hartmann K, Brockow K, Castells M, Sperr WR, Kluin-Nelemans HC, Hamdy NA, Lortholary O, Robyn J, van Doormaal J, Sotlar K, Hauswirth AW, Arock M, Hermine O, Hellmann A, Triggiani M, Niedoszytko M, Schwartz LB, Orfao A, Horny HP, Metcalfe DD: Standards and standardization in mastocytosis: consensus statements on diagnostics, treatment recommendations and response criteria. Eur J Clin Invest. 2007, 37: 435-453. 10.1111/j.1365-2362.2007.01807.x.
3. Homann J, Kolck UW, Ehnes A, Frieling T, Raithel M, Molderings GJ: Systemic mastocytosis - definition of an internal disease. Med Klin (Munich). 2010, 105: 544-553. 10.1007/s00063-010-1093-8.
4. Akin C, Valent P, Metcalfe DD: Mast cell activation syndrome: Proposed diagnostic criteria. J Allergy Clin Immunol. 2010, 126: 1099-1104. 10.1016/j.jaci.2010.08.035.
5. Hamilton MJ, Castells M, Greenberger NJ: Mast cell activation syndrome - a newly recognized cause of recurrent acute abdominal pain. Gastroenterology. 2010, 138 (Suppl 1): S89-
6. Alvarez-Twose I, González de Olano D, Sánchez-Muñoz L, Matito A, Esteban-López MI, Vega A, Mateo MB, Alonso Díaz de Durana MD, de la Hoz B, Del Pozo Gil MD, Caballero T, Rosado A, Sánchez Matas I, Teodósio C, Jara-Acevedo M, Mollejo M, García-Montero A, Orfao A, Escribano L: Clinical, biological, and molecular characteristics of clonal mast cell disorders presenting with systemic mast cell activation symptoms. J Allergy Clin Immunol. 2010, 125: 1269-1278. 10.1016/j.jaci.2010.02.019.
7. Molderings GJ, Kolck UW, Scheurlen C, Brüss M, Homann J, von Kügelgen I: Multiple novel alterations in Kit tyrosine kinase in patients with gastrointestinally pronounced systemic mast cell activation disorder. Scand J Gastroenterol. 2007, 42: 1045-1053. 10.1080/00365520701245744.
8. Molderings GJ, Meis K, Kolck UW, Homann J, Frieling T: Comparative analysis of mutation of tyrosine kinase kit in mast cells from patients with systemic mast

cell activation syndrome and healthy subjects. Immunogenetics. 2010, 62: 721-727. 10.1007/s00251-010-0474-8.

9. Horan RF, Austen KF: Systemic mastocytosis: retrospective review of a decade's clinical experience at the brigham and the women's hospital. Invest Dermatol. 1991, 96: 5S-14S. 10.1111/1523-1747.ep12468899.
10. Castells M: Mast cell mediators in allergic inflammation and mastocytosis. Immunol Allergy Clin North Am. 2006, 26: 465-485. 10.1016/j.iac.2006.05.005.
11. Hermine O, Lortholary O, Leventhal PS, Catteau A, Soppelsa F, Baude C, Cohen-Akenine A, Palmérini F, Hanssens K, Yang Y, Sobol H, Fraytag S, Ghez D, Suarez F, Barete S, Casassus P, Sans B, Arock M, Kinet JP, Dubreuil P, Moussy A: Case-control cohort study of patients' perceptions of disability in mastocytosis. PLoS ONE. 2008, 3: e2266-10.1371/journal.pone.0002266.
12. Alfter K, von Kügelgen I, Haenisch B, Frieling T, Hülsdonk A, Haars U, Rolfs A, Noe G, Kolck UW, Homann J, Molderings GJ: New aspects of liver abnormalities as part of the systemic mast cell activation syndrome. Liver Int. 2009, 29: 181-186. 10.1111/j.1478-3231.2008.01839.x.
13. Escribano L, Alvarez-Twose I, Sánchez-Muñoz L, Garcia-Montero A, Núñez R, Almeida J, Jara-Acevedo M, Teodósio C, García-Cosío M, Bellas C, Orfao A: Prognosis in adult indolent systemic mastocytosis: A long-term study of the Spanish Network on Mastocytosis in a series of 145 patients. J Allergy Clin Immunol. 2009, 124: 514-521. 10.1016/j.jaci.2009.05.003.
14. Lim KH, Pardanani A, Butterfield JH, Li CY, Tefferi A: Cytoreductive therapy in 108 adults with systemic mastocytosis: Outcome analysis and response prediction during treatment with interferon-alpha, hydroxyurea, imatinib mesylate or 2-chlorodeoxyadenosine. Am J Hematol. 2009, 84: 790-794. 10.1002/ajh.21561.
15. Lundequist A, Pejler G: Biological implications of preformed mast cell mediators. Cell Mol Life Sci. 2011, 68: 965-675. 10.1007/s00018-010-0587-0.
16. Akin C, Scott LM, Kocabas CN, Kushnir-Sukhov N, Brittain E, Noel P, Metcalfe DD: Demonstration of an aberrant mast cell population with clonal markers in a subset of patients with "idiopathic" anaphylaxis. Blood. 2007, 110: 2331-2333. 10.1182/blood-2006-06-028100.
17. Gonzalez de Olano D, de la Hoz Caballer B, Nunez Lopez R, Sanchez Munoz L, Cuevas Agustin M, Dieguez MC, Alvarez Twose I, Castells MC, Escribano Mora L: Prevalence of allergy and anaphylactic symptoms in 210 adult and pediatric patients with mastocytosis in Spain: a study of the Spanish network on mastocytosis (REMA). Clin Exp Allergy. 2007, 37: 1547-1555.
18. Brockow K, Jofer C, Behrendt H, Ring J: Anaphylaxis in patients with mastocytosis: a study on history, clinical features and risk factors in 120 patients. Allergy. 2008, 63: 226-232. 10.1111/j.1398-9995.2007.01569.x.
19. Sant GR, Kempuraj D, Marchand JE, Theoharides TC: The mast cell in interstitial cystitis: role in pathophysiology and pathogenesis. Urology. 2007, 69 (4 Suppl): 34-40. 10.1016/j.urology.2006.08.1109.

20. Enestrom S, Bengtsson A, Frodin T: Dermal IgG deposits and increase of mast cells in patients with fibromyalgia - relevant findings or epiphenomena?. Scand J Rheumatol. 1997, 26: 308-313. 10.3109/03009749709105321.

21. Lucas HJ, Brauch CM, Settas L, Theoharides TC: Fibromyalgia - new concepts of pathogenesis and treatment. Int J Immunopathol Pharmacol. 2006, 19: 5-9.

22. Kolck UW: Investigations on the pathogenesis of the systemic mast cell activation syndrome and its impact on heart function. Bonn, University, medical thesis. 2009, URN:nbn:de:hbz:5N-19064, [http://hss.ulb.uni-bonn.de/2009/1906/1906.htm]

23. Nickel JC, Tripp DA, Pontari MA, Moldwin RM, Mayer R, Carr LK, Doggweiler R, Yang CC, Whitcomb D, Mishra N, Nordling J: Phenotypic associations between interstitial cystitis/painfil bladder syndrome and irritable bowel syndrtome, fibromyalgia, chronis fatigue syndrome: a case control study. J Urology. 2009, 181 (Suppl): 19-10.1016/S0022-5347(09)60067-7.

24. Frieling T, Meis K, Kolck UW, Homann J, Hülsdonk A, Haars U, Hertfelder H-J, Oldenburg J, Seidel H, Molderings GJ: Evidence for mast cell activation in patients with therapy-resistant irritable bowel syndrome. Z Gastroenterol. 2011, 49: 191-194. 10.1055/s-0029-1245707.

25. Orfao A, Garcia-Montero AC, Sanchez L, Escribano L: REMA: Recent advances in the understanding of mastocytosis: the role of KIT mutations. Br J Haematol. 2007, 138: 12-30. 10.1111/j.1365-2141.2007.06619.x.

26. Bodemer C, Hermine O, Palmérini F, Yang Y, Grandpeix-Guyodo C, Leventhal PS, Hadj-Rabia S, Nasca L, Georgin-Lavialle S, Cohen-Akenine A, Launay JM, Barete S, Feger F, Arock M, Catteau B, Sans B, Stalder JF, Skowron F, Thomas L, Lorette G, Plantin P, Bordigoni P, Lortholary O, de Prost Y, Moussy A, Sobol H, Dubreuil P: Pediatric mastocytosis is a clonal disease associated with D(816) V and other activating c-KIT mutations. J Invest Dermatol. 2010, 130: 804-815. 10.1038/jid.2009.281.

27. Garcia-Montero AC, Jara-Acevedo M, Teodosio C, Sanchez ML, Nunez R, Prados A, Aldanondo I, Sanchez L, Dominguez M, Botana LM, Sanchez-Jimenez F, Sotlar K, Almeida J, Escribano L, Orfao A: KIT mutation in mast cells and other bone marrow hematopoietic cell lineages in systemic mast cell disorders: a prospective study of the Spanish Network on Mastocytosis (REMA) in a series of 113 patients. Blood. 2006, 108: 2366-2372. 10.1182/blood-2006-04-015545.

28. Lawley W, Hird H, Mallinder P, McKenna S, Hargadon B, Murray A, Bradding P: Detection of an activating c-kit mutation by real-time PCR in patients with anaphylaxis. Mutation Res. 2005, 572: 1-13. 10.1016/j.mrfmmm.2004.08.015.

29. Mayerhofer M, Gleixner KV, Hoelbl A, Florian S, Hoermann G, Aichberger KJ, Bilban M, Esterbauer H, Krauth MT, Sperr WR, Longley JB, Kralovics R, Moriggl R, Zappulla J, Liblau RS, Schwarzinger I, Sexl V, Sillaber C, Valent P: Unique effects of KIT D816V in BaF3 cells: induction of cluster formation, histamine synthesis, and early mast cell differentiation antigens. J Immunol. 2008, 180: 5466-5476.

30. Teodosio C, García-Montero AC, Jara-Acevedo M, Sánchez-Muñoz L, Alvarez-Twose I, Núñez R, Schwartz LB, Walls AF, Escribano L, Orfao A: Mast cells from different molecular and prognostic subtypes of systemic mastocytosis display distinct immunopheno-types. J Allergy Clin Immunol. 2010, 125: 719-726. 10.1016/j.jaci.2009.10.020.

31. Yang Y, Létard S, Borge L: Pediatric mastocytosis-associated KIT extracellular domain mutations exhibit different functional and signaling properties compared with KIT-phosphotransferase domain mutations. Blood. 2010, 116: 1114-1123. 10.1182/blood-2009-06-226027.

32. Gotlib J, Berubé C, Growney JD, Chen CC, George TI, Williams C, Kajiguchi T, Ruan J, Lilleberg SL, Durocher JA, Lichy JH, Wang Y, Cohen PS, Arber DA, Heinrich MC, Neckers L, Galli SJ, Gilliland DG, Coutré SE: Activity of the tyrosine kinase inhibitor PKC412 in a patient with mast cell leukemia with the D816V KIT mutation. Blood. 2005, 106: 2865-2870. 10.1182/blood-2005-04-1568.

33. Molderings GJ, Kolck U, Scheurlen C, Brüss M, Frieling T, Raithel M, Homann J: Systemic mast cell disease with gastrointestinal symptoms - a diagnostic questionnaire. Dtsch Med Wochenschr. 2006, 131: 2095-2100. 10.1055/s-2006-951337.

34. Theoharides TC, Kempuraj D, Tagen M, Conti P, Kalogeromitros D: Differential release of mast cell mediators and the pathogenesis of inflammation. Immunol Rev. 2007, 217: 65-78. 10.1111/j.1600-065X.2007.00519.x.

35. Roberts LJ, Oates JA: Biochemical diagnosis of systemic mast cell disorders. J Invest Dermatol. 1991, 96 (3 Suppl): 19S-24S. 10.1111/1523-1747.ep12468945.

36. Butterfield JH, Li C-Y: Bone marrow biopsies for the diagnosis of systemic mastocytosis: is one biopsy sufficient?. Am J Clin Path. 2004, 121: 264-267. 10.1309/2EWQKN00PG02JKY0.

37. Molderings GJ, Raithel M, Kratz F, Azemar M, Haenisch B, Harzer S, Homann J: Omalizumab treatment of systemic mast cell activation disease: experiences from four cases. Intern Med. 2011, 50: 1-5. 10.2169/internalmedicine.50.4640.

38. Droogendijk HJ, Kluin-Nelemans HJC, van Doormaal JJ, Oranje AR, van de Loosdrecht AA, van Daele PLA: Imatinib mesylate in the treatment of systemic mastocytosis - A phase II trial. Cancer. 2006, 107: 345-351. 10.1002/cncr.21996.

39. Gotlib J, George TI, Corless C, Linder A, Ruddell A, Akin C, DeAngelo DJ, Kepten I, Lanza C, Heinemann H, Yin O, Gallagher N, Graubert T: The Kit tyrosine kinase inhibitor midostaurine (PKC412) exhibits a high response rate in aggressive systemic mastocytosis (ASM): interim results of a phase II trial. Blood. 2008, 110: 1039A-

40. Verstovsek S, Tefferi A, Cortes J, O'Brien S, Garcia-Manero G, Pardanani A, Akin C, Faderl S, Manshouri T, Thomas D, Kantarjian H: Phase II study of dasatinib in Philadelphia chromosome-negative acute and chronic myeloid diseases, including systemic mastocytosis. Clin Cancer Res. 2008, 14: 3906-3915. 10.1158/1078-0432.CCR-08-0366.

41. Vega-Ruiz A, Cortes JE, Sever M, Manshouri T, Quintás-Cardama A, Luthra R, Kantarjian HM, Verstovsek S: Phase II study of imatinib mesylate as therapy for patients with systemic mastocytosis. Leuk Res. 2009, 33: 1481-1484. 10.1016/j.leukres.2008.12.020.

42. Parikh SA, Kantarjian HM, Richie MA, Cortes JE, Verstovsek S: Experience with everolimus (RAD001), an oral mammalian target of rapamycin inhibitor, in patients with systemic mastocytosis. Leuk Lymph. 2010, 51: 269-274. 10.3109/10428190903486220.

43. de Olano DG, Twose IA, Esteban López MI, Muñoz LS, Alonso Díaz de Durana MD, Castro AV, Montero AG, González-Mancebo E, González TB, Herrero Gil MD, Fernández-Rivas M, Orfao A, de la Hoz Caballer B, Castells MC, Mora LE: Safety and effectiveness of immunotherapy in patients with indolent systemic mastocytosis presenting with Hymenoptera venom anaphylaxis. J Allergy Clin Immunol. 2008, 121: 519-526. 10.1016/j.jaci.2007.11.010.

44. Ruëff F, Przybilla B, Biló MB, Müller U, Scheipl F, Aberer W, Birnbaum J, Bodzenta-Lukaszyk A, Bonifazi F, Bucher C, Campi P, Darsow U, Egger C, Haeberli G, Hawranek T, Körner M, Kucharewicz I, Küchenhoff H, Lang R, Quercia O, Reider N, Severino M, Sticherling M, Sturm GJ, Wüthrich B: Predictors of severe systemic anaphylactic reactions in patients with Hymenoptera venom allergy: importance of baseline serum tryptase-a study of the European Academy of Allergology and Clinical Immunology Interest Group on Insect Venom Hypersensitivity. J Allergy Clin Immunol. 2009, 124: 1047-1054.

45. Bonadonna P, Zanotti R, Müller U: Mastocytosis and insect venom allergy. Curr Opin Allergy Clin Immunol. 2010, 10: 347-353. 10.1097/ACI.0b013e32833b280c.

46. Valent P, Sperr WR, Akin C: How I treat patients with advanced systemic mastocytosis. Blood. 2010, 116: 5812-5817. 10.1182/blood-2010-08-292144.

47. Lim KH, Tefferi A, Lasho TL, Finke C, Patnaik M, Butterfield JH, McClure RF, Li CY, Pardanani A: Systemic mastocytosis in 342 consecutive adults: survival studies and prognostic factors. Blood. 2009, 113: 5727-5736. 10.1182/blood-2009-02-205237.

48. Simon J, Lortholary O, Caillat-Vigneron N, Raphael M, Martin A, Briere J, Barete S, Hermine O, Casussus P: Interest of interferon alpha in systemic mastocytosis. The french experience and review of the literature. Pathol Biol. 2004, 52: 294-299. 10.1016/j.patbio.2004.04.012.

49. Butterfield JH: Interferon treatment for hypereosinophilic syndromes ans systemic mastocytosis. Acta haematol. 2005, 114: 26-40. 10.1159/000085560.

50. Afrin LB: Polycythemia from mast cell activation disorder: lessons from incongruence of symptoms vs. test results. Am J Med Sci. 2011

51. Barete S, Assous N, de Gennes C, Grandpeix C, Feger F, Palmerini F, Dubreuil P, Arock M, Roux C, Launay JM, Fraitag S, Canioni D, Billemont B, Suarez F, Lanternier F, Lortholary O, Hermine O, Francès C: Systemic mastocytosis and bone involvement in a cohort of 75 patients. Ann Rheum Dis. 2010, 69: 1838-1841. 10.1136/ard.2009.124511.

52. Molderings GJ, Solleder G, Kolck UW, Homann J, Schröder D, von Kügelgen I, Vorreuther R: Ureteral stones due to systemic mastocytosis: diagnostic and therapeutic characteristics. Urol Res. 2009, 37: 227-229. 10.1007/s00240-009-0198-0.

13

CHAPTER

PAST, PRESENT AND FUTURE: OVERVIEW ON HISTOLOGY AND HISTOPATHOLOGY

Giuseppe musumeci

EDITORIAL

With sincere satisfaction and pride, I present this first editorial of the Journal of Histology and Histopathology edited by myself. I know this is a very challenging task, assuming the editorial coordination of this journal, targeted to enhance the work of so many esteemed international experts as well as dear colleagues, who work on morphological research. A special thanks goes to our current editorial team (Sherif M Karam, Xueyong Zhu, Gjumrakch Aliev, Khin Thway, Han-Seung yoon, Paul Evans, George Perry and Khush Mittal) and the publishing group (Herbert Publications) that, day after day, thanks to their valuable contribution, make possible the growth of this journal. Reviewing a manuscript is time-consuming and unpaid, and often reviewers are bombarded with requests to review simultaneously from several journals. I hope to increase the number of editors of the editorial board members (with different geographical origin), to assure a rapid publication. My aim and that of all the other editors is that this journal will constitute a valuable tool, of both learning and research, to understand how modern histology and histopathology can be a fundamental bridge between molecular and anatomicalphysiological disciplines and how the structural organization of cells in tissues is inextricably linked to the functions that the pathological and normal tissues

Citation: Musumeci G. Past, present and future: overview on histology and histopathology. J Histol Histopathol. 2014; 1:5. http://dx.doi.org/10.7243/2055-091X-1-5.

must perform. These concepts must constitute a significant part of imprinting training, necessary to help researchers to work in a more guided way, increasingly interested in a cellular approach to diseases and their related treatments. Finally, conscious of the fact that this journal can be considered a "system" subjected to the laws of evolution, we welcome criticism and suggestions for its improvement in the future. The purpose of this editorial was to explain my view on histology and histopathology of today, providing a brief overview from the past to the future.

HISTOLOGY

Histology and Histopathology are often discussed and described together. In fact, the concept of histopathology cannot be separated from that of histology since understanding of normal histology is essential for histo-pathological interpretation. It is indeed obvious and necessary to prepare histology slides of a sample or specimen and examine them first in order to find out if the cells or tissue are healthy or diseased. Moreover, expert histo-pathologists should also be able to inform histologists about normal variations of tissue morphology, improving in this way histo-pathological interpretations. We could state then, that histology and histopathology are inter-dependent. In the 19th century, histology was an eminent academic discipline in its own right and the first half of the 20th century was a very productive period for new staining techniques in histology and histopathology. Indeed the 1906 Nobel Prize in Physiology or Medicine was awarded to histologists Camillo Golgi and Santiago Ramon y Cajal. They had conflicting interpretations of the neural structure of the brain based on differing interpretations of the same images. Cajal was appreciated for his correct theory and Golgi for the staining technique that he invented. Many of the centenary staining techniques in cell biology and histopathology are still used and continue to provide valuable diagnostic information. Histology is the study of the microscopic details and structures of biological cells and tissues, using light, fluorescence or electron microscopes, examining a thin slice (called a "section") of tissues, that have been previously prepared using appropriate processes called "histological techniques". The first microscope had been constructed in 1591 but had several optical problems. In 1673 Anton van Leeuwenhoek developed a simple microscope with a single lense but with improved magnification and resolution. The first microtome suitable for sectioning animal tissues was constructed in 1848. During the 19th century paraffin wax was introduced for infiltration and support during sectioning. Over the years different laboratory substances were investigated for use as fixatives. Formalin was first used in 1893 and today is widely employed [1-3]. In order to better underline different biological structures, histological stains are often used to modify or enhance the colors of certain types of these biological structures differently from the others that may be located next to them or be in contact with them. There are many different histology stains selected according to the type of tissue to be observed. Some stains are more widely used, instead others are only used to study very specific types of biological tissues. One of the oldest stains was Prussian blue, introduced in 1774. Furthemore, Perl's reaction, discovered in 1867, is still widely used to localize intracellular iron and uses just Prussian blue for the histochemical localization of hemosiderin in tissues. Hematoxylin and eosin (H&E stain) is the most commonly used histology stain for light microscopy. Hematoxylin stains the nuclei within cells blue and eosin stains the cytoplasm of cells pink. H&E is a permanent histology stain, as opposed to a temporary stain. The hematoxylin and eosin staining techniques were first described in 1875–1878, with later modifications. Hematology took advantage from the introduction in the 1890s of Romanovsky-type staining for blood smears, including Giemsa's and May-Grunwald staining which are still fundamental in clinical practice. Louis B. Wilson was the first to develop a method using methylene dyes to stain fresh-frozen tissue of surgical specimens (1906). The periodic acid-Schiff (PAS) technique of McManus (1946) is still one of the most common diagnostic staining methods in histopathology, it superseded Best's carmine (1906) to stain polysaccharides and is widely used in liver and muscle disease [4-6]. Oil Red (ORO), introduced by French in 1926 highlights the presence of fat or lipids in fresh, frozen tissue sections. ORO is a fat soluble diazo dye, and is classified as one of the Sudan dyes used since the late 1800s. Feulgen stain (1924) is a staining technique used in histology to identify chromosomal material or DNA in cell specimens and has been the basis of many subsequent applications in cell biology. The Ziehl–Nielsen stain for Mycobacterium tuberculosis (1883) and Gram's stain for bacteria (1884) are examples of diagnostic bacteriological and pathological techniques, which are still used over a century since their discovery. Paul Ehrlich, who received the Nobel Prize in 1908 for his discovery and his work on "magic bullets", developed the use of dyes to combat disease i.e. methylene blue (1891) to fight malaria and trypan red (1904) against the trypanosomes. Trypan blue remains in widespread as a vital stain, particularly in highlighting cataracts during eye surgery [4-6]. These staining methods are generally inexpensive, reliable, fast, produce permanent preparations that are easy to interpret and archive, and deliver information for diagnoses that cannot be achieved by other means. For these reasons they remain useful and irreplaceable tools in the histology discipline.

HISTOPATHOLOGY

Histopathology regards biological tissues and cells with their microscopic changes or abnormalities that can be the causes or the result of diseases. The main application of histopathology in clinical medicine, is in the examination of a biopsy (i.e., a surgical sample or specimen taken from patients possibly for diagnosis and screening of various tumors) by a specialist physician called a pathologist. The pathologist may be more accurately referred to as a histopathologist. However, for some histopathologists the microscopic examination of diseased tissues may be only a relatively minor part of their overall professional responsibilities. A pathologist or histopathologist studies specimens of cells and tissue samples removed from the patients, processed using special histological techniques (histological slides and sections prepared and stained in order to make the sample ready for observation with a microscope). Either a light microscope or an electron microscope may be used to examine histology slides. The first book on the specialization of histopathology techniques, entitled, "On the Nature and Structural Characteristics of Cancer" was written in 1838 by Johannes Müller. Enzyme histochemistry, electron microscopy, and polarizing microscopy have all become diagnostic tools during the last 50 years. Actually, the use of electron microscopy is rare, except for specific contexts or disciplines such as renal pathology. The use of immunohistochemistry, still under development with new antibodies and biomarkers, began in the 1980s and has revolutionized cancer diagnosis [1-3]. The histology laboratory experienced several changes in the mid 20th century when cryostats, enclosed tissue processors, plastic cassettes, and disposable knives were introduced. The emergence of immunohistochemistry in the 1980s was a revolution among the histopathology methods [1-3] and made obsolete the necessity for the use of electron microscopy. New techniques include flow cytometry, fluorescence in situ hybridization (FISH), DNA and genetics studies, proteomics, telepathology, and digital imaging. The field of proteomics will be widened by the discovery of new biomarkers and new immunohistochemical tests. These new tests must be accepted by the medical community, and therefore histology laboratories in various hospitals will have to work together to standardize their protocols. Telepathology will be implemented for consultation and diagnosis. However, technicians will have to be sure that a slide prepared in one laboratory when sent as a scan to another laboratory for diagnosis conforms to certain criteria. Thus, specimen collection, fixation, and processing will need to be consistent between laboratories. In less-developed countries these telepathology techniques and equipment will be of benefit to patients [1-3].

CONCLUSION

We can be proud that basic histological, histochemical and immuohistochemical methods have a very long and productive history and continue to give us useful information. We have an enormous debt to the pioneers who discovered stains for coloring tissues and combating disease together with subsequent techniques. These old methodologies still continue to play an important role in the histopathology laboratory and remain at the forefront of research in these disciplines with an enormous long-term impact in cell biology and molecular biology. Histology is the tool for accessing a specific knowledge of the microscopic organization of the organs, microscopic anatomy, which is essential to understand the histopathology for a possible diagnosis. Although today in the research field these disciplines may seem displaced by the *in vitro* study of cell biology, molecular biology, genetics studies and proteomics, in my opinion, remain a key to help and sustain, with the *in vivo* study of tissue and organs, an efficient clinical practice. In confirmation, it is known that histopathology is an essential tool in diagnosis and the experience of the histopathologist is prime and irreplaceable for the correct interpretation of the data obtained. Although immunohistochemical analyses and molecular biology are useful for diagnostic purposes, light microscopy remains preeminent in cytological and histological diagnosis on a daily basis. Hematoxylin and eosin stain is still the gold standard for diagnosis, also in malignancy diagnosis that is based on the interpretation of cytological and architectural features, while immunohistochemistry and molecular biology are ancillary tools which can provide useful information in confirming histologically-based diagnosis.

ACKNOWLEDGEMENT

I thank Prof. Gaetano Magro from Department G.F. Ingrassia, Anatomic Pathology Section, University of Catania, Catania, Italy, for his kind support.

REFERENCES

1. TitfordM.AShortHistoryofHistopathologyTechnique.*JHistotechnol.*2006;29:99-110.
2. Titford M. Progress in the development of microscopical techniques for diagnostic pathology. *J Histotechnol.* 2009; 32:9-19.
3. Titford M and Bowman B. What May the Future Hold for Histotechnologists? *LabMedicine.* 2012; 43:5-10.
4. Coleman R. The impact of histochemistry--a historical perspective. *Acta Histochem.* 2000; 102:5-14.
5. Coleman R. The long-term contribution of dyes and stains to histology and histopathology. *Acta Histochem.* 2006; 108:81-3.
6. Coleman R. Eponyms in histology and histochemistry: do they still serve a purpose, or should they be abandoned in favor of standard non-eponymous terminology? *Acta Histochem.* 2006; 108:241-2.

14
CHAPTER

EFFECT OF HOMOCYSTEINE ON THE HISTOLOGICAL STRUCTURE OF FEMUR IN YOUNG MALE ALBINO RATS AND THE POSSIBLE PROTECTIVE ROLE OF FOLIC ACID

Rania A. Zidan and Heba M. Elnegris

Keywords: Homocysteine, femur, folic acid, growing rats

INTRODUCTION

Osteoporosis is a major health problem that is characterized by low bone mineral density, deterioration of bone microarchitecture and an increased risk of fracture [1].

Osteoporotic fractures are associated with increased level of morbidity and mortality and with substantial economic costs [2,3].

It has been hypothesized that the metabolism of homocysteine is involved in osteoporosis [4]. Homocystinuria, a rare autosomal recessive disease characterized by markedly elevated levels of plasma homocysteine, has several clinical manifestations involving the eyes, the vasculature, and the central nervous system. The presence of homocystinuria is associated with the early onset of generalized osteoporosis [5,6]. The underlying pathophysiological mechanism for the occurrence of early osteoporosis in patients who have homocystinuria is not completely understood [7].

Citation: Rania A. Zidan and Heba M. Elnegris, Effect of homocysteine on the histological structure of femur in young male albino rats and the possible protective role of folic acid, DOI : http://dx.doi.org/10.7243/2055-091X-2-16.

Several studies confirmed an association between homocysteine and bone mineral density in postmenopausal women [8,9], in patients with Crohn's disease [10], primary billiary cirrhosis [11], and hyperparathyroidism [12]. A high circulating homocysteine concentration has also been mentioned as an independent risk factor for several chronic conditions, including cardiovascular and Alzheimer disease [13]. It has been proved that the administration of homocysteine caused osteopenia in newborn rats [14]. Whereas, other studies failed to confirm such an association [15].

Homocysteine (HCY) is a sulfur-containing amino acid formed in the metabolic pathway between methionine and cysteine [16]. Elevated levels of homocysteine known as hyperhomocysteinemia (HHCY) are associated with various bone abnormalities, such as osteopenia and osteoporosis [17,18]. The thiol groups in Hcy undergo auto-oxidation, thus triggering oxidative stress. Methionine is condensed with ATP to form S-adenosylmethionine, the universal methyl donor in transmethylation reactions and the direct precursor of HCY *in vivo* [19].

Folate, vitamin B_6 and vitamin B_{12} are important enzymatic cofactors in the synthesis of methionine from homocysteine (Hcy), and an elevation of Hcy can be caused by insufficiency of folate, vitamin B_6 or vitamin B_{12}[20,21].

Numerous studies have linked high circulating Hcy levels and low concentrations of folate or vitamin B_{12} with increased risk of low bone mineral density (BMD) in non-diabetic subjects [22,23].

Supplementation with vitamin B_{12} and folate has recently been shown to decrease fracture risk in stroke patients [24].

Folic acid (FA) is a naturally occurring dietary component [25]. A lack of dietary folic acid leads to a folate deficiency [26].

Folic acid is essential to numerous body functions ranging from nucleotide biosynthesis to the remethylation of homocysteine [27,28]. Children and adults both require folic acid in order to produce healthy red blood cells and prevent anemia. Folic acid can be used to treat Alzheimer's disease, depression, and certain types of cancer [29].

Previous data indicated a higher bone turnover (resorption and formation) leading to decreased bone mineral density (BMD) among individuals with high Hcy levels. A high bone turnover may lead to lower BMD and is also a risk factor for fracture [30].

Osteoclasts are specialized cells that resorb bone, whereas osteoblasts are cells that synthesize new bone. The RANK ligand (RANKL), a protein expressed by the osteoblasts, plays an important role in osteoclast formation, function, and survival through its interaction with RANK on the osteoclast [31]. Osteoprotegerin (OPG), a natural inhibitor of RANKL, interferes with RANKL and RANK association and thereby regulates osteoclast activity and resorption in the bone [32,33]. Despite this considerable evidence that identifies homocysteine as a risk factor for osteoporosis, the molecular mechanisms of how bone remodeling is hampered during hyperhomocysteinemia still remain ambiguous.The aim of the present work is to investigate the structural changes that occur in the bone and epiphyseal plate of femur in young male albino rats after being treated with oral HCY and the possible protective role of folic acid.

MATERIALS AND METHODS

Experimental animals

Thirty six young male albino rats (aged 3 weeks, weighing 50-60gm at the beginning of experiment) were housed in stainless steel cages at Animal House, Faculty of Medicine, Zagazig University at room temperature, fed standard balanced diet and allowed water ad libitum. The experiment was performed in accordance with the "Guide for the Care and Use of Laboratory Animals" [34]. The experimental protocol was approved by the Ethical Committee of Zagazig University.

Chemicals

Homocysteine (HCY)

Was obtained from Sigma-Aldrich, USA. The drug was dissolved in distilled water as a vehicle.

Folic acid

Was obtained from El Nasr Pharmaceutical Chemicals Co. And was dissolved in normal saline to give a suspension.

Groups

Rats were classified into three equal groups (12 animals each).

Group I (Control)

Rats were further subdivided into three equal subgroups.

Subgroup IA (negative control group)

Rats were gavaged with 1 ml of distilled water once daily for 6 weeks.

Subgroup IB (saline positive control group)

Rats were gavaged with 1 ml of normal saline {solution of 0.90%w/v of NaCl, isotonic saline} (the solvent of folic acid) once daily for 6weeks [35].

Subgroup IC (folic acid positive control group)

Rats were gavaged with folic acid at a dose of 2 mg/kg dissolved in 1 ml of normal saline for 6weeks [35].

Group II (homocysteine treated group)

In which rats received daily Hcys at a dose of 0.6 mg/kg b.wt. dissolved in 1 ml distilled water [36] for 6 weeks through oral gavage [37].

Group III: (homocysteine+folic acid group) (protected group)

The animals in this group received concomitant administration of homocysteine at the same dose and duration as group II plus folic acid at the same dose and duration as group IC.

At the end of experiment, rats of all studied groups were anesthetized with 35mg/kg body weight sodium pentobarbital intraperitoneally [38].

Biochemical study

Blood samples were collected to undergo estimation of serum homocysteine by enzyme-linked immuno sorbent assay (ELISA) test.

With the use of a commercial enzyme-linked immunosorbent assay (ELISA kit) (Automated Chemiluminescent System, AUS: 180®, Bayer HealthCarc). Total HCY concentration was determined after protein-bound HCY was converted to free HCY, which was then enzymatically converted to S-adenosyl- L-HCY (SAH) by S-adenosylhomocysteine hydrolase enzyme. The enzyme is specific for the L-form of homocysteine, which is the only form present in the blood.

Histological study

Specimen preparation for light microscope examination

The right femurs were carefully dissected free of soft tissue. The distal part of each bone (including the diaphysis with distal metaphysis were obtained using a sharp blade) was immediately fixed in 10% neutral buffered formaldehyde for 2 days. After fixation, preparation of decalcified specimens was performed using the chelating agent ethylene diamine tetra acetic acid (EDTA) in the form of its disodium salt (5.5 g ethylene diamine tetra acetic acid in 90 ml distilled water and 10 ml formaldehyde 37-40%). Decalcification was carried out for 3 weeks, during this time the decalcifying solution was changed every day [39]. The decalcified specimens were dehydrated and processed to form paraffin blocks. Serial coronal sections (6 um thick) parallel to the long axis of the femur and extending from one-third to one-half the thickness of each bone were prepared and stained with hematoxylin and eosin (H&E) and Mallory trichrome stains [39].

The immunohistochemical staining for localization of osteoprotegerin protein was carried out by means of the avidin biotin-peroxidase complex method following the manufacturer's instructions. The slides were incubated with mouse monoclonal anti-OPG antibody 1:250, (MAb 8051, R&D Systems, Abingdon, UK) for 1 h, washed and incubated for 30 min with antimouse biotin-conjugated secondary antibody (30 μl/2 ml of casein solution diluted 1:50) (Vector Laboratories, Peterborough, UK). Slides were washed and developed using ABC Elite kit (Vector Laboratories), followed by diaminobenzidine (DAB) and a 20 sec counterstain with haematoxylin. Negative control sections were incubated with PBS instead of the primary antibody [40].

Positive reaction appeared as brownish granules mainly in the cytoplasm of cells of osteoblastic cell lineage and sometimes areas of the trabecular surface [41]. Positive reaction was also detected in maturative/hypertrophic chondrocytes, and early osteocytes [42].

Specimen Preparation for electron Microscope Examination

Small pieces from shaft of femur were immediately fixed in 2.5% glutaraldehyde buffered with 0.1 M phosphate buffer at pH 7.4 for 2 hours at 4°C and then washed with phosphate buffer, postfixed in 1% osmium tetraoxide in the same buffer for one hour at 4°C. The postfixed specimens were decalcified by EDTA solution in buffer for 3 successive days at 4°C. Then the specimens were washed in phosphate buffer and were dehydrated with ascending grades of ethanol. They were put in propylene oxide for 30 minutes at room temperature, impregnated in a mixture of propylene oxide and resin (1:1) for 24 hours and in a pure resin for another 24 hours. Then, the specimens were embedded in Embed-812 resin in BEEM capsules at 60°C for 24 hours [43].

Ultra-thin sections were obtained using Leica ultra cut UCT and stained with uranyl acetate and lead citrate [43] and were examined with JEOL JEM 1010 electron microscope in Electron Microscope Research Laboratory (EMRL) of Histology and Cell Biology Department, Faculty of Medicine, Zagazig University.

Morphometric and statistical study

The following parameters 'of the femur bone were quantified:

1. Outer cortical bone thickness (um) of diaphysis: (mean width of outer cortical bone). This was measured by drawing a perpendicular line from just beneath the periosteum to the endosteum. Cortical bone thickness or width (μm) were determined at five levels (0.5mm apart), starting 0.2 mm below the lowest point of the growth plate [44].
2. Trabecular bone thickness (um): the thickness of trabeculae in cancellous bone of distal metaphysis were measured at their midpoint away from their branching areas [45]. For estimation of outer cortical bone thickness and trabecular bone thickness, the mean values of ten non overlapping fields (at magnificationx200) from each of five different sections at different femur levels of 4 animals from each group were taken.
3. The number of osteoclasts was estimated/high power field (hpf). Osteoclasts were counted in ten random high power non overlopping fields in five sections obtained from each animal of 4animals in each group.

The standard deviation was calculated and statistical analysis was carried out. The image analyzer computer system Leica Qwin 500 (Leica Ltd, Cambridge, UK) at the Image Analyzing Unit of the Pathology Department, Faculty of Dentistry, Cairo University (Egypt), was used. using SPSS statistical program version 17.

Data were evaluated by using the one-way analysis of variance test. The probability values (P) less than 0.05 was considered significant and highly significant when the P values were less than 0.001.

RESULTS

Light microscopic observations

The light and electron microscopic examinations of subgroups Ia, Ib and Ic of the control group revealed similar morphological results; hence, we chose the results of subgroup Ia (negative control) to represent the control group.

Observations of H&E stained sections

The distal metaphysis of control femur showed a network of irregular bone trabeculae and bone marrow spaces between them. The osteocytes surrounded by their lacunae were present in the bone matrix (Figure 1A).

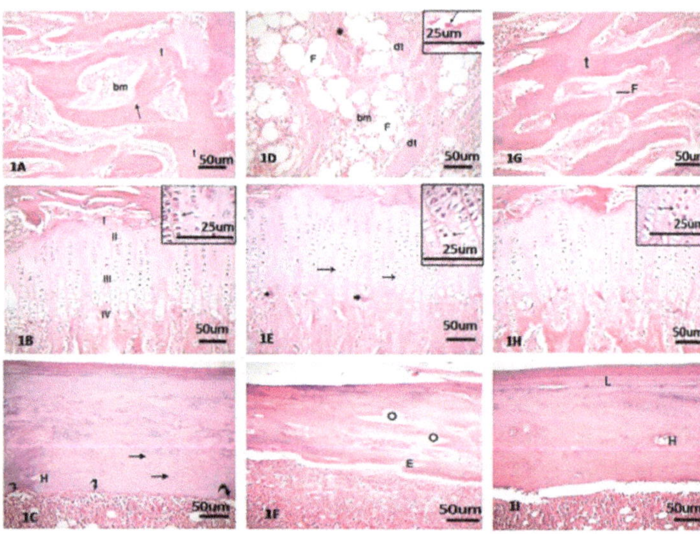

Figure 1: H&E stained sections of rat femur. Control group showing (A): A network of bone trabeculae (t) at the distal metaphysis separated by bone marrow spaces (bm). Osteocytes (arrows) surrounded by their lacunae are seen in the bone matrix. (B): Distal epiphyseal plate; showing the four well distinct zones of the epiphyseal plate; resting (I), proliferative (II), hypertrophied (III) and calcified (IV) Inset: highly organized chondrocytes (arrow). (C): Cortical bone of femur diaphysis with haversian canals (H) and osteocytes in their lacunae (arrows) Cuboidal basophilic osteoblasts on smooth endosteal bone surface (curved arrow) are also observed. Treated group showing (D): Thin widely separated disconnected trabeculae (dt) of distal metaphysis and wide bone marrow spaces in between trabeculae (bm) filled with many fat cells (F). Notice the congest-

ed blood sinusoids (*). Inset: is showing an acidophilic osteoclast (arrow) housed in the eroded bone surface. (E): Epiphyseal plate with disorganized chondrocyte column arrangement (arrow). Note the presence of many acidophilic oosteoclast (short thick arrow). Inset: most chondrocytes appear shrunken and atrophied with deeply stained nuclei. (F): Osteoporotic cavities (O) and multiple eroded (E) areas at the endosteal surface of the cortical bone. Protected group showing (G): The cancellous bone trabeculae (t) of femur metaphysis almost attaining their normal architecture as compared to group I with few fat cells (F) in marrow spaces. (H): The epiphyseal plate is almost identical with the control group in thickness. Inset: nearly preserved structure of chondrocytes. (I): Cortical bone of femur diaphysis: with observed reversal lines (L) and disappearance of osteoporotic cavities. (scale bar=50μm, inset scale bar=25μm).

The distal epiphyseal plate of control femur showed the four distinct zones of the epiphyseal growth plate with regular chondrocyte column arrangement. The growth plate showed columns of resting zone, proliferative zone, the prominent hypertrophic zone and the calcification zone, (Figure 1B). The cortical bone of femur diaphysis of the same group showed many haversian systems with well observed haversian canals and osteocytes in their lacunae. Basophilic osteoblasts on smooth endosteal bone surface were also noticed (Figure 1C).

Examination of H&E stained sections at the distal metaphysis of treated femur revealed thin widely separated disconnected trabeculae, wide bone marrow spaces filled with many fat cells and congested blood sinusoids (Figure 1D). Osteoclasts housed in the eroded bone surface were also seen (inset, Figure 1D).

Examination of H&E epiphyseal plate sections obtained from homocysteine treated rats revealed disorganized chondrocyte column arrangement, chondrocytes appeared shrunken atrophied with deeply stained nuclei. Also, many acidophilic osteoclasts were noticed (Figure 1E). As regard, sections of the femur diaphysis of this group; osteoprotic cavities (Resorption cavities) were observed in the cortical bone. Moreover, the endosteal surface of the cortical bone appeared irregularly eroded (Figure 1F).

Examination of H&E stained sections at the distal metaphysis of femur of protected group showed bone trabeculae almost attaining their normal architecture as compared with group I. Scattered adipocytes in marrow spaces were noticed. (Figure 1G). Whereas, the epiphyseal plate was almost identical with the control group in thickness and chondrocytes attain nearly preserved structure (Figure 1H). The femur diaphysis of this group showed cortical bone with disappearance of osteoporotic cavities and appearance of many reversal lines (Figure 1I).

Observations of mallory trichrome stained sections

Ttrabecular bone of control group showed high content of blue collagen fibers (Figure 2A). As regard the epiphyseal plate; the highly organized chondrocytes were embedded in an abundant bluish extracellular matrix (Figure 2B). Whereas; Cortical bone of femur diaphysis had many regularly arranged blue stained collagen fibers (Figure 2C). Mallory trichrome stained sections of treated group showed; few collagen fibers in the trabecular bone that appeared widely separated by bone marrow rich in fat cells (Figure 2D). The epiphyseal plate extracellular matrix had weak staining affinity so it appeared faint basophilic (Figure 2E). Femur diaphysis showed cortical bone with osteoporotic cavities, and few blue-stained collagen fibers. Note. Non homogenous matrix (Figure 2F).

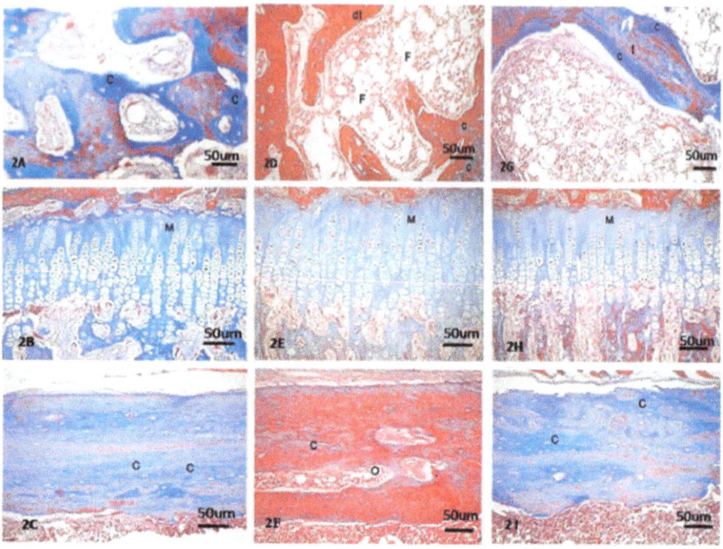

Figure 2: Mallory trichrome stained sections of rat femur. Control group showing. (A): High content of collagen fibers (C) in bone trabeculae of distal metaphysis. (B): Distal epiphyseal plate showing an abundant bluish extracellular matrix (M). (C): Cortical bone of femur diaphysis with many regularly arranged blue stained collagen fibers (C). Treated group showing. (D): Few collagen fibers (C) in the trabecular bone (dt) that appeared widely separated by bone marrow rich in fat cells (F). (E): Extracellular matrix (M) of epiphyseal plate has a weak staining affinity and appeared faint basophilic. (F): Cortical bone with osteoporotic cavities (O), and few blue-stained collagen fibers (C). Note: Non homogenous matrix. Protected group (as compared with control group) showing. (G): Nearly normal content and distribution of collagen fibers (C) in the trabecular bone (t). (H): Eepiphseal plate matrix (M) with a little reduced staining affinity in comparison with control group. (I): Cortical bone with nearly normal content and distribution of bluestained collagen fibers (C) with no cavity formation. (scale bar=50μm).

Mallory trichrome stained sections of protected group retained about normal content and distribution of collagen fibers in the trabecular bone in comparison with control group (Figure 2G). The epiphyseal plate matrix showed a little reduced staining affinity in comparison with control group (Figure 2H). Whereas, the cortical bone showed nearly normal content and distribution of blue-stained collagen fibers with no cavity formation (Figure 2I).

Osteoprotegerin immunohistochemistry

Control group of distal femur metaphysic revealed; osteoproteosteoprotegerin positive expression in the cytoplasm of most osteoblasts of endosteum. Some osteoprotegerin expression is also observed on the trabecular bone surface (Figure 3A). Examination of distal epiphyseal plate showed most hypertrophic chondrocytes and cartilage-bone interfaces are osteoprotegerin positive (Figure 3B). Whereas, cortical bone of diaphysis of the same group showed that most osteocytes were osteoprotegerin negative while few osteocytes were osteoprotegerin positive (Figure 3C).

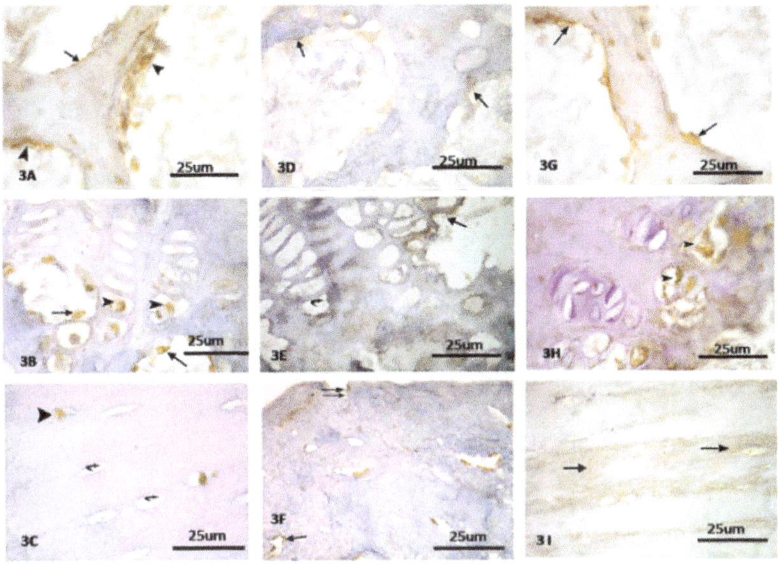

Figure 3: Osteoprotegerin stained sections of rat femur. Control group. (A): Distal metaphysis; showing the cytoplasm of most osteoblasts of endosteum are osteoprotegerin positive (arrowhead). Some osteoprotegerin expression is also observed on the trabecular bone surface (arrow) of distal metaphysis. (B): Epiphyseal plate showing most hypertrophic chondrocytes (arrow head) and cartilage-bone interfaces (arrow) are osteoprotegerin positive. (C): Cortical bone of diaphysis showing most osteocytes (curved arrow) are osteoprotegerin negative. Few osteocytes are osteoprotegerin positive (arrowhead). Treated group. (D): Trabecular bone showing weak osteoprotegerin expression in most of the cells covering the trabecular surface (arrow). (E): Epiphyseal plate revealing empty lacunae (curved arrow) and few cartilage-bone interfaces (arrow) are osteoprotegerin positive. (3): Cortical bone showing; few lining cells of osteoprotic cavities (arrow) and surface cells (double arrow) are osteoprotegerin positive. Protected group. (G): Trabecular bone showing some of the cells covering the trabecular surface are osteoprotegerin positive (arrow). (H). Epiphysal plate:a positive immunoreaction is observed in some hypertrophic chondrocytes (arrow head). (I): Cortical bone, revealing extracellular osteoprotegerin expression observed in bone matrix (arrow). (scale bar=25μm).

Examination of osteoprotegrin stained sections of treated group showed trabecular bone having weak osteoprotegerin expression in most of the cells covering the trabecular surface (Figure 3D). Examination of epiphyseal plate sections revealed empty lacunae with negative expression of osteoprotegerin whereas few cartilage-bone interfaces were osteoprotegerin positive (Figure 3E). As regard sections at femur diaphysis, lining cells of osteoprotic cavities were osteoprotegerin positive (Figure 3F).

Examination of osteoprotegrin stained sections of protected group: showed some of the cells covering the trabecular surface were osteoprotegerin positive (Figure 3G).

The epiphysal plate sections of the same group showed a positive immunoreaction observed in some hypertrophic chondrocytes (Figure 3H). Whereas; cortical bone revealed extracellular osteoprotegerin expression observed in bone matrix (Figure 3I).

Electron microscopic results

Considering examination of ultrathin sections from cortical bone of femur diaphysis of control rats revealed osteoprogenitor cells on bone surface, they contained euchromatic indented nuclei. The osteoblasts were present on the surface side by side, each cell showed many rough endoplasmic reticulum, and euochromatic nucleus with periphral heterochromatin (Figure 4A).

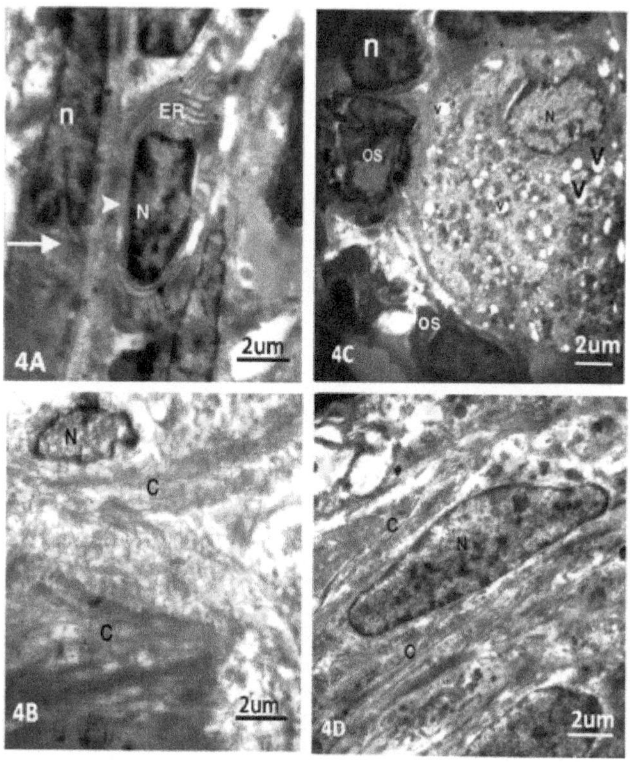

Figure 4: Electron micrographs of ultrathin sections of femur cortical bone (A) control group showing an osteoprogenitor cell (arrow) with euchromatic indented nucleus (n). An osteoblast (arrow head) is also seen having euchromatic nucleus (N) with peripheral heterochromatin and many rough endolasmic reticulum (ER). Treated group (B): Showing an osteocyt with irregular nucleus (N) containing condensed peripheral chromatin, and surrounded with many irregular collagen fibrils (C). (C): Showing an osteoclast with irregular nucleus (N). The cytoplasm contains many membrane bound-vacuoles (v) of different sizes. A row of osteoblasts, (OS) with heterochromatic nuclei (n) surrounding themselves within their osteoid product are also seen. (D): protected group showing an osteocyte with an oval nucleus (N). It is surrounded by few collagenous fibrils (C) in regular lamellae. (Scale bar=2 μm).

In treated group; osteocytes had irregular nuclei. They were surrounded by many irregular collagen fibrils (Figure 4B). The osteoclasts had irregular nuclei and many membrane bound vacuoles of different sizes. The cells were surrounded with row of osteoblasts within their osteoid product (Figure 4C). In protected group; osteocytes showed oval nuclei and were surrounded by few collagen fibrils in regular lamellae (Figure 4D).

Biochemical results

There was no significant difference between the biochemical results of group IA, group IB and IC.

There was a significant increase in the levels of serum homocysteine in treated group in comparison with the control group. On the other hand, the protected group showed a significant decrease in homocysteine level when compared with treated group. There was no significant change between the protected group and the control group (Table 1, Figure 5A).

Table 1: Mean values of serum homocysteine (μmol/l) in different groups

	Mean±SD				
	Group IA	**Group IB**	**Group IC**	**Group II (HCY treated)**	**Group III (HCY+folic acid) (protected)**
Serum homocysteine (μmol/l)	6.4±2.36	5.9±1.2[n]	6.3±1.25[n]	11.5±3.23[a]	7.2±2.26[b]

[n]non significant as compared with group IA
[a]significant as compared with group IA
[b]significant as compared with group II

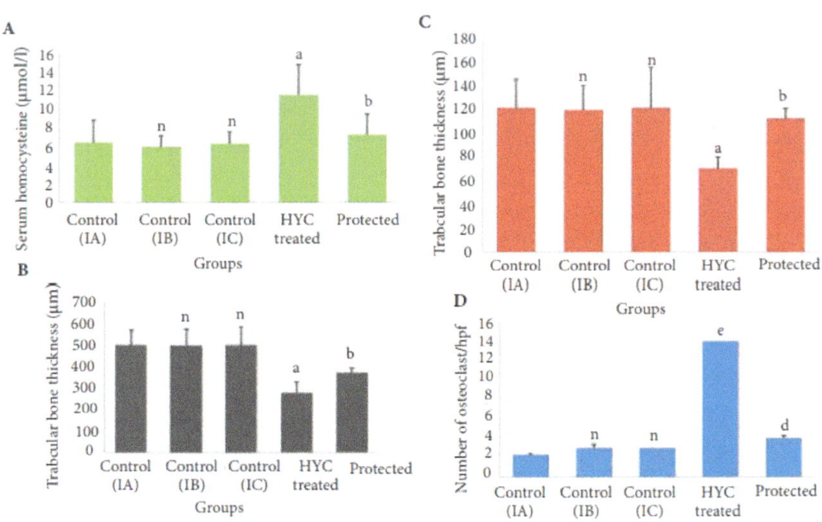

Figure 5: Histogram showing (A) the mean serum homocysteine (μmol/l), (B) outer cortical bone thickness (μm), (C) trabecular bone thickness (μm), (D) number of osteoclasts/hpf in different studied groups.

Morphometric results

There was no significant difference between the morphometric results of group IA, group IB and IC.

The mean cortical and trabecular bone thickness in group II (treated group) presented a significant decrease, ($p<0.05$) in comparison with the control group. both parameters showed a significant increase when comparing group III with group II (Table 2, Figures 5B and 5C). As regard the number of osteoclasts, there was a highly significant increase in treated group in comparison with the control group. whereas; there was a highly significant reduction in the number of osteoclasts ($P<0.001$) in protected group (III) as compared to group (II) (Table 2, Figure 5D).

Table 2: Showing the mean outer cortical bone thickness, the mean bone trabecular thickness and the number of osteoclasts/hpf in different groups

	Mean±SD				
	Group IA	Group IB	Group IC	Group II (HCY treated)	Group III (HCY+folic acid) (protected)
Outer cortical bone thickness(μm)	499.98±67.86	498±75.7^{n}	501±83.2^{n}	279.42±48.87^{a}	370.47±20.75^{b}
trabecular bone thickness(μm)	121.43±24.1	119.3±21.3^{n}	121.4±34.2^{n}	70.13±9.85^{a}	112.52±8.4^{b}
number of osteoclasts/hpf	2±0.1	3±0.37^{n}	3±0.32^{n}	14±0.26^{c}	4±0.27^{d}

[n]non significant as compared with group IA
[a]significant as compared with group IA
[b]significant as compared with group II
[c]highly significant as compared with group IA
[d]highly significant as compared with group II

DISCUSSION

Recent reports have indicated a higher risk of fractures among men and women with high levels of serum homocysteine (HCY) [46].

However, the mechanistic role of Hcy in osteoporosis is still unknown.

Regarding, the present histomorphometric results HCY treated group showed a significant reduction of cortical bone thickness with multiple cavity formation as well as a significant reduction in the trabecular bone thickness when compared with that of control rats of group I.

Previous researchers [48] have described osteoporosis as a syndrome of excessive skeletal fragility that results from both the loss of trabecular bone mass and trabecular bone connectivity.

Regarding the epiphyseal plate of HCy treated rats of the present study showed abnormal chondrocyte column cavity, shrunken atrophied chondrocytes with deeply stained nuclei. The extracellular matrix had weak staining affinity.

The observed results were in accordance with previous researcher findings [1] who demonstrated that homocysteine promoted growth in hypophysectomized rats, a finding, associated with increased thickness of epiphyseal plate.

In addition, other investigators [49] stated that HCY induced endoplasmic reticulum stress and reduced the secretion and expression of extracellular superoxide dismutase leading to an increase in the production of extracellular reactive oxygen species in vascular smooth muscle cells, leading to increased oxidative stress in the vascular wall [50,51].

In the present study, there was an accumulation of fat cells in the bone marrow of group II, Whereas, the protected group showed a decrease in marrow fat accumulation with the use of folic acid. Previous researchers [52] had reported an inverse relationship between fat and bone volume. This inverse relationship has been documented in bone obtained from animal models with high levels of marrow fat infiltration, such as osteoporosis and senescence-accelerated mouse. The mechanism suggested is through shifting of mesenchymal stem cells into fat cells at the expense of osteoblasts [53].

In the current work, osteoclasts of the treated group exhibited an increase in number as proved statitistically with subsequent bone erosions. Coinciding with these results, clinical studies have shown that adding homocysteine to chick-bud mesenchymal micromass culture caused matrix disorganization, decreased the ability of matrix to support mineralization, increased alkaline phosphatase activity, and abnormalities in collagen cross link formation [54]. Inhibition of collagen cross-linking [55], disturbance of osteoblast function [56], and increased osteoclast activity [57], were also observed in hyperhomocysteinemia.

Osteoprotegerin (OPG), is a member of the tumor necrosis factor receptor gene superfamily [58].

Osteoprotegerin (OPG) is secreted by stromal and osteoblastic lineage cells and inhibits osteoclastogenesis by preventing the interaction of receptor activator of nuclear factor-κB ligand (RANKL) with receptor activator of nuclear factor-κB (RANK) [41].

Ablation of OPG by targeted gene deletion in mice leads to early onset osteoporosis, demonstrating for the first time a critical requirement for endogenous OPG in the maintenance of normal postnatal bone mass and skeletal architecture [59].

In the current study, positive immunohistochemical expression of osteoprotegerin protein in control animals appeared mainly in the cytoplasm of the osteogenic cells and osteoblasts lining the trabecular surface, whereas epiphyseal plates showed positive reaction in maturative/hypertrophic chondrocytes. Most osteocytes of cortical bone appeared negative for osteoprotegerin. The distribution f OPG was previously demonstrated by previous studies [42].

In treated animals of the current work; the trabecular bone showed weak osteoprotegerin expression in most of the cells covering the trabecular surface. Whereas, negative expression of osteoprotegerin was demonstrated in maturative/hypertrophic chondrocytes of epiphyseal plate while treated cortical bone showed positive expression of OPG in few lining cells of osteoprotic cavities.

Similar observations were detected by previous studies [42] who also observed an extracellular immunolocalization of osteoprotegerin in the cement lines. The presence of osteoprotegerin in these site-specific areas of the trabecular bone matrix could be related to its protective action against the resorbing activity of osteoclasts.

An additional role for OPG in regulating remodeling within the cortical shafts of long bones and within bones of the skull was recorded in OPG-deficient mice [59].

It was found that osteoprotegerin administration inhibited trabecular bone loss and maintained the internal trabecular bone structure and volume in osteoprotegerin deficient mice [60].

In addition, osteoprotegerin administration in mice resulted in a decrease in the number of ostcoclasts together with absence of the ruffled border denoting reduced activity. The positive effect of osteoprotegerin on bone was most probably related to its antiosteoclastogenic capacity [61].

With reference to rats treated with HCY in the current study, electron microscopic examination revealed many degenerative changes in osteoblasts and osteocytes in the form of irregular nuclei with condensation of their chromatin. The matrix appears highly affected and its fibrils were irregularly arranged. On the other hand, the osteoclasts became more active, their cytoplasm contained many membrane-bound vesicles of various sizes that represent many lysosomes or ruffled border cut in many planes. Therefore, the osteoclasts were more active while osteoblasts and osteocytes were degenerated; reflecting that the bone resorption was more than bone formation with an inaccurate bone remdeling.

Previous experimental data have suggested that high HCY levels affected both osteoclasts and osteoblasts. It was suggested a dysbalance between osteoblasts and osteoclasts in favor of osteoclasts as a major mechanism for HCY-induced bone loss and reduced bone quality *in vivo* [4,6].

The ultrastructural results of the current work also showed that HCY treatment resulted in an irregular deposition of collagen fibrils in the extracellular compartment. This could be attributed to disruption of collagen cross-links with other agents which prevent the orderly arrangement of the extracellular matrix. The abnormal deposition of collagen in the extracellular matrix may lead to abnormal cell-matrix interactions [54].

In our study, rats of group III (protected with folic acid) had shown significant lower levels of homocysteine, histologically, these animals were protected from bone loss as compared with treated rats. However, it is not clear whether folic acid directly prevents bone loss or acts via its homocysteine lowering effect. This needs to be clarified in the next studies.

Prevention of bone loss and hyperhomocysteinemia by folic acid supplements in the present study are consistent with previous studies [62,63] which stated that the serum homocysteine level is inversely associated with folate level, and that folate supplements therapy can lower homocysteine level effectively.

Previous data suggested a role of folic acid in modulating the expression of the redox enzymes (Trx-1/NOX-4) disrupted by increased levels of HCY. These results also suggested that folic acid alleviates the oxidative stress [37].

CONCLUSION

The results of this study showed that hyperhomocysteinemia induced marked structural changes in the epiphyseal plate, trabecular and cortical bone of femur in young rats. These changes confirmed the association between increased homocysteine level and fracture risk. The suggested mechanism for these changes could be related to decreased osteoprotegerin expression as proved in our work.

Moreover, folic acid provided significant protection against bone changes induced by increased homocysteine levels. However, it is not clear whether folic acid directly prevents bone loss or acts via its homocysteine lowering effect. We recommend further research to clarify this point in the next studies. In addition, future research studies are needed to evaluate the potential clinical utility of folic acid as a therapeutic agent to prevent osteoporosis associated with hyperhomocysteinemia.

AUTHORS' CONTRIBUTIONS

Authors' contributions	RAZ	HMV
Research concept and design	√	√
Collection and/or assembly of data	√	√
Data analysis and interpretation	√	√
Writing the article	√	--
Critical revision of the article	--	√
Final approval of article	--	√
Statistical analysis	√	--

ACKNOWLEDGEMENT

We would like to thank Dr. Mona AboElkhair. For her aid in statistical results.

REFERENCES

1. Ray NF, Chan JK, Thamer M and Melton LJ, 3rd. Medical expenditures for the treatment of osteoporotic fractures in the United States in 1995: report from the National Osteoporosis Foundation. *J Bone Miner Res*. 1997; 12:24-35.
2. Center JR, Nguyen TV, Schneider D, Sambrook PN and Eisman JA. Mortality after all major types of osteoporotic fracture in men and women: an observational study. *Lancet*. 1999; 353:878-82.
3. Melton LJ, 3rd. Adverse outcomes of osteoporotic fractures in the general population. *J Bone Miner Res*. 2003; 18:1139-41.
4. van Meurs JB, Dhonukshe-Rutten RA, Pluijm SM, van der Klift M, de Jonge R, Lindemans J, de Groot LC, Hofman A, Witteman JC, van Leeuwen JP, Breteler MM, Lips P, Pols HA and Uitterlinden AG. Homocysteine levels and the risk of osteoporotic fracture. *N Engl J Med*. 2004; 350:2033-41.

5. Aubin JE, Liu F, Malaval L and Gupta AK. Osteoblast and chondroblast differentiation. *Bone*. 1995;17:77S-83S.
6. McLean R.R, Jacques P.F, Selhub J, Tucker K.L, Samelson E.J, Broe K.E and Kiel D.P. Homocysteine as a predictive factor for hip fracture in older persons. *N Engl J Med*. 2004; 350:2042-2049.
7. Sakamoto W, Fujie K, Isomura S, Kaga M, Kohgo T, Yamada N and Nishihira J. Secretion of macrophage migration inhibitory factor differs from interleukin-6 in hydrogen peroxide- and LPS-stimulated human fibroblasts. *Int Immunopharmacol*. 2002; 2:1123-31.
8. Cagnacci A, Baldassari F, Rivolta G, Arangino S and Volpe A. Relation of homocysteine, folate, and vitamin B12 to bone mineral density of postmenopausal women. *Bone*. 2003; 33:956-9.
9. Bucciarelli P, Martini G, Martinelli I, Ceccarelli E, Gennari L, Bader R, Valenti R, Franci B, Nuti R and Mannucci PM. The relationship between plasma homocysteine levels and bone mineral density in post-menopausal women. *Eur J Intern Med*. 2010; 21:301-5.
10. Roblin X, Phelip JM, Genevois M, Ducros V and Bonaz B. Hyperhomocysteinaemia is associated with osteoporosis in patients with Crohn's disease. *Aliment Pharmacol Ther*. 2007; 25:797-804.
11. Biagini MR, Tozzi A, Bongini E, Capanni M, Galli A, Milani S and Surrenti C. Association of plasma homocysteine with bone mineral density in postmenopausal women with osteoporosis or osteopenia affected by primary biliary cirrhosis. *J Clin Gastroenterol*. 2007; 41:635.
12. Alley RA, Chen EL, Beyer TD and Prinz RA. Does homocysteine contribute to bone disease in hyperparathyroidism? *Am J Surg*. 2008; 195:374-7.
13. Seshadri S, Beiser A, Selhub J, Jacques PF, Rosenberg IH, D›Agostino RB, Wilson PW and Wolf PA. Plasma homocysteine as a risk factor for dementia and Alzheimer's disease. *N Engl J Med*. 2002; 346:476-83.
14. Azizi ZA, Zamani A, Omrani LR, Omrani L, Dabaghmanesh MH, Mohammadi A, Namavar MR and Omrani GR. Effects of hyperhomocysteinemia during the gestational period on ossification in rat embryo.*Bone*. 2010; 46:1344-8.
15. McLean RR, Jacques PF, Selhub J, Fredman L, Tucker KL, Samelson EJ, Kiel DP, Cupples LA and Hannan MT. Plasma B vitamins, homocysteine, and their relation with bone loss and hip fracture in elderly men and women. *J Clin Endocrinol Metab*. 2008; 93:2206-12.
16. Dhonukshe-Rutten RA, Pluijm SM, de Groot LC, Lips P, Smit JH and van Staveren WA. Homocysteine and vitamin B12 status relate to bone turnover markers, broadband ultrasound attenuation, and fractures in healthy elderly people. *J Bone Miner Res*. 2005; 20:921-9.
17. Eberhardt RT, Forgione MA, Cap A, Leopold JA, Rudd MA, Trolliet M, Heydrick S, Stark R, Klings ES, Moldovan NI, Yaghoubi M, Goldschmidt-Clermont PJ,

Farber HW, Cohen R and Loscalzo J. Endothelial dysfunction in a murine model of mild hyperhomocyst(e)inemia. *J Clin Invest.* 2000; 106:483-91.

18. Dworakowski R, Anilkumar N, Zhang M and Shah AM. Redox signalling involving NADPH oxidase-derived reactive oxygen species. *Biochem Soc Trans.* 2006; 34:960-4.
19. Satta E, Perna A.F, Lombardi C, Acanfora F, Violetti E, Romano M.M, Capasso R, Pisano M, Paduano F and De Santo N.G. Hyperhomocyteinemia in chronic renal failure. *G. Ital. Nefrol.* 2006; 23:480-489.
20. Golbahar J, Hamidi A, Aminzadeh MA and Omrani GR. Association of plasma folate, plasma total homocysteine, but not methylenetetrahydrofolate reductase C667T polymorphism, with bone mineral density in postmenopausal Iranian women: a cross-sectional study. *Bone.* 2004; 35:760-5.
21. Morris MS, Jacques PF and Selhub J. Relation between homocysteine and B-vitamin status indicators and bone mineral density in older Americans. *Bone.* 2005; 37:234-42.
22. Stead LM, Brosnan ME and Brosnan JT. Characterization of homocysteine metabolism in the rat liver.*Biochem J.* 2000; 350 Pt 3:685-92.
23. Boushey CJ, Beresford SA, Omenn GS and Motulsky AG. A quantitative assessment of plasma homocysteine as a risk factor for vascular disease. Probable benefits of increasing folic acid intakes. *JAMA.* 1995; 274:1049-57.
24. Sato Y, Honda Y, Iwamoto J, Kanoko T and Satoh K. Effect of folate and mecobalamin on hip fractures in patients with stroke: a randomized controlled trial. *JAMA.* 2005; 293:1082-8.
25. Woo KS, Chook P, Lolin YI, Sanderson JE, Metreweli C and Celermajer DS. Folic acid improves arterial endothelial function in adults with hyperhomocystinemia. *J Am Coll Cardiol.* 1999; 34:2002-6.
26. Herrmann M, Taban-Shomal O, Muller S, Gunter L, Hubner U, Bohm M and Herrmann W.Hyperhomocysteinemia--the biochemical link between a weak heart and brittle bones? *Clin Lab.* 2006; 52:137-47.
27. Matte C, Scherer EB, Stefanello FM, Barschak AG, Vargas CR, Netto CA and Wyse AT. Concurrent folate treatment prevents Na+,K+-ATPase activity inhibition and memory impairments caused by chronic hyperhomocysteinemia during rat development. *Int J Dev Neurosci.* 2007; 25:545-52.
28. Bazzano LA. Folic acid supplementation and cardiovascular disease: the state of the art. *Am J Med Sci.* 2009; 338:48-9.
29. Zhu X, Smith MA, Honda K, Aliev G, Moreira PI, Nunomura A, Casadesus G, Harris PL, Siedlak SL and Perry G. Vascular oxidative stress in Alzheimer disease. *J Neurol Sci.* 2007; 257:240-6.
30. Gerdhem P, Ivaska KK, Isaksson A, Pettersson K, Vaananen HK, Obrant KJ and Akesson K. Associations between homocysteine, bone turnover, BMD, mortality, and fracture risk in elderly women. *J Bone Miner Res.* 2007; 22:127-34.
31. Boyce BF and Xing L. Biology of RANK, RANKL, and osteoprotegerin. *Arthritis*

Res Ther. 2007; 9 Suppl 1:S1.

32. Hofbauer LC and Schoppet M. Clinical implications of the osteoprotegerin/RANKL/RANK system for bone and vascular diseases. *JAMA*. 2004; 292:490-5.
33. Boyce BF and Xing L. Functions of RANKL/RANK/OPG in bone modeling and remodeling. *Arch Biochem Biophys*. 2008; 473:139-46.
34. Institute of Laboratory Animal Resources. Guide for the Care and Use of Laboratory Animals. *National Academy Press*. Washington, DC. 1996.
35. Ajeigbe KO, Olaleye SB, Oladejo EO and Olayanju AO. Effect of folic acid supplementation on oxidative gastric mucosa damage and acid secretory response in the rat. *Indian J Pharmacol*. 2011; 43:578-81.
36. Masse PG, Boskey AL, Ziv I, Hauschka P, Donovan SM, Howell DS and Cole DE. Chemical and biomechanical characterization of hyperhomocysteinemic bone disease in an animal model. *BMC Musculoskelet Disord*. 2003; 4:2.
37. Tyagi N, Kandel M, Munjal C, Qipshidze N, Vacek JC, Pushpakumar SB, Metreveli N and Tyagi SC.Homocysteine mediated decrease in bone blood flow and remodeling: role of folic acid. *J Orthop Res*. 2011; 29:1511-6.
38. Waynforth HB. Experimental and surgical techniques in the rat. London: Academic Press. 1980.
39. Bancroft JD and Gamble M. Theory and practice of histological techniques. 6th ed. London, NewYork, Philadelphia: Churchill Livingstone. 2008.
40. Cross SS, Yang Z, Brown NJ, Balasubramanian SP, Evans CA, Woodward JK, Neville-Webbe HL, Lippitt JM, Reed MW, Coleman RE and Holen I. Osteoprotegerin (OPG)--a potential new role in the regulation of endothelial cell phenotype and tumour angiogenesis? *Int J Cancer*. 2006; 118:1901-8.
41. Hofbauer LC and Heufelder AE. Clinical review 114: hot topic. The role of receptor activator of nuclear factor-kappaB ligand and osteoprotegerin in the pathogenesis and treatment of metabolic bone diseases. *J Clin Endocrinol Metab*. 2000; 85:2355-63.
42. Silvestrini G, Ballanti P, Patacchioli F, Leopizzi M, Gualtieri N, Monnazzi P, Tremante E, Sardella D and Bonucci E. Detection of osteoprotegerin (OPG) and its ligand (RANKL) mRNA and protein in femur and tibia of the rat. *J Mol Histol*. 2005; 36:59-67.
43. Singh D. Principle and Techniques. In Histology, Microscopy and Photography., 2003. 1st ed., CBS Puplishers and Distributers. New Delhy, Bangalore (India). 2003; 679-699.
44. Surve VV, Andersson N, Lehto-Axtelius D and Hakanson R. Comparison of osteopenia after gastrectomy, ovariectomy and prednisolone treatment in the young female rat. *Acta Orthop Scand*. 2001; 72:525-32.
45. Balena R, Toolan BC, Shea M, Markatos A, Myers ER, Lee SC, Opas EE, Seedor JG, Klein H, Frankenfield D and et al. The effects of 2-year treatment with the aminobisphosphonate alendronate on bone metabolism, bone histomorphometry, and bone strength in ovariectomized nonhuman primates. *J Clin Invest*.

1993; 92:2577-86.

46. Sato Y, Iwamoto J, Kanoko T and Satoh K. Homocysteine as a predictive factor for hip fracture in elderly women with Parkinson's disease. *Am J Med.* 2005; 118:1250-5.

47. Gerdhem P, Ivaska KK, Alatalo SL, Halleen JM, Hellman J, Isaksson A, Pettersson K, Vaananen HK, Akesson K and Obrant KJ. Biochemical markers of bone metabolism and prediction of fracture in elderly women. *J Bone Miner Res.* 2004; 19:386-93.

48. Lane NE, Yao W, Kinney JH, Modin G, Balooch M and Wronski TJ. Both hPTH(1-34) and bFGF increase trabecular bone mass in osteopenic rats but they have different effects on trabecular bone architecture. *J Bone Miner Res.* 2003; 18:2105-15.

49. Nonaka H, Tsujino T, Watari Y, Emoto N and Yokoyama M. Taurine prevents the decrease in expression and secretion of extracellular superoxide dismutase induced by homocysteine: amelioration of homocysteine-induced endoplasmic reticulum stress by taurine. *Circulation.* 2001; 104:1165-70.

50. Zhang Q, Zeng X, Guo J and Wang X. Effects of homocysteine on murine splenic B lymphocyte proliferation and its signal transduction mechanism. *Cardiovasc Res.* 2001; 52:328-36.

51. Zhang Q, Zeng X, Guo J and Wang X. Oxidant stress mechanism of homocysteine potentiating Con A-induced proliferation in murine splenic T lymphocytes. *Cardiovasc Res.* 2002; 53:1035-42.

52. Pei L and Tontonoz P. Fat's loss is bone's gain. *J Clin Invest.* 2004; 113:805-6.

53. Ng A and Duque G. Osteoporosis as a lipotoxic disease. *IBMS BoneKEy.* 2010; 7:108-123.

54. Khan M, Yamauchi M, Srisawasdi S, Stiner D, Doty S, Paschalis EP and Boskey AL. Homocysteine decreases chondrocyte-mediated matrix mineralization in differentiating chick limb-bud mesenchymal cell micro-mass cultures. *Bone.* 2001; 28:387-98.

55. Lubec B, Fang-Kircher S, Lubec T, Blom HJ and Boers GH. Evidence for McKusick's hypothesis of deficient collagen cross-linking in patients with homocystinuria. *Biochim Biophys Acta.* 1996;1315:159-62.

56. Sakamoto W, Isomura H, Fujie K, Deyama Y, Kato A, Nishihira J and Izumi H. Homocysteine attenuates the expression of osteocalcin but enhances osteopontin in MC3T3-E1 preosteoblastic cells. *Biochim Biophys Acta.* 2005; 1740:12-6.

57. Herrmann M, Widmann T, Colaianni G, Colucci S, Zallone A and Herrmann W. Increased osteoclast activity in the presence of increased homocysteine concentrations. *Clin Chem.* 2005; 51:2348-53.

58. Simonet WS, Lacey DL, Dunstan CR, Kelley M, Chang MS, Luthy R, Nguyen HQ, Wooden S, Bennett L and Boone T et al. Osteoprotegerin: a novel secreted protein involved in the regulation of bone density.*Cell.* 1997; 89:309-19.

59. Bucay N, Sarosi I, Dunstan CR, Morony S, Tarpley J, Capparelli C, Scully S, Tan HL, Xu W, Lacey DL, Boyle WJ and Simonet WS. osteoprotegerin-deficient mice develop early onset osteoporosis and arterial calcification. *Genes Dev.* 1998; 12:1260-8.

60. Yamazaki H and Sasaki T. Effects of osteoprotegerin administration on osteoclast differentiation and trabecular bone structure in osteoprotegerin-deficient mice. *J Electron Microsc (Tokyo)*. 2005; 54:467-77.

61. Gruber HE and Rude RK. Alterations in osteoclast morphology following osteoprotegerin administration in the magnesium-deficient mouse. *Biotech Histochem*. 2003; 78:231-6.

62. Manolagas SC. Birth and death of bone cells: basic regulatory mechanisms and implications for the pathogenesis and treatment of osteoporosis. *Endocr Rev.* 2000; 21:115-37.

63. Claes L, Schmalenbach J, Herrmann M, Olku I, Garcia P, Histing T, Obeid R, Schorr H, Herrmann W, Pohlemann T, Menger MD and Holstein JH. Hyperhomocysteinemia is associated with impaired fracture healing in mice. *Calcif Tissue Int*. 2009; 85:17-21.

15
CHAPTER

CHARACTERIZATION OF ADULT MALE ALBINO RAT MAMMARY GLAND: A HISTOLOGICAL AND SEROLOGICAL STUDY

Zienab A. Gouda, Samah M. Ahmed and Nabila M. Elghonaimy

Keywords: Male rat, mammary gland, growth factors, prolactin, progesterone, whole mount carmine alum

INTRODUCTION

The MG has been of great interest to generations of biologists from many disciplines. The structure of the male and female MG can provide a sensitive indicator of endocrinal disturbance [1]. This gland is particularly suited for studying developmental processes as it is readily amenable to experimental manipulation and can be easily accessed. Furthermore in animals, MG tissue is abundant because there are 6 pairs in each animal [2].

In females, a major part of MG development occurs postnatal, with distinct periods of intensive morphogenesis taking place at puberty and during pregnancy and lactation [3]. A course of ductal development includes multiple stages of proliferation and morphogenesis that are largely directed by concurrent alterations in key hormones and growth factors. Estrogen hormone is responsible for ductal elongation and bifurcation of MG [4]. While, progesterone hormone is responsible for lateral branching and alveologenesis of MG [5]. Further alveologenesis and differentiation of the luminal mammary epithelial cells into milk producing cells during late pregnancy require prolactin hormone [3]. EGF, IGF I and TGFα factors are potent mitogenic factors for

Citation: Gouda ZA, Ahmed SM and Elghonaimy NM. Characterization of adult male albino rat mammary gland: a histological and serological study. J Histol Histopathol. 2015; 2:5. http://dx.doi.org/10.7243/2055-091X-2-5.

both normal and transformed (neoplastic) mammary epithelium either *in vivo* [6] or *in vitro* [7].

Histologically, in virgin female animal, MG tissue contains epithelium and stroma. The mammary epithelial cells forming lactiferous ducts are bi-layered epithelium, with the inner luminal cells facing a central cavity and surrounded by the outer basal, myoepithelial cells. It also harbors stem and progenitor cells, which are the source of both luminal and myoepithelial cells [8]. The stroma includes fibrous connective tissue, and a wide variety of cell types, including inter- and intralobular fibroblasts, adipocytes, endothelial cells, and innate immune cells [9].

In male of most mammals, a rudimentary mammary structure is encountered; however the male albino rat MG is unique in displaying marked development (physiological *gynecomastia*) and in showing great sexual dimorphism [10]. *Gynecomastia* is a female like enlargement of the male breast resulting from increased parenchyma, stroma or fat. It is a common problem in the male population, particularly in young adults. Enlarged man breast can cause functional problems, psychosocial discomfort and fear of malignancy. So; it is the most common cause for seeking medical advice for a breast condition in men [11]. Despite the fact that there are no great quantitative differences between men and women either in progesterone secretion or serum progesterone levels, a little is known about the physiology, endocrinology, and pharmacology of progesterone and progestins in male gender or men especially in mammary gland development [12].

Being an organ designed to deliver nourishment and passive immunity to mammal's infants, most discussions of the functional and developmental anatomy and histology of the mammary gland focused on the female and not on the male one [13].

The aim of the present study was to detect causes and importance of mammary gland development in adult male albino rat to relate this normal appearance to *gynecomastia* in human. We hypothesized that histological examination of mammary glands in both sexes via whole mount carmine alum technique; H&E and MT stains will clarify structural differences. Moreover, analysis of serum levels of estrogen, progestrone and prolactin hormones and EGF, IGF I and TGFα tissue proteins and immune-staining for ER and PR could explain the causes of male mammary gland proliferation. We expected that the levels of tested steroid hormones and growth factors of both sexes may be equal or show slight differences.

MATERIALS AND METHODS

In this study, 28 adult albino rats of average weight 200-220 gm were used. The animals were obtained from the animal house, Faculty of Medicine, Zagazig University, Zagazig, Egypt. The animals were kept under strict care and cleaning measures. They were housed in hygienic cages according to the guidelines for animal research issued by the National Institute of Health and approved by Animal Ethics Committee, Zagazig University.

Chemicals

For whole mount carmine alum staining

Carmine (Aldrich Chemical Co Ltd, Gillingham Dorset England) and aluminum potassium sulfate (BDH Chemicals, Ltd, Poole, England) were purchased from Algomhuria co (Mohafza st, Zagazig, Egypt).

For hematoxylin and eosin staining

Harris hematoxylin (Park Scientific Limited, Northampton, UK) and Eosin (Sigma-Aldrich chemie, Steinheim, Germany) were purchased from Algomhuria Co (Mohafza st, Zagazig, Egypt).

For immunohistochemical staining

Anti-progesterone and estrogen antibodies, (Novacastra Laboratories Ltd, UK) were purchased from Sigma office (Egyptian International Center for Import, Cairo, Egypt). Mayer's hematoxylin (Sigma-Aldrich chemie, Steinheim, Germany)were purchased from Algomhuria co (Mohafza st, Zagazig, Egypt).

Experimental procedure

The rats were separated into two groups:

Female group: 14 rats.

Male group: 14 rats.

The female group was sacrificed at estrus stage under anesthesia by intraperitoneal injection of pentobarbitone sodium 60 mg/kg [14]. To determine the estrus stage in female rats, they were co-cycled for preparation of vaginal smears. The vaginal smears were taken via vaginal lavage with distilled water and were transferred to glass slides and allowed to dry at room temperature. Once dry, they were immediately stained with crystal violet stain. Microscopically, three types of cells could be recognized: epithelial cells, cornified cells and leukocytes. Prominence of cornified cells indicated the estrus stage [15].

Serological analysis of serum ERB, PRA and PRL hormones

Venous blood samples were withdrawn from the retro-orbital sinus by capillary tube and collected in clean glass centrifuge tubes. Blood samples were allowed to clot at room temperature for 30 minutes and then, the sera were stored at −20°C [16].

Histochemical analysis of EGF, IGF I and TGFα tissue protein

Small biopsies of the right mammary glands were weighed, homogenized in 20 volumes (wt/vol) of PBS at 37°C and centrifuged at 15,000 X gm for 20 min at 4°C; then, the supernatants were stored at −20°C [16]. Both serological and histochemical analyses were done in (Biochemistry Department, Faculty of Medicine, Cairo University, Egypt).

Whole mount carmine alum staining technique

The left dissected mammary glands were immediately spread on large glass slides, fixed in Carnoy's fixative (25% glacial acetic acid, 75% absolute ethanol), at room temperature in fume hood for 2 days then, washed in 70% ethyl alcohol for 1 hour, rinsed in distilled water (DW) for 30 min, stained in carmine alum stain for 2 days, dehydrated in ascending grades of alcohol and cleared in xylene at least for 2 days. To prepare carmine alum stain; 1 gm carmine and 2.5 gm aluminum potassium sulfate in 450 ml distilled water was boiled for 20 min. Final volume was adjusted to 500 ml with DW [17].

Histological study

In both sexes, the remaining parts of right fourth, fifth and sixth inguinal mammary glands were fixed overnight in 10% neutral buffered formalin and processed into paraffin blocks. They were cut into 5μm sections and stained with H&E, MT [18] and immunohistochemical procedure [19].

Immunohistochemistry technique

To examine the distribution of Progesterone and Estrogen receptors, streptavidin-biotin immunoperoxidase system was used. In brief, deparaffinized sections 3 μm thick were rehydrated in a descending graded alcohol series and washed twice with distilled water for 5 min each time. Antigen retrieval was conducted for all sections using heat–induced epitope retrieval, through immersion of tissue sections in citrate buffer, pH 6.0, autoclaved at 105°C, for 20 min. Endogenous peroxidase was blocked by incubating sections in 3% H_2O_2 in absolute methanol for 30 min at 4°C, followed by flushing with water. After blocking solution treatment (biotinylated rabbit anti-mouse secondary antibody),the sections were incubated overnight at 4°C with the primary antibody for ER and PR (monoclonal antibodies of estrogen and progesterone) diluted in 0.01 M phosphate buffered saline (PBS). The sections for negative controls were incubated in 0.01 M PBS without primary antibody. Finally, the mammary glands were visualized with 3,3'- diaminobenzidine tetrahydrochloride H_2O_2 solution for 3 min. Sections were washed in distilled water, and finally counterstained slightly with Mayer's hematoxylin [19].

Morphometric analysis

The image analyzer computer system Leica Qwin 500 (Leica Imaging system, Ltd, Cambridge, England) was used to measure the terminal ductules thickness using whole mount carmine alum stained slides (Pathology Department, Faculty of Dentistry, Cairo University, Cairo, Egypt).

Statistical analysis

Serum levels of steroid hormones, tissue levels of growth factors and terminal ductules thickness were statistically analyzed. The obtained data were expressed as mean values

±standard deviation and analyzed using unpaired student's T-test. Difference was considered to be significant at P<0.05 between groups.

RESULTS

Serological Results

The male group revealed a high statistically significant decrease of PRL hormone (P<0.001) and a statistically significant decrease of ERB hormone levels (P<0.05) in comparison to female group. Progesterone hormone serum level showed no statistically significant (P>0.05) difference between both groups (Table 1) and (Histogram 1). Statistically significant decreases regarding tissue EGF, IGF I and TGFα in male group were detected (Table 2) and (Histogram 2).

Table 1: Statistical analysis of serum levels of ERB, PRA and PRL hormones

Hormones	Female		Male		T test	P Value
	Mean±SD	Range	Mean±SD	Range		
Estradiol 17β (pg/ml)	40.2±10	19.2-55.8	8.9±2.3	4.6-11.1	9.9.65	0.013*
Progesterone (ng/ml)	32.4±16	14.8-64.4	29.7±9	11.4-39.8	8.18	0.554
Prolactin (pg/ml)	84.9±10	64.9-104.9	25.8±7	11.4-39.8	234.42	<0.001**

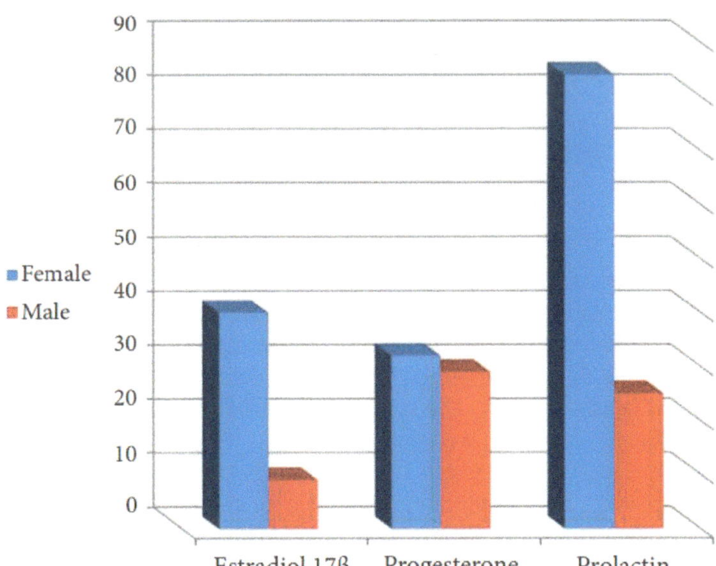

Histogram 1 : Mean values of serum Estradiol 17β, Progesterone and Prolactin hormones in both groups.

Table 2: Statistical analysis of tissue EGF, IGF I and TGFα in both groups

Factors	Female		Male		T test	P Value
	Mean±SD	Range	Mean±SD	Range		
EGF	0.48±0.1	0.28-0.68	0.24±0.01	0.22-0.26	7.55	0.023*
IGF I	0.63±0.1	0.23-1.03	0.53±0.1	0.33-0.73	5.0	0.036*
TGFα	0.25±0.04	0.21-0.33	0.12±0.01	0.1-0.14	9.97	0.01*

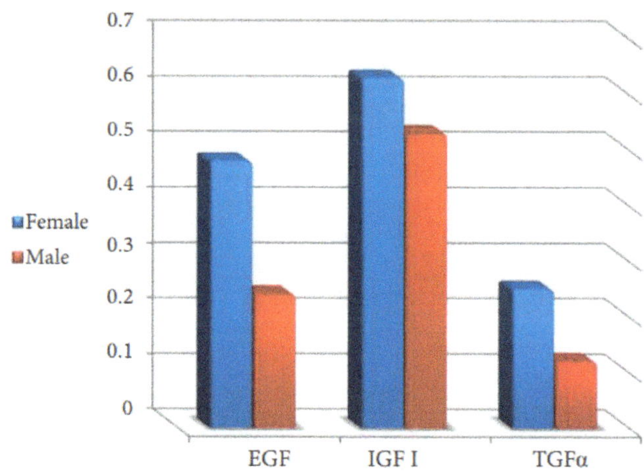

Histogram 2: Mean values of EGF, IGF I and TGFα in both groups.

Whole-mount Results

The whole-mount carmine alum stained slides showed that the ductal tree of the female MG reached the edge of the fat pad (Figure 1a). The ductal tree of male MG nearly filled half of the fat pad (Figure 1b). In the female mammary gland, extensively branched lactiferous duct in an apparent mass of fat pad was detected. The primary ducts were slightly thick and relatively short. The secondary ducts were thinner and longer than the primary ducts. The tertiary ducts were numerous, long, very thin and nearly formed the ductal tree (Figure 2a). A thin long tertiary duct bifurcated at its end into subtending duct that further bifurcates into long thin terminal ducts interlacing with large amount of fat pad (Figure 2b). In the male mammary gland, less extensively branched ductal tree in a little mass of fat pad was nearly reached the edge. The primary, secondary and tertiary ducts were indistinct from each other and nearly had the same thickness and length while the terminal ducts were well defined (Figure 2c). Arborization of apparently thick subtending ducts into irregular outlined short ducts showed small lobules at their ends and their walls had irregular shaped tiny lateral lobulation (Figure 2d). Smooth outlined terminal ducts, terminal end buds and lateral buds had thin stalks and bifurcated smooth bulbous structure at its ends were seen in female rat mammary gland (Figure 3). Large irregularly outlined lobules at the end of terminal ductules were characteristic to male mammary gland (Figure 4).

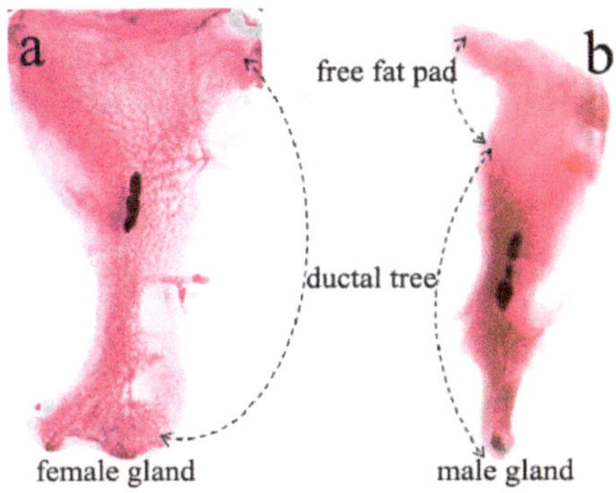

Figure 1. The ductal tree of female (a) and male (b) mammary glands according to whole-mount carmine alum stain. (a): The ductal tree nearly reaches the edge of the fat pad. [Carmine Alum stain]. (b): The ductal tree nearly fills half of the fat pad. [Carmine Alum stain].

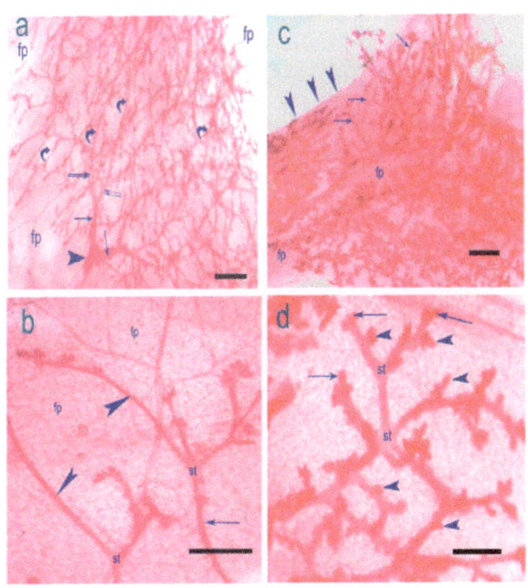

Figure 2 : The female (a,b) and male (c,d) mammary glands according to whole mount Carmine alum stain. (a): Showing extensively branching lactiferous duct (arrow head) in an apparent mass of fat pad (fp). The primary ducts (arrows) are slightly thick and relatively short. The secondary ducts (double arrows) are thin and long. The tertiary ducts (curved arrows) are numerous, long, very thin and nearly formed the ductal tree. [Carmine Alum stain, X10. Bar, 1.2mm]. (b): Showing a thin long tertiary duct (arrow) bifurcating into subtending ducts (st) which bifurcates into long thin terminal ducts (arrow heads) interlacing with fat pad (fp). [Carmine Alum stain, X40. Bar, 2.4mm]. (c): Showing less branched ductal tree in a little mass of fat pad (fp) nearly reached the edge(arrow heads). The primary, secondary and tertiary ducts are indistinct and nearly of the same thickness and length while the terminal ducts are well defined (arrows). [Carmine Alum stain, X10. Bar, 1.2mm]. (d): Showing thick subtending ducts (st) arborized into irregular outlined short ducts that end as small lobules (arrows). Their walls have irregular tiny lateral lobulation (arrow heads). [Carmine Alum stain, X40. Bar, 1.8mm].

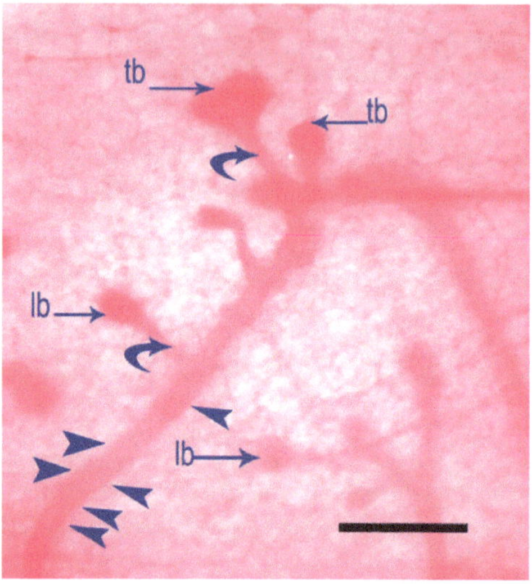

Figure 3: The mammary gland of female rat according to whole-mount carmine alum stain: Showing smooth outlined terminal ducts (arrow heads). The terminal bulbous end buds (tb) and lateral buds (lb) have thin stalks (curved arrows). [Carmine Alum stain, X80. Bar, 4.8mm].

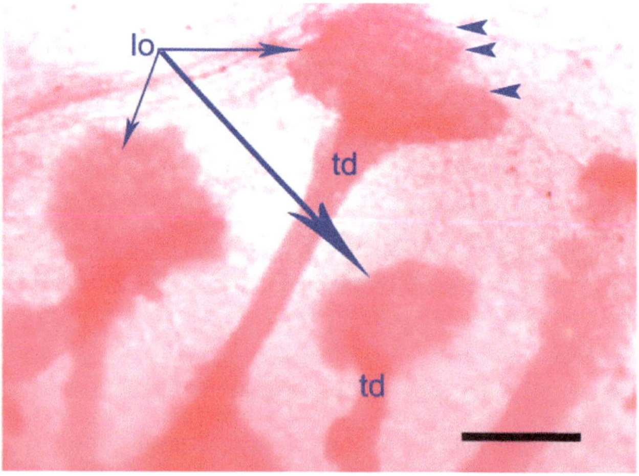

Figure 4: The mammary gland of male rat according to whole-mount carmine alum stain: Showing large irregularly outlined (arrow heads) lobules (lo) at the end of terminal ductules (td).

Histological results

H&E

Examination H&E stained sections of female gland showed thick capsule and vascular adipose connective tissue stroma containing ducts (Figure 5a). Scattered tubular duct system was surrounded by thick dense eosinophilic fibrous stroma which was full of fibroblasts (Figure 5b). The male gland showed less developed stroma, thin capsule and thin periductal fibrous stroma. Many alveoli and inguinal lymph node were also seen (Figure 5c). Lobulo-alveolar structures were predominant in male gland (Figure 5d).

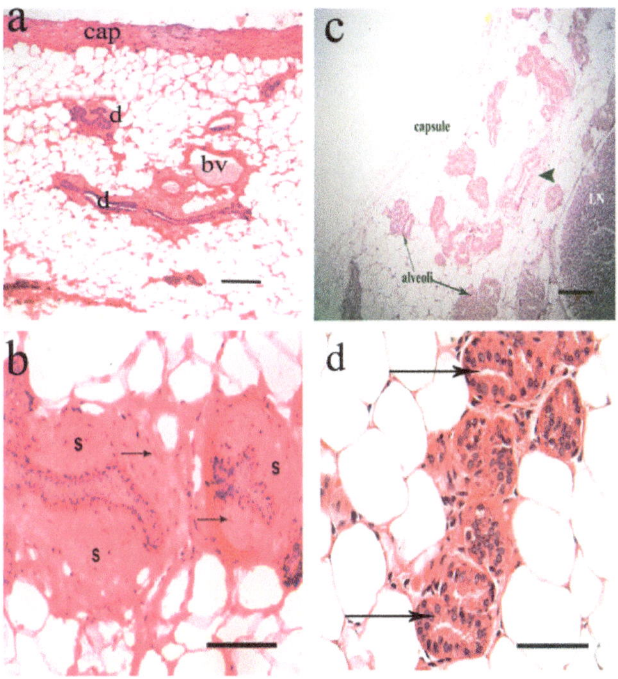

Figure 5: The structure of female (a,b) and male (c,d) mammary gland sections according to H&E stain. (a): Showing thick capsule (cap), vascular stroma (bv) and ducts (d). [H&E, X100. Bar, 100µm]. (b):Showing scattered duct system surrounded by dense eosinophilic stroma (s) which is full of fibroblasts (arrows). [H&E, X400. Bar, 100µm]. (c): Showing thin capsule, thin periductal fibrous stroma (arrow head), many alveoli and inguinal lymph node (LN). [H&E, X100. Bar,100µm]. (d): Showing lobulo-alveolar structure (arrows) predominant in male gland. [H&E, X400. Bar, 100µm].

The female mammary gland ducts were lined by stratified epithelium. The luminal cells were cuboidal and had large central rounded nuclei. The basal cells were flat with flat nuclei. Flat nuclei of fibroblasts were also seen in the fibrous stroma (Figure 6a). The male mammary gland large ducts were lined by multiple layers of large vacuolated luminal epithelial cells. Their nuclei were large and rounded. Luminal and ductal apoptotic cells and acidophilic secretion filling the lumen were detected. Thin layer of fibrous stroma around the ducts was seen. Thin outlined white unilocular adipocytes with large cytoplasmic fat droplets and peripheral nuclei surrounded the fibrous stroma (Figure 6b). Thick ductal fibrous stroma surrounded the small ducts and numerous small blood vessels were observed (Figure 6c). Very thin stroma and a few numbers of fibroblasts around the small ducts which were lined by two layers of vacuolated cells with rounded nuclei were seen. Deeply acidophilic secretion filling the lumen was also seen (Figure 6d).

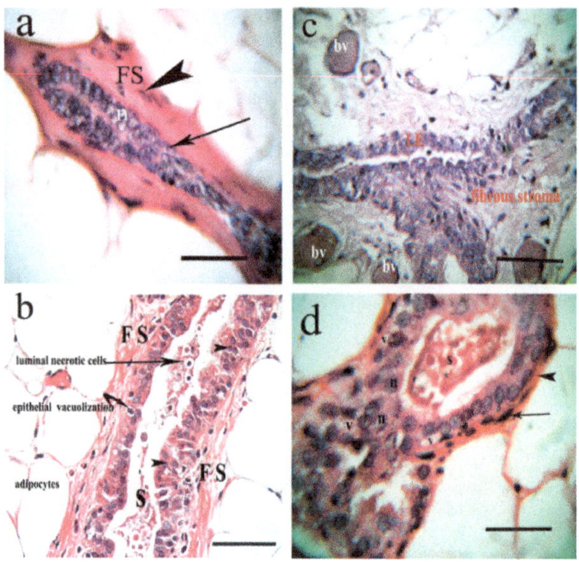

Figure 6: The structure of ducts of female (a) and male (b-d) mammary gland sections according to H&E stain. (a): Showing the duct is lined by stratified epithelium. The luminal cells are cuboidal with large central rounded nuclei (n). The basal cells are flat with flat nuclei (arrow). Flat nuclei of fibroblasts (arrow head) are seen in the fibrous stroma (FS). [H&E, X400. Bar, 100µm]. (b): Showing the large duct is lined by multiple layers of vacuolated large luminal epithelial cells (closed arrow) with large rounded nuclei (arrow heads). Luminal and ductal necrotic cells (arrows) and acidophilic secretion (S) are seen in the lumen. The fibrous stroma (FS) around the duct is thin. Large unilocular adipocytes surrounded the fibrous stroma are noted. [H&E, X400. Bar, 100µm]. (c): Showing the small duct (LE) is surrounded by thick fibrous vascularized stroma (bv). [H&E, X400. Bar, 100µm]. (d): Showing the subtending duct is lined by vacuolated cells (v) with rounded nuclei (n). Very thin stroma (arrow head), a few number of fibroblasts (arrow) and deeply acidophilic secretion (s) is seen. [H&E, X400. Bar, 100µm]

Masson's Trichrome

The female mammary gland showed thick layer collagen fibers around the blood vessels and ducts (Figure 7a). In male group, the alveoli were devoid of connective tissue. The collagen fibers around the ducts were thin while, around blood vessels were thick (Figures 7b and 7c).

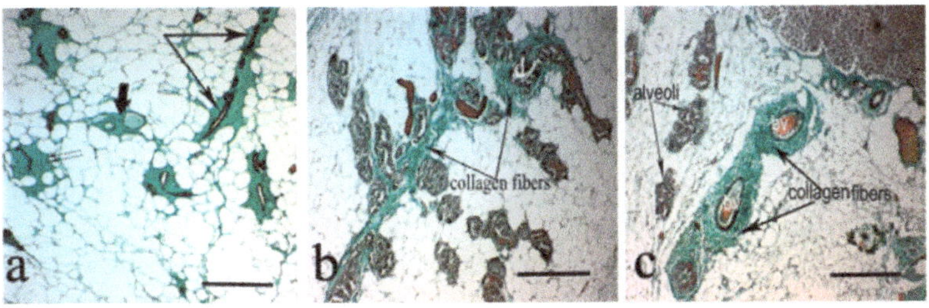

Figure 7: The female (a) and male (b,c) mammary gland sections according to MT stain. (a): Showing the fibrous stroma around the ducts (arrows) and the blood vessels (thick arrow) is thick collagenous. [Masson's trichrome, X100. Bar, 200μm]. (b): Showing a thin layer of collagen fibers around the ducts. [Masson's trichrome, X100. Bar, 200μm]. (c): Showing a thick layer of collagen fibers around blood vessels while, alveoli are devoid of connective tissue [Masson's trichrome, X100. Bar, 200μm].

Immunohistochemical Results

The female mammary gland showed positive reaction for progesterone in some ductal cells (Figure 8a) and a dense positive reaction for estrogen in most of ductal cells (Figure 8b). In male group, patchy distributed pattern was seen for progesterone positive reaction in some ductal epithelial cells, in luminal secretion and in fibroblastic stromal cells. A negative reaction for estrogen in the ductal epithelium and a weak positive reaction in periductal stroma were observed (Figures 8c and 8d).

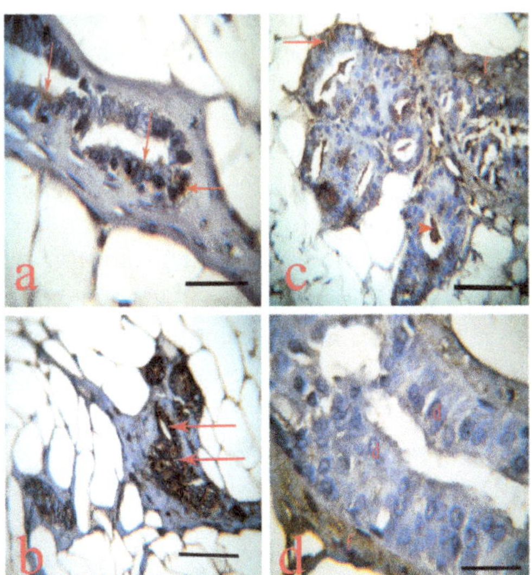

Figure 8: Immunodetection of progesterone and estrogen β receptors of female (a,b) and male (c,d) mammary gland sections. (a): A positive reaction for progesterone receptor in some ductal cells (arrows) is seen. [Progesterone receptor immunostaining, X400. Bar, 100μm]. (b): A tense

positive reaction for Estrogen β receptor in most of ductal cells (arrows) is seen. [Estrogen β receptor immunostaining, X400. Bar, 100μm]. (c): A patchy distributed pattern for progesterone receptor positive reaction in some ductal epithelial cells (arrow), in luminal secretion (arrow head) and in fibroblastic stromal cells (f) is noticed. [Progesterone receptor immunostaining, X400. Bar, 100μm]. (d): A negative reaction for estrogen β receptor immunostaining in the ductal epithelium (d) a weak positive in reaction in periductal stroma (f) is detected. [Estrogen β receptor immunostaining, X1000. Bar, 20μm].

DISCUSSION

In most mammals, the male mammary gland is regarded as a rudimentary organ without ascribed functions; as a result, research on the development and endocrine responses of male mammary glands has been limited [20]. In female, the MG is an important tool for examining some developmental, endocrinal and tumor biological aspects [21]. So, most discussions of the functional and developmental anatomy and histology of the mammary gland were focused on the female and not on the male [10].

Determination of estrous cycle stages is emerging as an important consideration when working on female animals in several research areas. In the present work, the time of sacrifice was at the estrus stage in the female group [15]. Unlike all other stages, during estrus stage, the rat serum prolactin was found to be the highest as determined by enzyme immunoassay. Additionally, it represents the most differentiated mammary gland state [21].

Necessity of Prolactin [22] and Progesterone [23] for lobuloalveolar development of female MG was reported. So, blood samples from both groups were collected to determine concentrations of hormones known to be involved in mammary gland growth and differentiation. Despite of a highly statistically significant decrease in Prolactin hormone and a non significant decrease in Progesterone serum levels in male rats, their mammary glands exhibited lobulo-alveolar secretory parenchyma. Knight and Peaker [24] referred this unique sex-specific morphology of rat male MG to tissue sensitivity that increases the susceptibility and responsiveness of mammary gland to various endogenous hormonal stimuli. Their explanation was confirmed by our data obtained from immunostained sections in male glands (intense positive immunoexpression to progesterone receptors in all parenchyma).

In the current study, EGF, IGF I and TGFα tissue protein, were measured as these factors were documented as potent mitogenic factors for both normal and neoplastic mammary epithelium either *in vivo* [7] or *in vitro* [8]. Interestingly, a significant increase in these factors was detected in female group in comparison to male group.

It is well known that both estrogen [25] and epidermal growth factor [26] are responsible for extensive branching and ductal elongation of the mammary glands. In addition, progesterone is responsible for lobulo-alveolar development [27]. In the current work, immuno-staining of PRA and ER β receptors were carried out aiming to reveal the exact causes of male mammary growth in rats. A striking observation was the strong positive expression of PR in male mammary luminal epithelial cells, luminal secretion and peri-alveolar stroma. Similar patterns of expression were observed for PRA in human female mammary gland [28]. The presence of PRA all over the mammary cells may provide a clue for lobuloalveolar predominance in male glands. In the male group of present work, the negative immunoexpression to ER in the luminal epithelium and the weak positive reaction to ER in periductal stroma can be correlated with the stunted ductal growth of the male mammary ductal tree [25].

Whole-mount technique is considered the most reliable technique used to visualize epithelial ductal and alveolar structures against a translucent fatty background as it readily reveals the extent of ductal elongation, branching, and alveolar development and allows strict quantitative measurements [17]. Based upon analysis of whole-mount slides, the male MG ducts were short, with irregular outline and nearly of the same thickness and length. The terminal ductules were well defined. These data were in accordance with Shyamala [23]. He recorded thick short ducts with extensive lateral branching and large numbers of terminal buds in transgenic mice with an excess PRA expression. Also, in knocked out estrogen receptor α animals, hypoplastic development of the epithelial tree was demonstrated [25]. The limited branching and length of male mammary ducts were related to decreased periductal collagenous connective tissue stroma [29]. Furthermore, estrogen drives extensive growth and branching of female mammary gland [25].

The development of the mammary ductal tree depends on stromal–epithelial interactions, and these interactions are important in embryonic and postnatal evolvement. The stromal compartment is composed of mesenchymal cells (fibroblasts and leukocytes) and extra-cellular matrix as laminin, fibronectin, collagen and proteoglycans [30]. In male albino rats, less developed stroma in the form of thin capsule and thin periductal stroma around the large ducts were in accordance with [1]. They suggested that extra-cellular matrix is involved in the interactions between the mammary cells and their environment.

The ducts of male mammary gland showed two different lining epithelium in relation to their size: the large ducts were lined by multiple layers of vacuolated luminal epithelial cells with large and rounded nuclei. The smaller ducts were lined by doubled layers of low epithelial cells. These features in male mammary gland structure were documented [31]. These features referred probably to a higher sensitivity of male rat mammary tissue to steroid hormones than other male mammals e.g., mice [32]. A completely different picture of male mammary glands in other male rodents was recorded. Their mammary glands were described as a rudimentary mammary glandular tissue [3].

The cells lined large male mammary ducts were characterized by abundant foamy eosinophilic cytoplasm containing distinct variable sized vacuoles. Their lumina were mostly contained evidence of secretory activity with apoptotic bodies and fragmented epithelial cells. These histological changes were identified in rats' female mammary gland after Dehydroepiandrosterone (DHEA) treatment [33]. They showed that, the potent stimulatory effects of androgens on lobuloalveolar as well as ductal development in the female rat mammary gland are due to intracrine conversion of DHEA into active sex steroids with predominant or even possibly exclusive androgenic activity in the mammary gland. They added that local formation of androgen and estrogen through intracrine activity in rats plays a major role in these histological features.

Masson's trichrome staining revealed that the male periductal stroma was much reduced relative to that in female, especially around small ducts and alveoli. The previous hypotheses proposed that the mammary gland development and branching is partially dependent on the amount of extracellular matrix [34,35].

Gynecomastia is a proliferation of the glandular component of the male breast. In most cases, it is a pathological condition in response to increased level of estrogen or decreased level of testosterone [36], drugs e.g., ethionamide [37], spironolactone, cimetidine and ketoconazole [38] or increased endogenous Prolactin [39]. In the current work, evaluated steriodal hormones were within normal levels in both groups.

CONCLUSION

The results of the present study concluded that proliferation of male albino rat MG occurred despite of normal levels of its serum steroid hormones and without drug supplementation or any endocrinal disturbance. This condition can provide fundamental information about a physiological type of *gynecomastia* that does not need hormonal correction and may need only cosmetic surgical intervention. We recommended immuno-staining of breast biopsy in diagnosed cases of *gynecomastia* in men. In addition, further serological and histological investigations of male rat mammary tissue are needed to strengthen our data.

COMPETING INTERESTS

The authors declare that they have no competing interests.

AUTHORS' CONTRIBUTIONS

Authors' contributions	ZAG	SMA	NME
Research concept and design	√	--	--
Collection and/or assembly of data	√	--	--
Data analysis and interpretation	√	√	√
Writing the article	√	√	√
Design of figures	√	--	√
Critical revision of the article	√	√	√
Final approval of article	√	√	√
Statistical analysis	--	√	--

ACKNOWLEDGEMENT

We would like to thank Prof. Dr. Fadia Khalid Abdo for her English language editing and reviewing of the manuscript, Prof.Dr.Dalia Elrobi for morphometrical aid and Dr.Eman Elshahate for statistical aid.

REFERENCES

1. Lucas JN, Rudmann DG, Credille KM, Irizarry AR, Peter A and Snyder PW. The rat mammary gland: morphologic changes as an indicator of systemic hormonal perturbations induced by xenobiotics.*Toxicol Pathol.* 2007; 35:199-207.
2. Brisken C and O'Malley B. Hormone action in the mammary gland. *Cold Spring Harb Perspect Biol.* 2010;2:a003178.
3. Richert MM, Schwertfeger KL, Ryder JW and Anderson SM. An atlas of mouse mammary gland development. *J Mammary Gland Biol Neoplasia.* 2000; 5:227-41.
4. Forster C, Makela S, Warri A, Kietz S, Becker D, Hultenby K, Warner M and Gustafsson JA. Involvement of estrogen receptor beta in terminal differentiation of mammary gland epithelium. *Proc Natl Acad Sci U S A.* 2002; 99:15578-83.
5. Beleut M, Rajaram RD, Caikovski M, Ayyanan A, Germano D, Choi Y, Schneider P and Brisken C. Two distinct mechanisms underlie progesterone-induced proliferation in the mammary gland. *Proc Natl Acad Sci U S A.* 2010; 107:2989-94.
6. Vonderhaar BK. Local effects of EGF, alpha-TGF, and EGF-like growth factors on lobuloalveolar development of the mouse mammary gland in vivo. *J Cell Physiol.* 1987; 132:581-4.
7. Valverius EM, Bates SE, Stampfer MR, Clark R, McCormick F, Salomon DS, Lippman ME and Dickson RB.Transforming growth factor alpha production and epidermal growth factor receptor expression in normal and oncogene transformed human mammary epithelial cells. *Mol Endocrinol.* 1989; 3:203-14.
8. Visvader JE. Keeping abreast of the mammary epithelial hierarchy and breast tumorigenesis. *Genes Dev.* 2009; 23:2563-77.
9. Sternlicht MD. Key stages in mammary gland development: the cues that regulate ductal branching morphogenesis. *Breast Cancer Res.* 2006; 8:201.
10. Vandenberg LN, Schaeberle CM, Rubin BS, Sonnenschein C and Soto AM. The male mammary gland: a target for the xenoestrogen bisphenol A. *Reprod Toxicol.* 2013; 37:15-23.
11. Arvind A, Khan MA, Srinivasan K and Roberts J. Gynaecomastia correction: A review of our experience.*Indian J Plast Surg.* 2014; 47:56-60.
12. Oettel M and Mukhopadhyay AK. Progesterone: the forgotten hormone in men? *Aging Male.* 2004; 7:236-57.
13. Masso-Welch PA, Darcy KM, Stangle-Castor NC and Ip MM. A developmental atlas of rat mammary gland histology. *J Mammary Gland Biol Neoplasia.* 2000; 5:165-85.
14. Ozmen J, Bobryshev YV, Lord RS and Ashwell KW. Identification of dendritic cells in aortic atherosclerotic lesions in rats with diet-induced hypercholesterolaemia. *Histol Histopathol.* 2002;17:223-37.
15. McLean AC, Valenzuela N, Fai S and Bennett SA. Performing vaginal lavage,

crystal violet staining, and vaginal cytological evaluation for mouse estrous cycle staging identification. *J Vis Exp.* 2012; e4389.

16. Ingman WV, Wyckoff J, Gouon-Evans V, Condeelis J and Pollard JW. Macrophages promote collagen fibrillogenesis around terminal end buds of the developing mammary gland. *Dev Dyn.* 2006;235:3222-9.
17. de Assis S, Warri A, Cruz MI and Hilakivi-Clarke L. Changes in mammary gland morphology and breast cancer risk in rats. *J Vis Exp.* 2010.
18. Bancroft JD and Layton C. The Hematoxylin and eosin. In: Suvarna SK, Layton C and Bancroft JD editors.Theory and Practice of histological techniques. 7th ed., ChurchillLivingstone of El Sevier. Philadelphia. Ch 10 and 11. 2013; 172–214.
19. Jackson P and Blythe D. Immunohistochemical techniques. In: Suvarna SK, Layton C and Bancroft JD editors.Theory & Practice of histological techniques. 7th ed., Churchill Livingstone of El Sevier. Philadelphia. Ch. 18. 2013; 381–434.
20. Wang XJ, Bartolucci-Page E, Fenton SE and You L. Altered mammary gland development in male rats exposed to genistein and methoxychlor. *Toxicol Sci.* 2006; 91:93-103.
21. Fata JE, Leco KJ, Voura EB, Yu HY, Waterhouse P, Murphy G, Moorehead RA and Khokha R. Accelerated apoptosis in the Timp-3-deficient mammary gland. *J Clin Invest.* 2001; 108:831-41.
22. Das R and Vonderhaar BK. Prolactin as a mitogen in mammary cells. *J Mammary Gland Biol Neoplasia.* 1997; 2:29-39.
23. Shyamala G. Progesterone signaling and mammary gland morphogenesis. *J Mammary Gland Biol Neoplasia.* 1999; 4:89-104.
24. Knight CH and Peaker M. Development of the mammary gland. *J Reprod Fertil.* 1982; 65:521-36.
25. Feng Y, Manka D, Wagner KU and Khan SA. Estrogen receptor-alpha expression in the mammary epithelium is required for ductal and alveolar morphogenesis in mice. *Proc Natl Acad Sci U S A.* 2007;104:14718-23.
26. Walczak M, Pawlus B, Kędzia A and Walkowiak J. Active synthesis of epidermal growth factor in human mammary glands. *Acta scientiarum polonorum technologia alimentaria.* 2010; 9:237-241.
27. Aupperlee MD and Haslam SZ. Differential hormonal regulation and function of progesterone receptor isoforms in normal adult mouse mammary gland. *Endocrinology.* 2007; 148:2290-300.
28. Li S, Han B, Liu G, Ouellet J, Labrie F and Pelletier G. Immunocytochemical localization of sex steroid hormone receptors in normal human mammary gland. *J Histochem Cytochem.* 2010; 58:509-15.
29. Kass L, Erler JT, Dembo M and Weaver VM. Mammary epithelial cell: influence of extracellular matrix composition and organization during development and tumorigenesis. *Int J Biochem Cell Biol.* 2007;39:1987-94.

30. Couldrey C, Moitra J, Vinson C, Anver M, Nagashima K and Green J. Adipose tissue: a vital in vivo role in mammary gland development but not differentiation. *Dev Dyn.* 2002; 223:459-68.

31. Cardy RH. Sexual dimorphism of the normal rat mammary gland. *Vet Pathol.* 1991; 28:139-45.

32. Neumann F. Early indicators for carcinogenesis in sex-hormone-sensitive organs. *Mutat Res.* 1991;248:341-56.

33. Sourla A, Martel C, Labrie C and Labrie F. Almost exclusive androgenic action of dehydroepiandrosterone in the rat mammary gland. *Endocrinology.* 1998; 139:753-64.

34. Wiseman BS and Werb Z. Stromal effects on mammary gland development and breast cancer. *Science.*2002; 296:1046-9.

35. Muschler J and Streuli CH. Cell-matrix interactions in mammary gland development and breast cancer.*Cold Spring Harb Perspect Biol.* 2010; 2:a003202.

36. Nordt CA and DiVasta AD. Gynecomastia in adolescents. *Curr Opin Pediatr.* 2008; 20:375-82. | Article |PubMed

37. Dixit R, George J, Sharma AK, Chhabra N, Jangir SK and Mishra V. Ethionamide-induced gynecomastia. *J Pharmacol Pharmacother.* 2012; 3:196-9.

38. Deepinder F and Braunstein GD. Drug-induced gynecomastia: an evidence-based review. *Expert Opin Drug Saf.* 2012; 11:779-95.

39. Carlson HE. Approach to the patient with gynecomastia. *J Clin Endocrinol Metab.* 2011; 96:15-21.

16
CHAPTER

EFFECT OF TOPICAL ALOE VERA ON THE PROCESS OF HEALING OF FULL-THICKNESS SKIN BURN: A HISTOLOGICAL AND IMMUNOHISTOCHEMICAL STUDY

Ahmed A.M. Abdel Hamid and Mona FM Soliman

Keywords: Full-thickness skin burn, aloe vera, pericytes, inflammation, healing

INTRODUCTION

Skin burn wound injury is ranked fourth in all injuries [1]. It can severely affect not only the skin but the whole body according to their depth and extension [2]. Although there are advances in its treatment the incidence of scarring remains high [3] and the deaths are over 300,000 each year throughout the world [1].

Healing of burn wound is essentially dependent on the angiogenesis which is the mainstay in the granulation tissue formation [4]. Apart from that they are considered as progenitor/stem cells, pericytes are bone marrow-derived cells (BMDC) embedded within the basement membrane of capillaries [5,6]. During the process of angiogenesis, there is a very intimate interaction between endothelial cells and pericytes [7,8]. Furthermore, pericytes play a key role not only in the proliferation and migration of the endothelium and but also in their stabilization [5]. In addition, the transmigrated inflammatory cells interact with the endothelial basement membrane to enter the site of injury [4].

Several natural substances had been tried to improve burn healing; honey is claimed to delay healing in both partial- and full-thickness burns [9]. On the other hand,

Citation: Ahmed A.M. Abdel Hamid and Mona FM Soliman, Effect of topical aloe vera on the process of healing of full-thickness skin burn: a histological and immunohistochemical study, DOI : http://dx.doi.org/10.7243/2055-091X-2-3.

topical application of curcumin showed beneficial effects in the acceleration of partial-thickness burns healing [10].

Aloe vera (AV) is a cactus-like perennial succulent that belongs to the Liliaceae Family that is usually cultivated in tropical areas [11]. It is the one of oldest medicinal substances that was used in wound healing [12]. AV has a potentially significant anti-inflammatory effect, therefore it could be used in treating: gingivitis [12-14], skin wound [15-17] and first to second degree burns [18,19]. Topical application of AV has been demonstrated to have a promising effect on the wound healing process [15]. It might have greater efficacy over silver sulfadiazine cream for treating second-degree burns [18]. However, other study claimed that AV did not increase burn healing [11] or even delayed the healing process of the burn compared with silver sulfadiazine cream [20]. In addition, it might increase production of human fibroblasts 6-8 folds faster than conventional, improve their structure and accelerate their collagen production [21].

The aim of this study was to explore the effect of AV on the process of healing specially angiogenesis in full thickness (FT) skin burn and to find out whether it improves this healing or not and the mechanism by which it acts.

MATERIAL AND METHODS

Animals

In the current study, 70 adult male albino rats weighing 180-200 gm were provided by Animal Housing of the Mansoura Faculty of Pharmacy. The animals were placed in standard plastic cages (2 animals per cage) for 12 days under 12/12 hours light/dark cycle with 23-25°C room temperature. All animals were received standard laboratory animal's chow and water ad labitum during the whole period of experiment. The experiment was performed according to the guide for the care and use of laboratory animals (Institute for Laboratory Animal Research, National Research Council, Washington, DC: National Academy Press, no. 85-23, revised 1996).

Experimental procedure

For the experiment, animals received general anesthesia by intramuscular injection of Ketamine hydrochloride (Ketalar®, Parke-Davis), 85 mg/kg of body weight, and Xylazine hydrochloride (Rompun®, Bayer), 6 mg/kg of body weight each. Then the hair on the back of the dorsal region was removed. FT skin burns were produced to each animal by using a cone-shaped, stainless steel specially-made metal instrument (purchased from Hisham Medical Company, Mansoura, Egypt), equipped with a control thermometer and heated to 1000C in a pot of boiling water for 5 seconds. Then this instrument was applied on the upper back of the rat to produce a FT burn of an area of about 2-3 cm^2. A dry dressing was applied to the wound of each, after inducing the burn, Daily monitoring of the animals and the burned wound were done.

Aloe vera gel preparation Plant leaves of AV were obtained from and processed in the Department of Pharmacognosy and Medicinal Plants, Mansoura Faulty of Pharmacy. After cleaning and disinfection, the gel was extracted by an incision in the plant leaves, which then was exposed to heat at 50°C and filtered. Glycerin and triethanolamine were added to achieve purity of AV gel of 95% which was administrated at a concentration of 200 mg/kg [22,23].

Experimental design

Group A: control group contained 10 animals. Group B: 30 animals were left to spontaneous healing. The animals were randomly divided into three subgroups of 10 animals each. Under general anesthesia, from each subgroup the burnt skin area was collected, at 4, 8, 12 days postburn. Group C: 30 animals had topical AV gel application once daily at a concentration of 200 mg/kg on the burnt skin. Then animals were randomly divided into three subgroups of ten animals each. Under general anesthesia, from each subgroup the burnt skin area was collected at 4, 8, 12 days postburn.

Histological study

Specimens were taken from the burnt skin of spontaneouslyhealed animals as well as from AV treated ones. Specimens were processed for light microscopic examination and fixed in 10% neutral-buffered formalin. They were then processed for preparation of serial paraffin sections (5 μm thick). Then, these sections were stained with H&E and MT stains [24].

Immunohistochemical study

Sections of 3 μm-thick were cut and collected on poly-L-lysine coated slides for the immunohistochemical study. Then the slides were left for 24 hours to dry at 37°C for ideal adhesion of the specimens to the surface of the slide. Following deparaffinization, hydration and antigen retrieval, sections were cooled down to room temperature. Next, they were incubated for 30 minutes in 1% H_2O_2 solution and washed in PBS, then followed by blocking in 2% skim milk for 30 minutes. The slides were incubated with the primary antibodies at 40°C for a night, and the next day, a peroxidase polymer-based secondary detection system (Dako, Heliopolis, Cairo, Egypt) was used for 30 minutes for signal amplification. 3, 3'-diaminobenzidine (DAB) (Dako, Egypt) was used for signal detection and the slides were counterstained by Hematoxylin then coverslipped. The mouse anti-α-SMA primary antibodies (Dako, Egypt) were used at dilution 1:100 for the immunohistochemical study according to the standard guidelines. They stain pericytes of blood capillaries, meanwhile the endothelium cells do not show α-SMA positivity [25,26].

Morphometric study

The sections were imaged with a microscope (Olympus, Japan) equipped with a digital camera connected to a computer and were randomly evaluated by two 8-year experience histologists under blindfold conditions.

Qualitative assessment of the phases of healing was done by employing a scoring system (0–3) for each section in various groups. This system is basically dependent on specific selected parameters which are: the inflammatory cells, the collagen deposition, the angiogenesis and the granulation tissue (Table 1) [10,27,28]. The extent of collagen deposition was qualitatively evaluated by MT stain, while the other parameters were qualitatively assessed using H&E stained sections.

Table 1: Histological scoring system for skin burn healing evaluation according to the listed specific parameters

	0	1	2	3
Inflammatory cells	None	Minimal	Mild	Evident
Collagen deposition	None	Minimal	Mild	Evident
Angiogenesis	None	Minimal	Mild	Evident
Granulation tissue	None	Minimal	Mild	Evident

Quantitative assessment of the neovascularization during the healing process in the GT was carried out. Four images from areas of maximum density of vessels(NFC) were captured in each specimen that stained by anti-α-SMA (with an x20 objective) in each group. Then, they were digitally imported to a professional image analyzer software (Image Pro Plus 6.0, Media Cybernetics, Bethesda, MD). Both the areas and numbers (densities) of the neovascularization in the GT in the specimens of each group were assessed.

The average of all values measured from images of the same slide was used, and the results were expressed as average vascular areas/1000 μm^2, and average vessel numbers/1 mm^2 respectively [7].

Statistical Analysis

All statistical data analysis and graphs were carried out using SPSS 16.0 (SPSS, Chicago, IL, USA) and Microsoft Excel 13. Data were presented in mean(±)standard deviations (SD) by using ANOVA test for dual comparisons between groups, except the scoring system of healing which was evaluated by Mann–Whitney U test. The differences were considered significant when probability (P) was less than 0.05.

RESULTS

By H&E stain in the control group, the skin was formed of dermis and epidermis. The dermis was divided into papillary layer and reticular layer. The papillary layer contained dermal papillae, blood vessels and loose connective tissue (CT) with fine collagen fibers, while the reticular layer contained dense CT with coarse collagen fibers which stained blue by MT (Figures 1A-1C). Minimal α-SMA expression could be detected in the capillaries of the papillary layer of the dermis (Figure 1D).

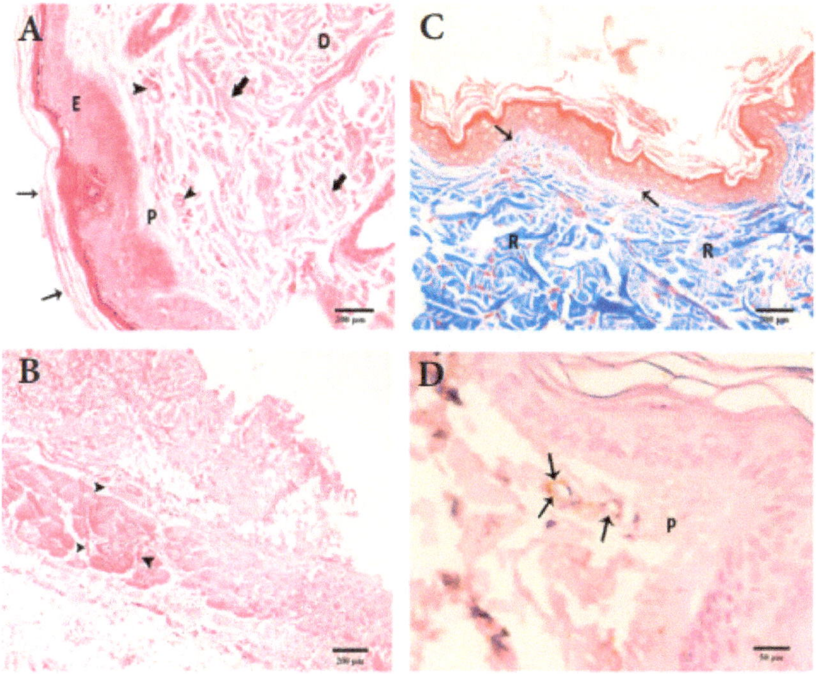

Figure 1: Photomicrographs of thin skin sections. (A) A section in thin skin of control group showing the two layers of the skin; epidermis (E) and dermis (D). The epidermis is formed of stratified squamous keratinized epithelium (arrows) covered by a thin layer of keratin. The dermis is formed of papillary layer containing abundant blood vessels (arrowheads) surrounded fine collagen while the reticular layer is formed mainly of coarse collagen (thick arrows). (H&E, x200, Scale bar=200 μm). (B) A section in thin skin 4 days post burn involving the whole layers of the skin in the form of tissue loss of the epidermis and coagulation necrosis of the dermis with infiltration of the deep dermis with mononuclear cell infriltrate (arrowheads) extending to the muscle layer. (H&E, x200, Scale bar=200 μm). (C) A section in thin skin of control group showing fine collagen fibers in the papillary layer stained light blue (arrows) while the reticular layer (R) contains more dense collagen bundles stained deep blue. (MT, x200, Scale bar=200 μm). (D) A section in thin skin of control group showing negative to weak positive α-SMA expression (arrows) in the blood capillaries in the papillary layer (P) of the dermis. (α-SMA immunostaining, x1000, Scale bar=50 μm).

After 4 days from inducing FT burn, sections in the skin stained by H&E stain showed coagulative necrosis involving the whole thickness of the skin with tissue loss of the epidermis and superficial layer of dermis fibers (Figure 1B). By higher magnification, there were severely congested blood vessels and marked infiltration of the dermis by significant mononuclear inflammatory cells in the GT appeared at base of the burnt area. This GT was formed of collagen fibers and NFC. Fibroblasts were the predominant cells between the collagen fibers (Figure 2A). On the other hand, in sections of 4 days skin burn treated with AV, there were less inflammatory cells infiltrate in the GT deposited at the base of the burnt area (Figure 2B).

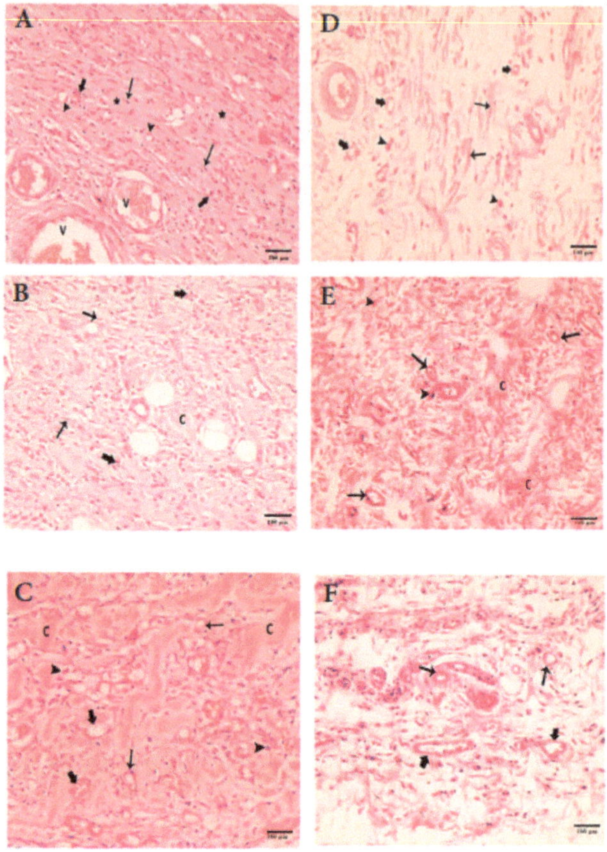

Figure 2: Photomicrographs of a H&E (x400) sections. (A) A section in thin skin 4 days post burn showing inflitration of the deep dermis with GT contining both collagen fibres (*) and NFC (arrowheads). Larger sized blood vessels (V) appear congested and surrounded by mononuclear inflammatory cells (thick arrows) together with other CT cells mainly fibroblasts (arrows). (H&E, x400, Scale bar=100 μm). (B) A section in thin skin 4 days post burn treated with AV showing GT containing abundant less coarse collagen bundles (C) with abundant CT cells specially fibroblasts (arrows) in between. Fewer inflammatory cells (thick arrows) are seen compared with 4-d skin burn per se group. (H&E, x400, Scale bar=100 μm). (C): A section in thin skin 8 days post burn showing increased number of immature NFC (arrows) which have sometimes incomplete wall (thick arrows) with a relatively decreased number of inflammatory cells (arrowheads) lying between the coarse collagen bundles (C). (H&E, x400, Scale bar=100 μm). (D) A section in thin skin 8 days post burn treated with AV showing increased number of NFC (thick arrows) and marked decrease in the inflammatory cells (arrowheads) lying in fine collagen fibers (arrows). (H&E, x400, Scale bar=100 μm). (E) A section in thin skin 12 days post burn showing increased GT formation in the form of increased density of the numerous NFC (arrows) lying in the abundant irregular collagen fibers (C) which enclose less mononuclear inflammatory cells (arrowheads). (H&E, x400, Scale bar=100 μm). (F) A section in thin skin 12 days post burn treated with AV showing increase of the NFC (arrows) with appearance of larger-sized blood vessels (thick arrows) in the GT. (H&E, x400, Scale bar=100 μm).

After 8 and 12 days from inducing FT burn, in sections of the skin stained by H&E stain, the GT showed porgessive significant increase in the vascularity by appearance of more NFC toghther with deposition of significantly more collagen rather than inflammatory cells (Figures 2C and 2E) (Histograms 2 and 3). On the other hand, in skin sections of 8,12 days skin burn treated with AV, the inflammatory cells infiltrate were decreased significantly in the deposited GT compared with burn per se group (Figures 2D and 2F); (Histogram 1).

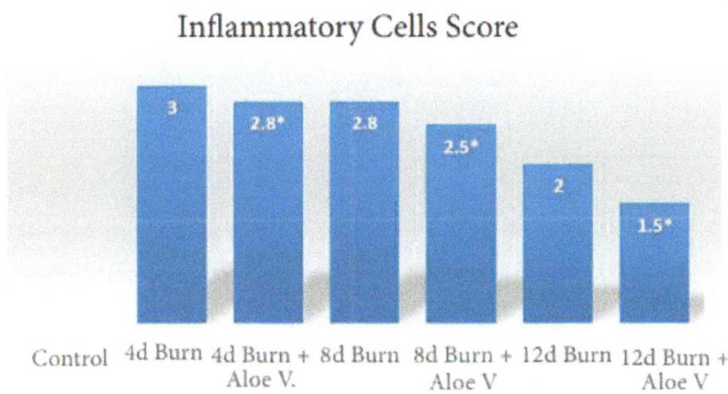

Histogram 1: Inflammatory cells score. It shows qualitative assessment of healing taking the inflammatory cells as one parameter of this assessment. *Significant difference between the means of all the groups (p<0.05).

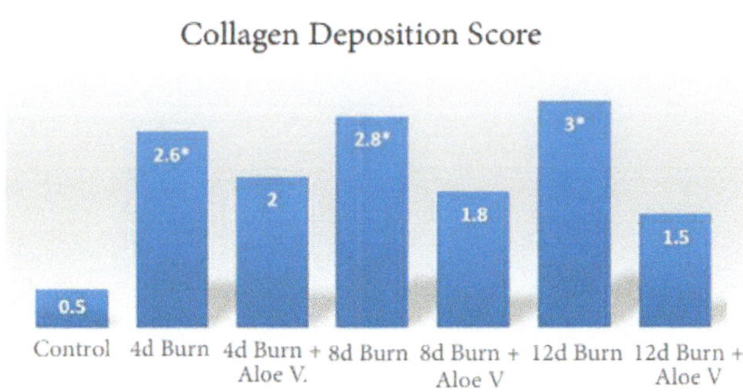

Histogram 2: Collagen deposition score. It shows qualitative assessment of healing taking thecollagen deposition as one parameter of this assessment. *Significant difference between the means of all the groups (p<0.05).

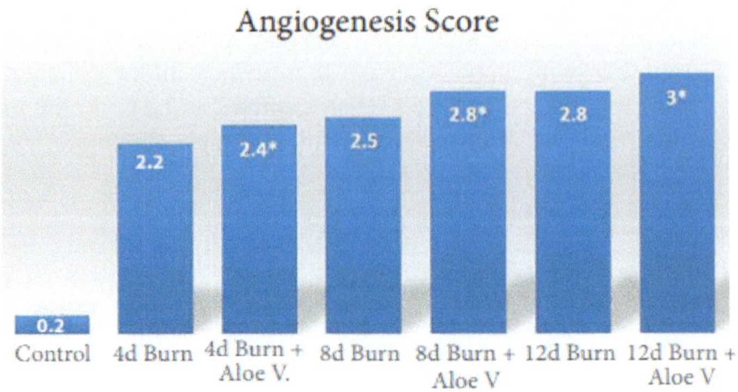

Histogram 3: Angiogenesis score. It shows qualitative assessment of healing taking the degree of angiogenesis as one parameter of this assessment. *Significant difference between the means of all the groups ($p<0.05$).

By MT stain, after 4 days of the burn, skin sections showed collagen deposition which appeared blue in color which progressively increased on 8th and 12th day sections (Figures 3A, 3C and 3E). On the other hand, in the groups treated with AV after 4, 8 and 12 days of the burn, skin sections showed much fine, less dense and more well-remodeled bluish collagen fibers compared with burn per se groups (Figures 3B, 3D and 3F); (Histograms 2 and4).

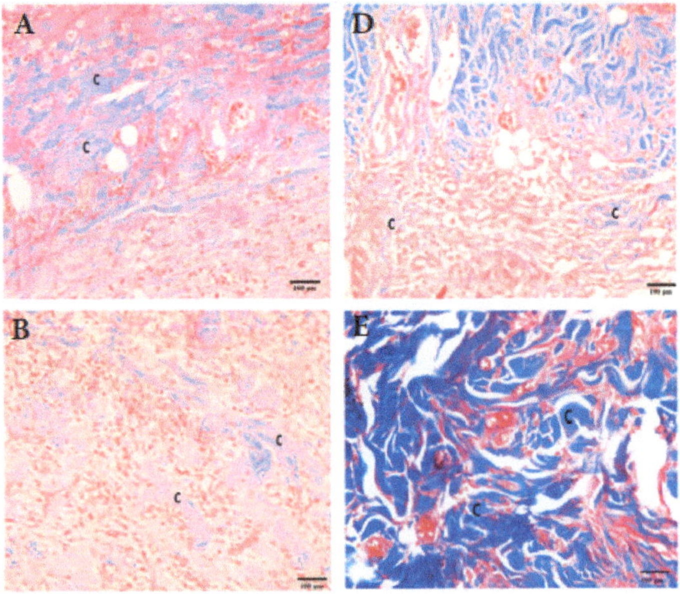

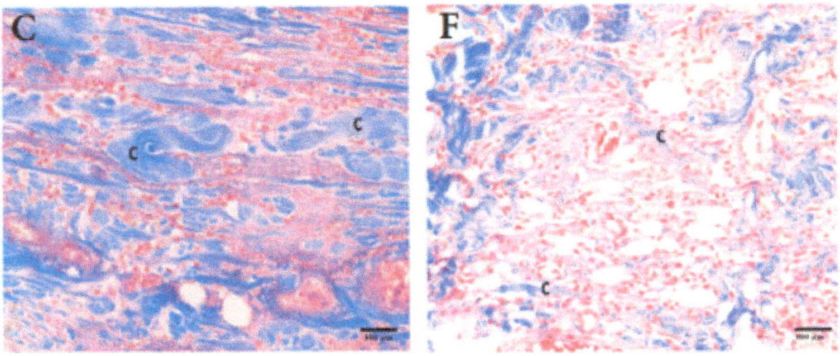

Figure 3: Photomicrographs of MT (x400) sections. (A) A section in thin skin 4 days post burn showing coarse thick bundles of collagen (C) stained blue. (MT, x400, Scale bar=100 μm). (B) A section in thin skin 4 days post burn treated with AV showing much more fine collagen bundles (C) compared with A. (MT, x400, Scale bar=100 μm). (C) A section in thin skin 8 days post burn showing excessive irregular dense collagen deposition (C). (MT, x400, Scale bar=100 μm). (D) A section in thin skin 8 days post burn treated with AV showing finer and more regular collagen fibers (C) in the GT compared with C. (MT, x400, Scale bar=100 μm). (E) A section in thin skin 12 days post burn showing increased the deposition of coarse collagen fibers (C) in the GT of the dermis. (MT, x400, Scale bar=100 μm). (F) A section in thin skin 12 days post burn treated with AV showing well-formed collagen deposition (c) in the dermis. (MT, x400, Scale bar=100 μm).

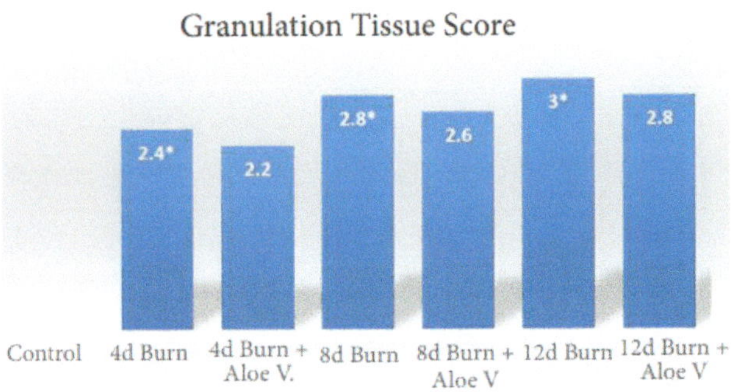

Histogram 4: Granulation tissue score. It shows qualitative assessment of healing taking the granulation tissue as one parameter of this assessment. * Significant difference between the means of all the groups ($p<0.05$).

By α-SMA immunostain, in the 4 and 8 days burn per se group, skin sections showed progressive increase in the α-SMA expression in the pericytes surrounding the immature variable size NFC in the GT. This expression become less detected on 12th day sections postburn per se. The immaturity of NFC appeared both in their size and shape; some of these NFC were small in size while the other are larger. Many of the NFC were multilayered and their lumen sometimes ranged from obliterated to partially- to fully-lumenized NFC. This NFC immaturity appeared on 4th and reached maximum on 8th day postburn per se then they become more mature in both size and shape on the 12th day sections as most these NFC were luminized with disappearance of the multilayered wall. In addition, the endothelium lining of these NFC showed always negative α-SMA expression in all sections (Figures 4A, 4C and4D).

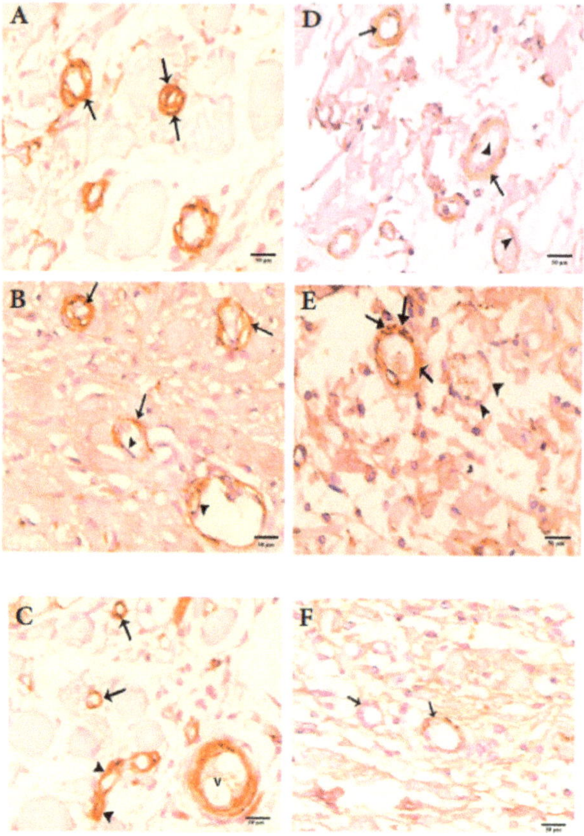

Figure 4: Photomicrographs of α-SMA immune-stained (x1000) sections. (A) A section in thin skin 4 days post burn showing increased number of immature multilayered NFC with strong positive α-SMA-stained pericytes (arrows). (α-SMA immunostaining, x1000, Scale bar=50 μm). (B) A section in thin skin 4 days post burn treated with AV showing immature variable size NFC made up of two rows of cells: internal negative α-SMAstained endothelial cell (arrowheads) and external positive α-SMA-stained pericytes (arrows) surrounding the lumen which appears partially obliterated in some and fully canalized in others. (α-SMA immunostaining, x1000, Scale bar=50 μm). (C) A section in thin skin 8 days post burn showing increased density of the immature variable-sized NFC surrounded by positive α-SMA-stained pericytes (arrows). Blood vessels sometimes appear as partially erupted cord (arrowheads) and occasionally acquire more layers to form a larger vessel (V). (α-SMA immunostaining, x1000, Scale bar=50 μm). (D) A section in thin skin 8 days post burn treated with AV showing more mature NFC with patent lumen lined by negative α-SMA-stained endothelium (arrowheads) surrounded by moderately positive α-SMA-stained pericytes (arrows). (α-SMA immunostaining, x1000, Scale bar=50 μm). (E) A section in thin skin 12 days post burn showing two NFC; one shows a moderately positiveα-SMA expression (arrows)while in the other no α-SMA expression could be detected (arrowheads). (α-SMA immunostaining, x1000, Scale bar=50 μm). (F) A section in thin skin 12 days post burn treated

with AV showing more mature NFC with negative α-SMA immunostaining in most of the pericytes (arrows). (α-SMA immunostaining, x1000, Scale bar=50 μm).

In sections of 4, 8 and 12 days skin burn treated with AV, the α-SMA expression was less detected and moderate in intensity compared with burn per se groups, then this expression decreased progressively on the 8th day till it became minimally detected in most of the pericytes on the 12th day postburn (Figure 4B). Moreover, in sections of 8 and 12 days skin burn treated with AV, NFC size as well as lumen was relatively more uniform, reflecting more mature NFC compared with burn per se groups (Figures 4B, 4E and 4F). In addition, there was a significant increase in vascular numbers (densities) as well as areas on 4th , 8th and 12th day postburn groups treated with AV compared with non treated groups (Tables 2 and 3).

Table 2: Average vascular areas in different groups. Average vascular areas/1000 μm^2

	FT Burn per se	FT Burn+AV
4d	42±4	48±3*
8d	71±5	78±2*
12d	87±4	96±1*

*Significant difference between the means of all the groups ($p<0.05$).

Table 3: Average vascular numbers (densities) in different groups/mm^2

	FT Burn per se	FT Burn+AV
4d	86±4	94±2*
8d	154±6	168±3*
12d	189±6	197±5*

*Significant difference between the means of all the groups ($p<0.05$).

DISCUSSION

After 4 days from inducing FT skin burn, there was coagulative necrosis which is healed by GT appeared at base of the burnt area. On 8th and until 12th day from inducing the FT skin burn, the vascularity of the GT is increased by appearance of more NFC together with deposition of more collagen rather that inflammatory cells. These results were in agreement with previous studies [7,29]. Fibroblasts were always the predominant CT cells in the GT regardless the stage of healing. The core function of fibroblasts is the formation of collagen, which is a supportive protein that responsible for the skin to be firm [21]. Therefore, these non-inflammatory BMDCs are essential for homeostasis and healing of the skin [30]. Moreover, fibroblasts crosstalk with monocytes/macrophages that infiltrate the site of injury and orchestrate the healing process and tissue repair. Monocytes dynamically react with selected extracellular matrix (ECM) components secreted by the fibroblasts. In addition, monocytes decreased fibroblast interleukin (IL)-1α and transforming growth factor-alpha (TGF)-α, however they highly increased fibroblast matrix metalloproteinase (MMP)-2 and granulocyte-macrophage colony-stimulating factor (GM-CSF) [31].

In this study, there was heavy infiltration mononuclear inflammatory cells especially initially after 4 days of inducing the burn which became milder later, when the GT acquired collagen rather than inflammatory cells. This was in agreement with other researchers [2], who claimed that macrophages initially increased by about 3 folds, then decreased gradually with maturation of the GT. Monocytes/macrophages are crucial regulatory inflammatory cells as well as the immediate arm of the innate immunity [32-34], therefore their influx into the tissue plays a critical role in the healing process. In addition, it was demonstrated that depletion of macrophages in early inflammatory phase of the healing, significantly reduced GT formation [35].

In the present study, there was significant progressive increase in the number as well as area of NFC. Macrophages, which are also BMDC, secrete proangiogenic cytokines, ECMremodeling proteases and provide physical support to the growing NFC [6,36]. Therefore, they could be responsible for the increased angiogenesis more than 10% in severe inflammatory reactions as in FT burns [2]. This may explain the significant increase in the vascularity from 4th to 12th in this study and its induction by the severity of the inflammation especially in the early reparatory phase of the burn healing.

In this experiment, in the 4 days burn per se group, skin sections showed α-SMA positive expression in the pericytes surrounding the immature variable size NFC in the GT. Then after 8 days from inducing the burn there was increase of the α-SMA expression in the pericytes. This might indicate increased immaturity of the NFC till 8 days post burn, then became less detected 12 days post burn specimens. These results were in agreement with previous studies [7] which demonstrated that during the process of angiogenesis, there was an intimate relationship between pericytes (α-SMApositive) and endothelial cells. These BMDCs, stimulated by PDGFR (platelet-derived growth factor receptors)-β, can promote mechanical support and signaling to maintain the NFC by direct interaction with endothelial cells [6]. Moreover, they could transdifferentiate into other mesenchymal cell types, including fibroblasts, smooth muscle cells or even osteoblasts. Furthermore, the increased expression of these α-SMA-positive investing pericytes could mediates sprouting as well as remodeling new vessels [37]. This might explain how essential the abundant expression of these α-SMA-positive progenitor cells specially early in 4th to 8th day post-burn rather than 12th day post-burn as they might transdifferentiate into a rather mature clone of cells in the wall of the vessel.

In skin sections of 4, 8 and 12 days skin burn treated with AV there were a significantly less inflammatory cells infiltrate in the GT compared with 4, 8 and 12 skin burn per se specimens respectively. These might be attributed to the potentially significant anti-inflammatory effect of AV [12-14]. Other researchers reported that in addition to its anti-inflammatory effect, AV acts as immunomodulator as well as scavenger of free radicals [38]. Moreover, previous studies demonstrated that AV inhibited the cyclooxygenase pathway and reduced prostaglandin E2 which might be attributed to an anti-inflammatory compound called C-glucosyl chromone isolated from

AV [38,39]. In addition, recent studies suggest that a bradykinase isolated from AV could break down bradykinin, an inflammatory substance that induces pain and inflammation [21] and this might disclose the mechanisms by which AV acts as anti-inflammatory.

The collagen fibers in skin sections of 4, 8 and 12 days skin burn treated with AV there were less dense, thinner and more remodeled compared with 4, 8 and 12 skin burn per se specimens respectively. This was in agreement with previous studies, which postulated that AV induced more rapid maturation of collagen [40]. Some researchers attributed this action to glucomannan, a mannose-rich polysaccharide [41,42]. On the other hand, other researchers claimed that gibberellin, a growth hormone, interacts with receptor on the fibroblasts, thereby stimulating its activity and proliferation, which in turn accelerated collagen synthesis after topical or oral application of AV [43]. Other studies suggest that AV is an inhibitor of collagenase which might be responsible for the better remodeled collagen in the AV-treated groups [38].

In the present study, in skin sections of 4, 8 and 12 days treated with AV there were gradual decrease in α-SMA expression together with gradual significant increase in density and area as well as the maturity of NFC compared with specimens of 4, 8 and 12 d skin burn without AV respectively. This was in concurrence with other researchers who postulated that AV improved healing by increasing angiogenesis and thereby oxygenation [44,45]. This could be attributed to acemannan, a polysaccharide in AV, which was shown to activate macrophages, an effect that improved healing in a rat model [46,47]. In addition, it was reported that AV stimulated blood vessel formation in the vascular chorioallantoic membrane in chicken by a glycoprotein which could promote the stimulation of endothelial cells proliferation *in vitro* and induced them to interact with collagen [48]. However, other studies postulated that AV reduced both the vascularity and mast cells number of inflamed synovial membrane to about the half [49].

Therefore, the neovascularization effect of AV might be multifactorial from tissue to other, affected not only by the hypoxia but also by the cellular interactions and molecular alterations promoted by the injury.

CONCLUSION

In full-thickness skin burn, aloe vera shows a beneficial effect by reducing the inflammation significantly and providing a more mature granulation tissue which could accelerate healing and might produce a sound well-remodeled scar. Based on the significantly positive results of this study, it is recommended to carry out further experimental research as well as clinical trials to standardize aloe vera as a biological treatment in skin burn.

AUTHORS' CONTRIBUTIONS

Authors contributions	AAMAH	MFMS
Research concept and design	√	--
Collection and/or assembly of data	√	--

Data analysis and interpretation	√	--
Writing the article	√	√
Critical revision of the article	√	√
Final approval of article	√	√
Statistical analysis	√	--

REFERENCES

1. Peck MD. Epidemiology of burns throughout the world. Part I: Distribution and risk factors. *Burns.*2011; 37:1087-100.
2. Busuioc CJ, Popescu FC, Mogosanu GD, Parvanescu H, Streba L and Mogoanta L. Histological and immunohistochemical study of cutaneous angiogenesis process in experimental third-degree skin burns treated with allograft. *Rom J Morphol Embryol.* 2012; 53:1061-7.
3. Penn JW, Grobbelaar AO and Rolfe KJ. The role of the TGF-beta family in wound healing, burns and scarring: a review. *Int J Burns Trauma.* 2012; 2:18-28.
4. Li J, Zhang YP and Kirsner RS. Angiogenesis in wound repair: angiogenic growth factors and the extracellular matrix. *Microsc Res Tech.* 2003; 60:107-14.
5. Ribatti D, Nico B and Crivellato E. The role of pericytes in angiogenesis. *Int J Dev Biol.* 2011; 55:261-8.
6. Ding Y, Song N and Luo Y. Role of bone marrow-derived cells in angiogenesis: focus on macrophages and pericytes. *Cancer Microenviron.* 2012; 5:225-36.
7. Busuioc CJ, Popescu FC, Mogosanu GD, Lascar I, Pirici I, Pop OT and Mogoanta L. Angiogenesis assessment in experimental third degree skin burns: a histological and immunohistochemical study.*Rom J Morphol Embryol.* 2011; 52:887-95.
8. Siemerink MJ, Klaassen I, Vogels IM, Griffioen AW, Van Noorden CJ and Schlingemann RO. CD34 marks angiogenic tip cells in human vascular endothelial cell cultures. *Angiogenesis.* 2012; 15:151-63.
9. Jull AB, Rodgers A and Walker N. Honey as a topical treatment for wounds. *Cochrane Database Syst Rev.* 2008; CD005083.
10. Kulac M, Aktas C, Tulubas F, Uygur R, Kanter M, Erboga M, Ceber M, Topcu B and Ozen OA. The effects of topical treatment with curcumin on burn wound healing in rats. *J Mol Histol.* 2013; 44:83-90.
11. Dat AD, Poon F, Pham KB and Doust J. Aloe vera for treating acute and chronic wounds. *Cochrane Database Syst Rev.* 2012; 2:CD008762.
12. Ajmera N, Chatterjee A and Goyal V. Aloe vera: It›s effect on gingivitis. *J Indian Soc Periodontol.* 2013;17:435-8.
13. Karim B, Bhaskar DJ, Agali C, Gupta D, Gupta RK, Jain A and Kanwar A. Effect of Aloe vera mouthwash on periodontal health: triple blind randomized control trial. *Oral Health Dent Manag.* 2014; 13:14-9.

14. Gupta RK, Gupta D, Bhaskar DJ, Yadav A, Obaid K and Mishra S. Preliminary antiplaque efficacy of aloe vera mouthwash on 4 day plaque re-growth model: randomized control trial. *Ethiop J Health Sci.* 2014;24:139-44.

15. Khan AW, Kotta S, Ansari SH, Sharma RK, Kumar A and Ali J. Formulation development, optimization and evaluation of aloe vera gel for wound healing. *Pharmacogn Mag.* 2013; 9:S6-S10.

16. Feily A and Namazi MR. Aloe vera in dermatology: a brief review. *G Ital Dermatol Venereol.* 2009; 144:85-91.

17. Mendonca FA, Passarini Junior JR, Esquisatto MA, Mendonca JS, Franchini CC and Santos GM. Effects of the application of Aloe vera (L.) and microcurrent on the healing of wounds surgically induced in Wistar rats. *Acta Cir Bras.* 2009; 24:150-5.

18. Khorasani G, Hosseinimehr SJ, Azadbakht M, Zamani A and Mahdavi MR. Aloe versus silver sulfadiazine creams for second-degree burns: a randomized controlled study. *Surg Today.* 2009; 39:587-91.

19. Maenthaisong R, Chaiyakunapruk N, Niruntraporn S and Kongkaew C. The efficacy of aloe vera used for burn wound healing: a systematic review. *Burns.* 2007; 33:713-8.

20. Kaufman T, Kalderon N, Ullmann Y and Berger J. Aloe vera gel hindered wound healing of experimental second-degree burns: a quantitative controlled study. *J Burn Care Rehabil.* 1988; 9:156-9.

21. Ahmadi A. Potential prevention: Aloe vera mouthwash may reduce radiation-induced oral mucositis in head and neck cancer patients. *Chin J Integr Med.* 2012; 18:635-40.

22. Rajasekaran S, Sivagnanam K, Ravi K and Subramanian S. Hypoglycemic effect of Aloe vera gel on streptozotocin-induced diabetes in experimental rats. *J Med Food.* 2004; 7:61-6.

23. Daburkar M, Lohar V, Rathore AS, Bhutada P and Tangadpaliwar S. An in vivo and in vitro investigation of the effect of Aloe vera gel ethanolic extract using animal model with diabetic foot ulcer. *J Pharm Bioallied Sci.* 2014; 6:205-12.

24. Bancroft JD and Layton C. The Hematoxylin and eosin. In: Suvarna SK, Layton C and Bancroft JD editors. Theory & Practice of histological techniques. 7th ed., Churchill Livingstone of El Sevier. Philadelphia. Ch.10 and 11. 2013; 173-214.

25. Jackson P and Blythe D. Immunohistochemical techniques. In: Suvarna SK, Layton C and Bancroft JD editors. Theory & Practice of histological techniques. 7th ed., Churchill Livingstone of El Sevier. Philadelphia. Ch. 18. 2013; 381-434.

26. Busuioc CJ, Mogosanu GD, Popescu FC, Lascar I, Parvanescu H and Mogoanta L. Phases of the cutaneous angiogenesis process in experimental third-degree skin burns: histological and immunohistochemical study. *Rom J Morphol Embryol.* 2013; 54:163-71.

27. Schlager A, Oehler K, Huebner KU, Schmuth M and Spoetl L. Healing of

burns after treatment with 670-nanometer low-power laser light. *Plast Reconstr Surg.* 2000; 105:1635-9.

28. Karadag CA, Birtane M, Aygit AC, Uzunca K and Doganay L. The efficacy of linear polarized polychromatic light on burn wound healing: an experimental study on rats. *J Burn Care Res.* 2007;28:291-8.

29. Nassar MA, Eldien HM, Tawab HS, Saleem TH, Omar HM, Nassar AY and Hussein MR. Time-dependent morphological and biochemical changes following cutaneous thermal burn injury and their modulation by copper nicotinate complex: an animal model. *Ultrastruct Pathol.* 2012; 36:343-55.

30. Wu Y, Zhao RC and Tredget EE. Concise review: bone marrow-derived stem/progenitor cells in cutaneous repair and regeneration. *Stem Cells.* 2010; 28:905-15.

31. Chung AS and Kao WJ. Fibroblasts regulate monocyte response to ECM-derived matrix: the effects on monocyte adhesion and the production of inflammatory, matrix remodeling, and growth factor proteins. *J Biomed Mater Res A.* 2009; 89:841-53.

32. Geissmann F, Manz MG, Jung S, Sieweke MH, Merad M and Ley K. Development of monocytes, macrophages, and dendritic cells. *Science.* 2010; 327:656-61.

33. Popescu FC, Mogosanu GD, Busuioc CJ, Parvanescu H, Lascar I and Mogoanta L. Macrophage response in experimental third-degree skin burns treated with allograft. Histological and immunohistochemical study. *Rom J Morphol Embryol.* 2012; 53:1027-36

34. Mannon RB. Macrophages: contributors to allograft dysfunction, repair, or innocent bystanders?*Curr Opin Organ Transplant.* 2012; 17:20-5.

35. Lucas T, Waisman A, Ranjan R, Roes J, Krieg T, Muller W, Roers A and Eming SA. Differential roles of macrophages in diverse phases of skin repair. *J Immunol.* 2010; 184:3964-77.

36. Nucera S, Biziato D and De Palma M. The interplay between macrophages and angiogenesis in development, tissue injury and regeneration. *Int J Dev Biol.* 2011; 55:495-503.

37. Gerhardt H and Betsholtz C. Endothelial-pericyte interactions in angiogenesis. *Cell Tissue Res.* 2003;314:15-23.

38. Hutter JA, Salman M, Stavinoha WB, Satsangi N, Williams RF, Streeper RT and Weintraub ST.Antiinflammatory C-glucosyl chromone from Aloe barbadensis. *J Nat Prod.* 1996; 59:541-3.

39. Yagi A, Kabash A, Mizuno K, Moustafa SM, Khalifa TI and Tsuji H. Radical scavenging glycoprotein inhibiting cyclooxygenase-2 and thromboxane A2 synthase from aloe vera gel. *Planta Med.* 2003;69:269-71.

40. Reynolds T and Dweck AC. Aloe vera leaf gel: a review update. *J Ethnopharmacol.* 1999; 68:3-37.

41. Tai-Nin Chow J, Williamson DA, Yates KM and Goux WJ. Chemical characterization of the immunomodulating polysaccharide of Aloe vera L. *Carbohydr Res.* 2005; 340:1131-42.

42. Gupta VK and Malhotra S. Pharmacological attribute of Aloe vera: Revalidation through experimental and clinical studies. *Ayu.* 2012; 33:193-6.

43. Heggers JP, Kucukcelebi A, Listengarten D, Stabenau J, Ko F, Broemeling LD, Robson MC and Winters WD.Beneficial effect of Aloe on wound healing in an excisional wound model. *J Altern Complement Med.*1996; 2:271-7.

44. Yagi A, Egusa T, Arase M, Tanabe M and Tsuji H. Isolation and characterization of the glycoprotein fraction with a proliferation-promoting activity on human and hamster cells in vitro from Aloe vera gel. *Planta Med.* 1997; 63:18-21.

45. Davis RH and Maro NP. Aloe vera and gibberellin. Anti-inflammatory activity in diabetes. *J Am Podiatr Med Assoc.* 1989; 79:24-6.

46. Rodriguez Rodriguez E, Darias Martin J and Diaz Romero C. Aloe vera as a functional ingredient in foods. *Crit Rev Food Sci Nutr.* 2010; 50:305-26.

47. Jittapiromsak N, Sahawat D, Banlunara W, Sangvanich P and Thunyakitpisal P. Acemannan, an extracted product from Aloe vera, stimulates dental pulp cell proliferation, differentiation, mineralization, and dentin formation. *Tissue Eng Part A.* 2010; 16:1997-2006.

48. Davis RH, Donato JJ, Hartman GM and Haas RC. Anti-inflammatory and wound healing activity of a growth substance in Aloe vera. *J Am Podiatr Med Assoc.* 1994; 84:77-81.

49. Davis RH, Stewart GJ and Bregman PJ. Aloe vera and the inflamed synovial pouch model. *J Am Podiatr Med Assoc.* 1992; 82:140-8.

17

CHAPTER

CYTOGENOMICS OF FELINE CANCERS: ADVANCES AND OPPORTUNITIES

Rachael Thomas

Keywords: Cat, feline, genomics, chromosome, cytogenomics, cancer, comparative, fibrosarcoma, lymphoma, mammary carcinoma

INTRODUCTION

The domestic cat offers a diverse range of opportunities to contribute to the "One Health" concept, which capitalizes on the integration of complementary human and veterinary biomedical research efforts for synergistic gain. Cats continue to grow in popularity as family-owned pets and benefit from increasingly comprehensive medical surveillance [1]. It has been estimated that one in three U.S. households owns at least one cat, equating to a total U.S. cat population of approximately 74 million and a total annual expenditure of approximately $7.4 billion on veterinary services [2]. Cats exhibit approximately 200 genetic diseases that are considered analogous to human disorders, many of which are rarely encountered in any other widely studied species [3]. The cat has served as a particularly powerful model system for studying facets of neuroscience, reproduction and both heritable and infectious disease, and the field of feline oncology offers several novel angles to the comparative medicine arena. The ability to explore these attributes from a molecular standpoint has become possible only relatively recently through intensive efforts to characterize domestic cat genome organization in detail. The combination of data from complementary approaches now allows us to

Citation: Rachael Thomas, Cytogenomics of Feline Cancers: Advances and Opportunities, doi:10.3390/vetsci2030246.

explore the cat genome directly in context with that of humans and other key players in comparative biomedical research. In turn we may now begin to investigate in earnest the causes and consequences of genomic abnormalities associated with heritable and spontaneous disease in our feline companions.

GROSS KARYOTYPIC ORGANIZATION IN THE DOMESTIC CAT

The genome of the domestic cat (*Felis catus*, FCA) is organized into 18 pairs of autosomes and two sex chromosomes. Unlike in other mammals, where autosomes are numbered consecutively in descending order of size, standardized nomenclature in the cat takes into account both chromosome size and morphology. The karyotype comprises six autosomal subgroups termed A-F, with between two and four members in each. All but two autosomal pairs, cat chromosomes (FCA) F1 and F2, are biarmed, as are both sex chromosomes. There is substantial variation in chromosome size throughout the karyotype, from the largest (FCA A1, 240Mb) to the smallest (FCA E3, 43Mb) [4,5]. This marked diversity in size and morphology, broadly comparable to that of the human karyotype, means that chromosome identification in the cat is generally less challenging than in other key model species that exhibit more limited karyotypic variation. Gross similarity in the architecture of the human and domestic cat karyotypes has long been evident through direct comparison of their chromosome banding patterns [6,7]. These observations were reinforced by a series of molecular cytogenetic studies that indicated a remarkably limited degree of divergent evolution between the human and domestic cat genomes over the 92 million years since they shared a common ancestor, compared to the more extensive reshuffling evident in other model species [4,8,9,10,11]. The passage towards development of whole genome sequence assemblies for diverse mammals has since provided a far more comprehensive appreciation of conserved genome organization and potential mechanisms for karyotypic evolution.

GENERATION OF A REFERENCE CAT GENOME SEQUENCE ASSEMBLY

The potential role of the domestic cat in comparative biomedical research was boosted substantially by the generation of a light (~two-fold) coverage feline genome sequence assembly of "Cinnamon", a female Abyssinian, which captured ~65% of euchromatic sequence [12]. This formed part of a broader initiative funded by the National Human Genome Research Institute (NHGRI) to aid interpretation of the human genome sequence assembly, and to investigate patterns of sequence conservation, divergence and rearrangement between rodents, primates and other carnivores [13]. These studies showed that genome evolution in canine, ursine and murine lineages was driven strongly by interchromosomal translocation events, while intrachromosomal inversions were predominant in felids and also most primates [10,12]. A ~14x coverage whole genome assembly has recently become available for "Cinnamon", spanning 2.35 Gb, with sequence annotation for almost 22,000 putative protein-coding cat genes [4,5]. This resource affords a fascinating insight into the genomic factors that provide the unique phenotypic attributes of the domestic cat, and firmly equips the cat to contribute to, and benefit from, a "One Health" approach to biomedical research. Among the most rapid and exciting advances in feline molecular medicine are now being made in the area of oncology.

FUNDAMENTALS OF CANCER CYTOGENOMICS

It is well established that the onset of a malignant phenotype is associated with the accumulation of both random and non-random genomic abnormalities [14,15]. Molecular characterization of numerous diverse human cancers has identified vast numbers of recurrent somatic abnormalities, of which a proportion have been shown to correlate with discrete clinicopathologic criteria [16]. The ability to screen individual patients for these genomic markers has revolutionized diagnostic and prognostic capabilities, refining historically broad tumor classifications into clinically predictive subcategories and paving the way towards personalized disease management strategies. "Genomic profiling" also provides insight into the molecular pathogenesis of disease, identifying gene dosage imbalances associated with functional disruption of regulatory pathways, revealing key mechanistic processes underlying neoplastic transformation and progression and highlighting opportunities for targeted therapeutics.

Techniques for molecular cytogenomic evaluation of tumors fall broadly into two categories (see [17] for a detailed review). Direct techniques, such as fluorescence *in situ* hybridization (FISH) analysis, enable both structural and numerical assessment of small numbers of discrete genomic loci (typically < five) within individual cells. In contrast, indirect methods, such as comparative genomic hybridization (CGH) analysis, permit semi-quantitative measurement of mean DNA copy number within a tumor cell population at many thousands of defined intervals selected throughout the genome, but cannot detect balanced structural rearrangements. Since cancers typically exhibit a combination of both structural and numerical aberrations coupled with cell-to-cell heterogeneity, these highly complementary approaches are often used in tandem. Modified protocols allow their application to challenging specimens, such as those where the availability of clinical material is limited, or where the integrity of the sample is compromised, such as archived histologic specimens. This opens up a multitude of possibilities for retrospective studies of case materials for which detailed clinical histories are available.

The concepts of cancer cytogenomics are well established in human medicine, and enormous strides have been made in translating the same fundamental principles to domestic dog cancers. This has revealed remarkable conservation of discrete molecular alterations in human and canine counterparts of the same cancer (reviewed in [18,19]), providing strong evidence in support of a shared pathogenesis. Progress in the feline field is now gaining momentum, particularly in those areas in which the cat offers a novel perspective that has not been explored in other model species.

INJECTION-SITE SARCOMA

It is now 25 years since concerns were first raised over the increasing number of reports of malignant lesions arising at routine vaccination sites in cats [20]. The masses, predominantly fibrosarcomas, were observed most commonly in association with inflammatory reactions following the use of adjuvanted vaccines against rabies and feline leukemia virus. Vaccine-site sarcomas typically exhibit a rapid, aggressive clinical course and a bleak long-term prognosis. Treatment often involves radical surgical intervention due to the highly invasive nature of the disease, despite which localized post-surgical recurrence is common [21]. Since wide surgical margins markedly reduce the risk of tumor regrowth, there has been widespread encouragement for a transition away from traditional interscapular and femoral vaccination sites where adequate resection is highly challenging. The introduction of non-adjuvanted vaccines has also gone some way to limit the impact of vaccine-site sarcoma; however it remains a substantial clinical concern in feline medicine [22].

Interestingly, histopathologically similar tumors have also been described, infrequently, in dogs, ferrets and rabbits [23,24]. Furthermore, this phenomenon is not restricted to vaccination, since there are reports, albeit rare, of apparently related tumors manifesting in conjunction with injection of other fluids, in response to non-absorbable suture materials and even following microchipping procedures [21]. This has led to increased usage of the term "injection-site sarcoma" (ISS). Additionally, ISS shares many features with lesions occurring following ocular trauma in cats, and also with tumors arising in people in response to prolonged contact with foreign materials, such as artificial implants [22,25]. Taken in combination, these observations provide intriguing evidence for an association between persistent inflammation and malignant transformation. More than two decades after the first description of ISS, however, there remains no solid, detailed explanation for their underlying etiology, and they remain somewhat of an enigma [26,27].

Recognition of the etiology, incidence and impact of feline ISS has been challenged by difficulty in conclusive distinction between these sarcomas and those arising spontaneously without an apparent underlying injection-related origin. ISS typically are more locally invasive and prone to local recurrence than fibrosarcomas of spontaneous origin (non-ISS). Consequently, ISS generally warrant highly extensive surgical margins followed by regular and meticulous monitoring for recurrence, while non-ISS tumors may respond favorably to more conservative clinical management [27,28]. The ability to distinguish ISS from non-ISS at diagnosis therefore has far-reaching implications for patient, owner and clinician; however their extensive clinicopathologic similarity often confounds prompt and unequivocal identification. Distinction between these subtypes currently involves combinatorial consideration of multiple histopathologic features in context with clinical history and anatomical location, and often remains subjective and inconclusive. Currently there are no robust and broadly consistent diagnostic features for distinction between these subtypes. Advances in feline genomics now offer a potential molecular means to address this need and comprehend the factors that underlie the differences in their biological behavior.

Prior to the genomics era, conventional cytogenetic studies identified highly disrupted karyotypic organization in feline fibrosarcomas, with frequent hyperdiploidy and broad cell-to-cell heterogeneity [29,30,31,32]. A putative link has since been reported between amplification of feline satellite DNA sequences and the onset of genomic instability in fibrosarcomas, likely through disruption of normal centromere activity and the formation of aberrant marker chromosomes [33]. A subsequent study of five established ISS cell lines by classical enumeration of banded chromosome preparations also showed tremendously complex karyotypic reorganization, with a range of 19 to 155 chromosomes per cell, as compared to the normal 2n = 38 [34]. None of these studies, however, included detailed assessment of the composition of these aberrant chromosome structures.

Towards this goal, a microarray platform was developed to permit CGH-based identification of recurrent genomic DNA copy number aberrations (CNAs) in feline tumors [35]. This "aneuploidy array" comprised 210 large-insert clones representing loci anchored at ~15 Mb intervals throughout the initial 2x-coverage cat genome sequence assembly. Microarray-based profiling of 46 retrospective primary feline fibrosarcomas identified an extensive range of highly recurrent CNAs, consistent with the high level of genomic instability identified in earlier chromosome-based studies. Targeted FISH analysis of tumor chromosome preparations demonstrated broad heterogeneity in the patterns of structural and numerical aberrations evident both within and between cases. Remarkably, combined CGH and FISH analyses showed that a subset of genomic regions exhibited in excess of 30 copies within individual tumor cells, which were distributed across as many as ten different chromosome structures. Also of note, ISS cases showed non-random reorganization of FCA E1 in conjunction with copy number amplification of a discrete region on FCA E1p12 [35], consistent with the location of a nucleolar organizing region (NOR) [36]. Elevated argyrophilic nucleolar organizing region (AgNOR) scores, as defined by silver staining analysis, are common indicators of increased cellular proliferation, and have been associated with decreased overall survival for canine soft tissue sarcomas [37]. It is tempting to consider that this may reflect the inferior outcome that is typically associated with ISS. Statistical comparison of genomic profiles across the cohort identified two subchromosomal regions that showed significant differences in DNA copy number status in ISS *versus* non-ISS cases. While providing support for molecular discrimination, the limited resolution capabilities of the aneuploidy array confounded the ability to refine the boundaries of these regions and in turn to assess their gene content [35].

A higher-density second-generation cat CGH microarray platform has since been developed utilizing the 14x coverage cat genome sequence assembly, comprising ~110,000 oligonucleotide probes distributed at mean intervals of ~21kb. This provides a >300-fold increase in resolution over the aneuploidy array, bringing feline resources closely in line with those of other model systems for the first time. Evaluation of the same cohort of feline fibrosarcomas with this more comprehensive platform [38] identified homozygous deletions of the tumor-suppressor gene *PTEN* and recurrent amplifications of the *KIT*proto-oncogene. Elevated *KIT* protein expression has been reported as a persistent finding in both ISS and non-ISS tumors [39]; however it is not yet clear whether upregulation is a direct consequence of increased *KIT* gene dosage, nor whether this confers potential for utilizing targeted therapies directed towards this receptor tyrosine kinase. ISS and non-ISS tumors showed grossly comparable profiles of DNA copy number imbalance; however ISS cases exhibited elevated levels of global genomic disruption, consistent with their typically more aggressive behavior and poorer outcome. Among these lay a subset of discrete regions with promise as discriminatory markers [38]. With focus on the most clinicopathologically compelling genomic regions, in combination with assessment of transcriptional and translational status, there is great promise for a more detailed definition of the molecular pathogenesis of feline fibrosarcomas, and in turn, for refinement of diagnostic and therapeutic modalities for both subtypes. In a broader sense, genomic characterization of ISS also may aid elucidation of molecular mechanisms involved in the passage from chronic inflammation to neoplastic transformation, which continues to challenge human medicine.

LYMPHOMA

Lymphoma is the most common hematopoietic malignancy of cats and the third most common feline cancer overall, comprising approximately one third of all cancer diagnoses. Moreover, cats are considered to show the highest relative incidence of lymphoma among all species studied to date (reviewed in [40]), offering another promising angle for comprehending key facets of tumor biology. Historically, cytogenetic studies of feline lymphomas have focused heavily on established cell lines, primarily those developed from tumors associated with infection by feline leukemia virus, which often are nodal or mediastinal in origin. Common observations from these reports include hyperdiploidies resulting from low amplitude copy number increases of a variety of chromosomes, with no strongly recurrent features. These investigations have greatly expanded our understanding of the mechanisms by which clonal proviral integration into a host genome can initiate tumorigenesis and genomic instability through oncogenic activation [41,42]. With the diminished incidence of retrovirus-associated feline lymphoma since the 1980's, as a result of increased testing, vaccination and global vigilance, the focus has since shifted toward subtypes that offer opportunities for a more comparative approach.

Extensive volumes of clinically predictive cytogenomic data are accumulating for nodal lymphomas in human patients, and more recently also in dogs [43,44]. In contrast, gastrointestinal (GI) lymphoma, which represents the most common extranodal form in people and comprises more than 50% of all feline lymphomas, remains vastly understudied at the molecular level [45,46,47,48]. Given the high incidence of the disease in cats there is an opportunity for feline studies to pave the way forward for mutual benefit. In cats, the overall survival time for low-grade small-cell GI-lymphomas is generally four-fold greater than for high-grade large-cell tumors, following standard of care chemotherapy [45,49]. The relative frequency of these histologic subtypes in different anatomical locations varies widely in prior reports [40,45,50,51,52], in part due to the logistical challenges of performing diagnostic evaluation of GI lesions by surgical biopsy [40,53]. This invites assessment of a genomic approach for comprehensive DNA-based subclassification. Initial observations from microarray-based CGH analysis have indicated that feline GI-lymphoma exhibits a relatively subtle degree of genomic copy number instability, with no evidence for recurrent high-level amplifications or homozygous deletions. The majority of aberrations are shared by fewer than 30% of cases, and include defects involving key cancer-associated genes, such as elevated copy number of the *MYC* proto-oncogene and deletion of *PTEN*. Efforts to identify candidates for molecular distinction between histologic and immunophenotypic subtypes are now underway [54].

MAMMARY CARCINOMA

Mammary tumors represent the third most commonly diagnosed feline neoplasm, the vast majority of which (in contrast to dogs) are malignant, primarily simple carcinomas. Feline mammary carcinomas (FMCs) generally are highly aggressive, infiltrative and metastatic and show extensive heterogeneity in outcome that is not readily predicted at the time of diagnosis [55]. FMC shares extensive clinicopathologic, demographic and epidemiological similarity with human breast carcinoma (HBC), the most frequently diagnosed cancer in women [56]. While there is evidence for steroid hormone involvement in some FMCs, 80%–90% are estrogen- and progesterone-receptor negative [57,58,59]. FMC therefore offers a particularly powerful spontaneous model of the ~30% of "basal-like" late-stage HBCs that are highly aggressive and unresponsive to hormone-antagonist therapies, with a lack of targeted treatments and a poor prognosis.

Diagnostic and prognostic descriptions for FMC frequently are limited in detail since there is little evidence to associate specific histomorphologic subtypes with outcome. In HBC histologic grade, typically defined using the Elston and Ellis scoring system, is one of the most robust prognostic factors [60]. Although inconclusive in dogs, it has been shown recently, using this same grading system, that invasive FMC also shows a significant incremental association between histologic grade and outcome [61]. In both human and feline patients, intermediate grade tumors show the lowest concordance in routine diagnosis and the broadest heterogeneity in outcome [60,61], and thus the greatest need for improved subclassification.

Genome-wide surveys of HBC have identified discrete genomic signatures that define clinically predictive subtypes, leading to effective treatment strategies based on molecular pathogenesis [62]. Assessment of evidence for corresponding molecular subtypes in FMC may confer potential to extrapolate these advances rapidly to feline patients. To date, the search for prognostic factors for FMC from a molecular perspective has been targeted to individual candidate genes known to be associated with HBC. Of particular note, approximately 25% of HBCs exhibit upregulation of the *ERBB2* gene encoding the receptor tyrosine kinase HER2/neu, of which >90% exhibit DNA copy number amplification of this region [63]. This aberration, historically considered to be an indicator of poor prognosis, also confers susceptibility to Trastuzamab (Herceptin®), a monoclonal antibody targeted against the HER2/neu receptor. Published estimates of HER2-positive FMCs by immunohistochemistry show tremendous variation between studies, largely due to the use of diverse patient cohorts and contrasting analytical techniques [64]. Consequently the true frequency of HER2-positive FMC, and the relationship between protein expression and gene copy number, is yet to be determined.

At the genome-wide level, early conventional chromosome banding studies of FMC identified highly disrupted karyotypes, including recurrent deletions of FCA B2 and gains of FCA E3 [65,66]. These long predated the "genomics era", precluding detailed interpretation in terms of their significance in disease pathogenesis. Microarray-based molecular profiling of FMC is now yielding more substantial insight. Preliminary results with the second-generation CGH array have demonstrated moderate DNA copy number instability in FMC that is distributed broadly throughout the genome, with very few CNAs shared by more than 50% of cases surveyed [67]. Overall, higher-grade tumors exhibit an elevated incidence of genomic imbalance, suggesting that increased chromosome instability may itself represent an indicator of inferior outcome. Interestingly, copy number gain of *ERBB2* was >3-fold more common in high-grade *versus* intermediate-grade tumors. The incidence of *PTEN* deletion was also increased in high-grade tumors, correlating with an earlier study that showed inferior outcome in FMC cases with decreased PTEN protein expression [68]. Gain of *ERBB2* and deletion of *PTEN* are among the most recurrent genomic imbalances in HBC and are associated with concomitant disregulation of gene expression and anti-apoptotic activity, and in turn with inferior outcome [69]. Continued efforts should offer new insight into the degree to which the clinicopathologic similarities between HBC and FMC are recapitulated at the genomic level, highlighting disrupted pathways and potential therapeutic targets for FMC.

CONCLUSIONS

The domestic cat is becoming increasingly well placed to stimulate new advances in molecular medicine. The unique range and distribution of cancers diagnosed in our feline companions fills a series of critical niches that have confounded progress in human medicine. Included among this diverse spectrum are those with direct human counterparts that have remained understudied due to their rarity in people, while others offer a means to study discrete facets of tumor biology that are largely peculiar to the cat. We are now in a position to perform rapid and comprehensive interrogation of normal and aberrant feline genomes and to interpret our observations directly in terms of gene content and potential dysfunction. In turn we have the ability to extrapolate with relative ease between the genomes of different species in the search for conserved molecular features that suggest a common disease mechanism. Given the gross similarity in the structural organization and evolutionary history of the human and cat genomes, it is conceivable that an integrated cytogenomic approach may help to reveal as yet unrecognized mechanisms of tumor-associated chromosome instability.

The field of personalized medicine continues to make tremendous strides in the human field, and opportunities to integrate similar concepts into the veterinary arena are gradually becoming a reality. Cytogenomic techniques are continuing to evolve, with increases in resolution, sensitivity, flexibility, throughput and cost-effectiveness, coupled with the ability to combine related techniques into single platforms that allow synergistic acquisition of data from complementary approaches in a single experiment. In the human field, cancer cytogenomic discovery is gradually transitioning from chromosome- and microarray-based techniques toward the use of next generation sequencing approaches [17]. These strategies provide substantially increased resolution capabilities and have the advantage of permitting concomitant assessment of both structural and numerical aberrations in conjunction with detection of sequence mutations. At the present time, however, their integration into the veterinary arena is constrained by high costs and intensive computational needs, and limited access to dedicated reagents and analytical tools for non-human species. Ten years ago, the same limitations applied to the use of microarray-based technologies such as those described here. Given that the field of veterinary molecular oncology is now well established, and its comparative and translational value is continually being proven, one must hope that the delay in widespread introduction of next generation sequencing strategies for use in companion animal medicine will be less profound.

REFERENCES

1. Cannon, C. Cats, cancer and comparative oncology. *Vet. Sci.* 2015, *2*, 111–126.
2. American Veterinary Medical Association (AVMA). *U.S. Pet Ownership and Demographics Sourcebook*; AVMA: Schaumburg, IL, USA, 2012.
3. Online Mendelian Inheritance in Animals (OMIA). Faculty of Veterinary Science, University of Sydney. Available online: http://omia.angis.org.au (accessed on 28 May 2015).
4. Montague, M.J.; Li, G.; Gandolfi, B.; Khan, R.; Aken, B.L.; Searle, S.M.; Minx, P.; Hillier, L.W.; Koboldt, D.C.; Davis, B.W.; *et al.* Comparative analysis of the domestic cat genome reveals genetic signatures underlying feline biology and domestication. *Proc. Natl. Acad. Sci. USA* 2014, *111*, 17230–17235.
5. Tamazian, G.; Simonov, S.; Dobrynin, P.; Makunin, A.; Logachev, A.; Komissarov, A.; Shevchenko, A.; Brukhin, V.; Cherkasov, N.; Svitin, A.; *et al.* Annotated features of domestic cat-*Felis catus* genome. *Gigascience* 2014, *3*.
6. Nash, W.G.; O'Brien, S.J. Conserved regions of homologous G-banded chromosomes between orders in mammalian evolution: Carnivores and primates. *Proc. Natl. Acad. Sci. USA* 1982, *79*, 6631–6635.
7. Yang, F.; Graphodatsky, A.S.; O'Brien, P.C.; Colabella, A.; Solanky, N.; Squire, M.; Sargan, D.R.; Ferguson-Smith, M.A. Reciprocal chromosome painting illuminates the history of genome evolution of the domestic cat, dog and human. *Chromosome Res.* 2000, *8*, 393–404.
8. Rettenberger, G.; Klett, C.; Zechner, U.; Bruch, J.; Just, W.; Vogel, W.; Hameister, H. Zoo-FISH analysis: Cat and human karyotypes closely resemble the putative ancestral mammalian karyotype. *Chromosome Res.* 1995, *3*, 479–486.
9. Stanyon, R.; Yang, F.; Cavagna, P.; O'Brien, P.C.; Bagga, M.; Ferguson-Smith, M.A.; Wienberg, J. Reciprocal chromosome painting shows that genomic rearrangement between rat and mouse proceeds ten times faster than between humans and cats. *Cytogenet. Cell Genet.* 1999, *84*, 150–155.
10. O'Brien, S.J.; Johnson, W.; Driscoll, C.; Pontius, J.; Pecon-Slattery, J.; Menotti-Raymond, M. State of cat genomics.*Trends Genet.* 2008, *24*, 268–279.
11. Graphodatsky, A.S.; Trifonov, V.A.; Stanyon, R. The genome diversity and karyotype evolution of mammals. *Mol. Cytogenet.* 2011, *4*.
12. Pontius, J.U.; Mullikin, J.C.; Smith, D.R.; Lindblad-Toh, K.; Gnerre, S.; Clamp,

M.; Chang, J.; Stephens, R.; Neelam, B.; Volfovsky, N.; *et al.* Initial sequence and comparative analysis of the cat genome. *Genome Res.* 2007, *17*, 1675–1689.

13. Lindblad-Toh, K.; Garber, M.; Zuk, O.; Lin, M.F.; Parker, B.J.; Washietl, S.; Kheradpour, P.; Ernst, J.; Jordan, G.; Mauceli, E.; *et al.* A high-resolution map of human evolutionary constraint using 29 mammals. *Nature* 2011, *478*, 476–482.
14. Bernheim, A. Cytogenomics of cancers: From chromosome to sequence. *Mol. Oncol.* 2010, *4*, 309–322.
15. Sandberg, A.A.; Meloni-Ehrig, A.M. Cytogenetics and genetics of human cancer: Methods and accomplishments.*Cancer Genet. Cytogenet.* 2010, *203*, 102–126.
16. Mitelman, F.; Johansson, B.; Mertens, F. Mitelman Database of Chromosome Aberrations and Gene Fusions in Cancer. Available online: http://cgap.nci.nih.gov/chromosomes/mitelman (accessed on 31 May 2015).
17. Le Scouarnec, S.; Gribble, S.M. Characterising chromosome rearrangements: Recent technical advances in molecular cytogenetics. *Heredity (Edinb)* 2012, *108*, 75–85.
18. Breen, M. Comparative Cytogenetics. Available online: http://www.els.net (accessed on 22 July 2015).
19. Schiffman, J.D.; Breen, M. Comparative oncology: What dogs and other species can teach us about humans with cancer. *Phil. Trans. Roy. Soc. B-Biol. Sci.* 2015, *370*.
20. Hendrick, M.J.; Goldschmidt, M.H. Do injection site reactions induce fibrosarcomas in cats? *J. Amer. Vet. Med. Assoc.*1991. Avaiable online: http://europepmc.org/abstract/med/1748617 (accessed 28 August 2015).
21. Martano, M.; Morello, E.; Buracco, P. Feline injection-site sarcoma: Past, present and future perspectives. *Vet. J.* 2011,*188*, 136–141.
22. Woodward, K.N. Origins of injection-site sarcomas in cats: The possible role of chronic inflammation—A review.*ISRN Vet. Sci.* 2011, *2011*.
23. Munday, J.S.; Stedman, N.L.; Richey, L.J. Histology and immunohistochemistry of seven ferret vaccination-site fibrosarcomas. *Vet. Pathol.* 2003, *40*, 288–293.
24. Vascellari, M.; Melchiotti, E.; Bozza, M.A.; Mutinelli, F. Fibrosarcomas at presumed sites of injection in dogs: Characteristics and comparison with non-vaccination site fibrosarcomas and feline post-vaccinal fibrosarcomas. *J. Vet. Med. A-Physiol. Pathol. Clin. Med.* 2003, *50*, 286–291.
25. Moizhess, T.G. Carcinogenesis induced by foreign bodies. *Biochemistry (Mosc.)* 2008, *73*, 763–775.
26. Hendrick, M.J. Musings on feline injection site sarcomas. *Vet. J.* 2011, *188*, 130–131.
27. Ladlow, J. Injection site-associated sarcoma in the cat: Treatment recommendations and results to date. *J. Feline Med. Surg.* 2013, *15*, 409–418.
28. Dobson, J.M.; Demetriou, J.; Seguin, B. Chapters 20: Skin tumors and 22: Injection site sarcomas. In *Feline Soft Tissue and General Surgery*, 1st ed.; Langley-Hobbs,

S., Demetriou, J., Ladlow, J., Eds.; Saunders Elsevier: Philadelphia, PA, USA, 2013; pp. 209–242.

29. Kalat, M.; Mayr, B.; Schleger, W.; Wagner, B.; Reifinger, M. Chromosomal hyperdiploidy in a feline sarcoma. *Res. Vet. Sci.* 1991, *51*, 227–228.

30. Mayr, B.; Bockstahler, B.; Loupal, G.; Reifinger, M.; Schleger, W. Cytogenetic variation between four cases of feline fibrosarcoma. *Res. Vet. Sci.* 1996, *61*, 268–270.

31. Mayr, B.; Eschborn, U.; Kalat, M. Near triploidy in a feline fibrosarcoma. *Zentralbl. Veterinarmed. A* 1991, *38*, 617–620.

32. Mayr, B.; Hofstadler, E.; Schleger, W.; Reifinger, M.; Eisenmenger, E. Trisomy D1, marker F1: New cytogenetic findings in two cases of feline fibrosarcoma. *Zentralbl. Veterinarmed. A* 1994, *41*, 197–201.

33. Santos, S.; Chaves, R.; Adega, F.; Bastos, E.; Guedes-Pinto, H. Amplification of the major satellite DNA family (FA-SAT) in a cat fibrosarcoma might be related to chromosomal instability. *J. Hered.* 2006, *97*, 114–118.

34. von Erichsen, J.; Hecht, W.; Lohberg-Gruene, C.; Reinacher, M. Cell lines derived from feline fibrosarcoma display unstable chromosomal aneuploidy and additionally centrosome number aberrations. *Vet. Pathol.* 2012, *49*, 648–657.

35. Thomas, R.; Valli, V.E.; Ellis, P.; Bell, J.; Karlsson, E.K.; Cullen, J.; Lindblad-Toh, K.; Langford, C.F.; Breen, M. Microarray-based cytogenetic profiling reveals recurrent and subtype-associated genomic copy number aberrations in feline sarcomas. *Chromosome Res.* 2009, *17*, 987–1000.

36. Szczerbal, I.; Michalak, E. FISH-localization of the nucleolar organizer region on the feline E1p12 chromosome. *Anim. Genet.* 2003, *34*, 386–387.

37. Ettinger, S.N.; Scase, T.J.; Oberthaler, K.T.; Craft, D.M.; McKnight, J.A.; Leibman, N.F.; Charney, S.C.; Bergman, P.J. Association of argyrophilic nucleolar organizing regions, Ki-67, and proliferating cell nuclear antigen scores with histologic grade and survival in dogs with soft tissue sarcomas: 60 cases (1996–2002). *J. Am. Vet. Med. Assoc.* 2006, *228*, 1053–1062.

38. Thomas, R.; Pontius, J.; Borst, L.; Lamm, C.; Breen, M. Development Of A Genome-Anchored Microarray Platform for Identification of Clinically Predictive Somatic DNA Copy Number Aberrations in Feline Cancers. In Proceedings of the 7th International Conference on Advances in Canine and Feline Genomics and Inherited Diseases, Cambridge, MA, USA, 23–27 September 2013.

39. Smith, A.J.; Njaa, B.L.; Lamm, C.G. Immunohistochemical expression of c-KIT protein in feline soft tissue fibrosarcomas. *Vet. Pathol.* 2009, *46*, 934–939.

40. Moore, P.F.; Rodriguez-Bertos, A.; Kass, P.H. Feline gastrointestinal lymphoma: Mucosal architecture, immunophenotype, and molecular clonality. *Vet. Pathol.* 2011, *49*, 658–668.

41. Wu, F.Y.; Iijima, K.; Tsujimoto, H.; Tamura, Y.; Higurashi, M. Chromosomal translocations in two feline T-cell lymphomas. *Leuk. Res.* 1995, *19*, 857–860.

42. Fujino, Y.; Ma, Z.; Satoh, H.; Mizuno, T.; Hisasue, M.; Baba, K.; Masuda, K.;

Ohno, K.; Onishi, T.; Tsujimoto, H. Characterization of a newly established nonproducer lymphoma cell line for feline leukemia virus. *Vet. Immunol. Immunopathol.* 2004, *102*, 429–439.

43. Breen, M.; Modiano, J.F. Evolutionarily conserved cytogenetic changes in hematological malignancies of dogs and humans—Man and his best friend share more than companionship. *Chromosome Res.* 2008, *16*, 145–154.
44. Thomas, R.; Seiser, E.L.; Motsinger-Reif, A.; Borst, L.; Valli, V.E.; Kelley, K.; Suter, S.E.; Argyle, D.; Burgess, K.; Bell, J.;*et al.* Refining tumor-associated aneuploidy through "genomic recoding" of recurrent DNA copy number aberrations in 150 canine non-Hodgkin lymphomas. *Leuk. Lymphoma* 2011, *52*, 1321–1335.
45. Wilson, H.M. Feline alimentary lymphoma: Demystifying the enigma. *Top. Companion Anim. Med.* 2008, *23*, 177–184.
46. Vail, D.M. Chapter 324: Hematopoetic tumors. In *Textbook of Veterinary Internal Medicine*, 7th ed.; Ettinger, S.N., Feldman, E.C., Eds.; Saunders: Philadelphia, PA, USA, 2009; p. 2148.
47. Rissetto, K.; Villamil, J.A.; Selting, K.A.; Tyler, J.; Henry, C.J. Recent trends in feline intestinal neoplasia: An epidemiologic study of 1129 cases in the veterinary medical database from 1964 to 2004. *J. Am. Anim. Hosp. Assoc.*2011, *47*, 28–36.
48. Jasdanwala, S.; Pitchumoni, C. Epidemiological spectrum of gastrointestinal lymphoma. *Pract. Gastroenterol.* 2014, *38*, 8–28.
49. Moore, P.F.; Woo, J.C.; Vernau, W.; Kosten, S.; Graham, P.S. Characterization of feline T cell receptor gamma (TCRG) variable region genes for the molecular diagnosis of feline intestinal T cell lymphoma. *Vet. Immunol. Immunopathol.*2005, *106*, 167–178.
50. Waly, N.E.; Gruffydd-Jones, T.J.; Stokes, C.R.; Day, M.J. Immunohistochemical diagnosis of alimentary lymphomas and severe intestinal inflammation in cats. *J. Comp. Pathol.* 2005, *133*, 253–260.
51. Briscoe, K.A.; Krockenberger, M.; Beatty, J.A.; Crowley, A.; Dennis, M.M.; Canfield, P.J.; Dhand, N.; Lingard, A.E.; Barrs, V.R. Histopathological and immunohistochemical evaluation of 53 cases of feline lymphoplasmacytic enteritis and low-grade alimentary lymphoma. *J. Comp. Pathol.* 2011, *145*, 187–198.
52. Pohlman, L.M.; Higginbotham, M.L.; Welles, E.G.; Johnson, C.M. Immunophenotypic and histologic classification of 50 cases of feline gastrointestinal lymphoma. *Vet. Pathol.* 2009, *46*, 259–268.
53. Scott, K.D.; Zoran, D.L.; Mansell, J.; Norby, B.; Willard, M.D. Utility of endoscopic biopsies of the duodenum and ileum for diagnosis of inflammatory bowel disease and small cell lymphoma in cats. *J. Vet. Intern. Med.* 2011, *25*, 1253–1257.
54. Thomas, R.; *et al.* Genomic profiling of feline gastrointestinal lymphoma (To be submitted).

55. Hughes, K.; Dobson, J.M. Prognostic histopathological and molecular markers in feline mammary neoplasia. *Vet. J.*2012, *194*, 19–26.

56. Siegel, R.; Naishadham, D.; Jemal, A. Cancer statistics, 2013. *CA Cancer J. Clin.* 2013, *63*, 11–30.

57. Burrai, G.P.; Mohammed, S.I.; Miller, M.A.; Marras, V.; Pirino, S.; Addis, M.F.; Uzzau, S.; Antuofermo, E. Spontaneous feline mammary intraepithelial lesions as a model for human estrogen receptor- and progesterone receptor-negative breast lesions. *BMC Cancer* 2010, *10*.

58. Gimenez, F.; Hecht, S.; Craig, L.E.; Legendre, A.M. Early detection, aggressive therapy: Optimizing the management of feline mammary masses. *J. Feline Med. Surg.* 2010, *12*, 214–224.

59. Zappulli, V.; De Zan, G.; Cardazzo, B.; Bargelloni, L.; Castagnaro, M. Feline mammary tumours in comparative oncology. *J. Dairy Res.* 2005, *72*, 98–106.

60. Rakha, E.A.; Reis-Filho, J.S.; Baehner, F.; Dabbs, D.J.; Decker, T.; Eusebi, V.; Fox, S.B.; Ichihara, S.; Jacquemier, J.; Lakhani, S.R.; *et al.* Breast cancer prognostic classification in the molecular era: The role of histological grade. *Breast Cancer Res.* 2010, *12*, 207.

61. Seixas, F.; Palmeira, C.; Pires, M.A.; Bento, M.J.; Lopes, C. Grade is an independent prognostic factor for feline mammary carcinomas: A clinicopathological and survival analysis. *Vet. J.* 2011, *187*, 65–71.

62. Curtis, C.; Shah, S.P.; Chin, S.F.; Turashvili, G.; Rueda, O.M.; Dunning, M.J.; Speed, D.; Lynch, A.G.; Samarajiwa, S.; Yuan, Y.; *et al.* The genomic and transcriptomic architecture of 2000 breast tumours reveals novel subgroups. *Nature*2012, *486*, 346–352.

63. Kiyose, S.; Igarashi, H.; Nagura, K.; Kamo, T.; Kawane, K.; Mori, H.; Ozawa, T.; Maeda, M.; Konno, K.; Hoshino, H.; *et al.* Chromogenic *in situ* hybridization (CISH) to detect HER2 gene amplification in breast and gastric cancer: Comparison with immunohistochemistry (IHC) and fluorescence *in situ* hybridization (FISH). *Pathol. Int.* 2012, *62*, 728–734.

64. Rasotto, R.; Caliari, D.; Castagnaro, M.; Zanetti, R.; Zappulli, V. An immunohistochemical study of HER-2 expression in feline mammary tumours. *J. Comp. Pathol.* 2011, *144*, 170–179.

65. Mayr, B.; Jugl, M.; Brem, G.; Reifinger, M.; Loupal, G. Cytogenetic variation in six cases of feline mammary tumours.*Zentralbl. Veterinarmed. A* 1999, *46*, 367–377.

66. Mayr, B.; Ortner, W.; Reifinger, M.; Loupal, G. Loss of chromosome B2-material in three cases of feline mammary tumours. *Res. Vet. Sci* 1995, *59*, 61–63.

67. Thomas, R.; Seixas, F.; Borst, L.; Breen, M. Landscapes of Genomic Copy Number Aberrations in Feline Mammary Cancer. In Proceedings of the 8th International Conference on Advances in Canine and Feline Genomics and Inherited Diseases, Cambridge, UK; Available online: http://www.caninefelinegenomicsconference.org/ (accessed on 22–26 June 2015).

68. Ressel, L.; Millanta, F.; Caleri, E.; Innocenti, V.M.; Poli, A. Reduced pten protein expression and its prognostic implications in canine and feline mammary tumors. *Vet. Pathol.* 2009, *46*, 860–868.

69. Curtis, C.; Lynch, A.G.; Dunning, M.J.; Spiteri, I.; Marioni, J.C.; Hadfield, J.; Chin, S.F.; Brenton, J.D.; Tavare, S.; Caldas, C. The pitfalls of platform comparison: DNA copy number array technologies assessed. *BMC Genom.* 2009, *10*.

INDEX

G

H

I

L

M

N

O

P

R

S

T

W